T0235918

Perspectives in Comparative Politics

Series Editor: Kay Lawson
Published by Palgrave Macmillan

The Struggle against Corruption: A Comparative Study
    Edited by Roberta Ann Johnson
Women, Democracy, and Globalization in North America: A Comparative Study
    By Jane Bayes, Patricia Begne, Laura Gonzalez, Lois Harder,
    Mary Hawkesworth, and Laura Macdonald
Politics and Ethnicity: A Comparative Study
    By Joseph Rudolph
Immigration Policy and the Politics of Immigration: A Comparative Study
    By Martin Schain
Politics, Policy, and Health Care: A Comparative Study
    By Paul Godt
Social Movements in Politics, Second Edition
    By Cyrus Ernesto Zirakzadeh
The Development of Institutions of Human Rights: A Comparative Study
    Edited by Lilian A. Barria and Steven D. Roper
The Changing Basis of Political Conflict in Advanced Western Democracies:
The Politics of Identity in the United States, Belgium, and the Netherlands
    Edited by Alan Arwine and Lawrence Mayer
The Politicized Ethnicity: A Comparative Perspective
    By Anke Weber, Wesley Hiers, and Anaïd Flesken
Reforming Health Care in the United States, Germany, and
South Africa: Comparative Perspectives on Health
    By Susan Giaimo

Previous Publications by Susan Giaimo

"Interest Groups, Think Tanks, and Health Care Policy, 1960s–present." In *The CQ Guide to U.S. Health and Health Care Policy*, edited by Thomas Oliver. New York: DWJ Books, 2014, pp. 375–392.

"Behind the Scenes of the Patient Protection and Affordable Care Act: The Making of a Health Care Co-op." *Journal of Health Politics, Policy and Law* (2013) 38 (3) June: 599–610.

"Importing Our Own Best Ideas on Health Care," op-ed piece. *Milwaukee Journal Sentinel*, February 7, 2014.

Comparative Politics: Structures and Choices, Lowell Barrington, primary author. Boston: Wadsworth, Cengage Learning, 2010. Contributor; author of German sections.

"Look to Germany for Reform Model," op-ed piece. *Milwaukee Journal Sentinel* September 12, 2009.

Markets and Medicine: The Politics of Health Care Reform in Britain, Germany, and the United States. Ann Arbor: University of Michigan Press, 2002.

"Who Pays for Health Care Reform?" In *The New Politics of the Welfare State*, edited by Paul Pierson. Oxford: Oxford University Press, 2001.

"New Labour and the Uncertain Futures of Progressive Politics," by Stuart White and Susan Giaimo. In *New Labour: The Progressive Future?* edited by Stuart White. Basingstoke: Macmillan, 2001.

"Adapting the Welfare State: The Case of Health Care Reform in Britain, Germany, and the United States," by Susan Giaimo and Philip Manow. *Comparative Political Studies* (1999) 32 (8) December: 967–1000.

"Institutions and Ideas into Politics: Health Care Reform in Britain and Germany," by Susan Giaimo and Philip Manow. In *Health Policy Reform, National Variations and Globalization*, edited by Christa Altenstetter and James Warner Björkman. London and New York: Macmillan and St. Martin's Press, 1997, pp. 175–202.

"Health Care Reform in Britain and Germany: Recasting the Political Bargain with the Medical Profession." *Governance* (1995) 8 (3) July: 354–379.

"Cost Containment vs. Solidarity in the Welfare State: The Case of German and American Health Care Reform." American Institute for Contemporary German Studies, Johns Hopkins University, Washington, DC, Policy Papers No. 6, 1998.

Reforming Health Care in the United States, Germany, and South Africa

Comparative Perspectives on Health

Susan Giaimo

palgrave
macmillan

First published 2016 by
PALGRAVE MACMILLAN

The author has asserted their right to be identified as the author of this work in accordance with the Copyright, Designs and Patents Act 1988.

Palgrave Macmillan in the UK is an imprint of Macmillan Publishers Limited, registered in England, company number 785998, of Houndmills, Basingstoke, Hampshire, RG21 6XS.

Palgrave Macmillan in the US is a division of Nature America, Inc., One New York Plaza, Suite 4500, New York, NY 10004-1562.

Palgrave Macmillan is the global academic imprint of the above companies and has companies and representatives throughout the world.

Hardback ISBN: 978–0–230–33887–6
Paperback ISBN: 978–1–349–57087–4
E-PUB ISBN: 978–1–137–23607–4
E-PDF ISBN: 978–1–137–10717–6
DOI: 10.1057/9781137107176

Distribution in the UK, Europe and the rest of the world is by Palgrave Macmillan®, a division of Macmillan Publishers Limited, registered in England, company number 785998, of Houndmills, Basingstoke, Hampshire RG21 6XS.

Library of Congress Cataloging-in-Publication Data

Giaimo, Susan, author.
    Reforming health care in the United States, Germany, and South Africa : comparative perspectives on health / Susan Giaimo.
        p. ; cm.—(Perspectives in comparative politics)
    Includes bibliographical references and index.
    ISBN 978–0–230–33887–6

        I. Title. II. Series: Perspectives in comparative politics.
        [DNLM: 1. Health Care Reform—Germany. 2. Health Care Reform—South Africa. 3. Health Care Reform—United States. 4. Delivery of Health Care—Germany. 5. Delivery of Health Care—South Africa. 6. Delivery of Health Care—United States. WA 540.1]
RA395.A3
362.1'0425—dc23   2015021288

A catalogue record for the book is available from the British Library.

For all the uninsured and those who otherwise lack access to good health care

CONTENTS

List of Illustrations   ix

Series Editor's Foreword   xi

Acknowledgments   xiii

List of Abbreviations   xv

One   The Intersection of Health and Politics   1

Two   The United States: An Ambivalent Journey
          toward Universal Coverage   35

Three   Germany: Modernizing Social Health Insurance
          to Meet New Challenges   95

Four   South Africa: Confronting the Legacies of
          Apartheid   143

Five   Conclusions and Prospects   183

Notes   211

Bibliography   249

Index   267

ILLUSTRATIONS

Figures

1.1 Health care spending per capita and as a share of public
    and private sources, 2011 (or nearest year)   6
1.2 Health care spending as a percentage of GDP, 2011
    (or nearest year)   7
3.1 Corporatist structure of German social health insurance   105
3.2 Financing flows in German social health insurance
    since 2009   132

Tables

1.1 Leading causes of death by country income group, 2012   24
2.1 Main Provisions of the PPACA of 2010   61

SERIES EDITOR'S FOREWORD

Reforming Health Care in the United States, Germany and South Africa: Comparative Perspectives on Health by Susan Giaimo presents a timely topic in contemporary politics, as do all the books in the Palgrave series, *Perspectives in Comparative Politics.* Like them, this book offers an introductory overview, followed by three case studies, and concludes by summarizing the findings and what they suggest for the future work of scholars and for today's makers of policy. Throughout these books there also runs a quiet subtext: note what we can learn when we compare cases that are vastly different in some respects and strikingly similar in others, recognize the power of this kind of comparative study.

The topic of this particular book, the politics of health care reform in the United States, Germany, and South Africa, is unusually timely and vital. Professor Giaimo reviews in well-documented detail these three nations' efforts to bring about massive reforms in the quality and quantity of health care available to their citizens. She shows us three sets of problems, daunting in every case, and three paths of reform. In all three cases the paths have been—and to a greater or lesser extent still are—fraught with peril. The dangers include more than inadequate resources, the outbreak of a powerful epidemic, and the difficulties of achieving democratic consensus when opinions honestly differ as to what works best for whom. They also include past histories and present narratives of racially based inequalities of access, policies based on misinformation, bureaucratic and scientific inefficiencies, and outright corruption. They include politics.

And yet the three stories are also stories of victories and triumphs, and these too are the fruit of politics. Perhaps only governments could get it so wrong, but it is also true that only governments can put things right in ways that apply to all and have a chance of enduring beyond the lifetimes of individuals and administrations. As we observe the torturous road forward to passage and implementation of the Affordable Care Act (still menaced with dismantlement), the twists and turns the German path has taken through compromise after compromise in region after region to resolve problem after problem, and the heartbreaking journey South Africans have been forced to travel through prejudice, poverty, and plague, we cannot but marvel at the fortitude of those who have endured, resisted, and finally prevailed, using political power to achieve what progress they could, significant progress that has changed the lives—*preserved* the lives—of millions.

Professor Giaimo tells these stories clearly and well, in scholarly depth and with compassion. I welcome her and her work to the series and urge her readers on to valuable new understandings of one of the most difficult and most important problems facing governments throughout the world.

KAY LAWSON,
Series Editor,
Perspectives in Comparative Politics

ACKNOWLEDGMENTS

This book has been a long time coming and would not have been possible without the following people. First and foremost, my thanks go to Kay Lawson, who asked me to write the book for her series, *Perspectives in Comparative Politics*. Many times I thought of abandoning this project, but her firm support and encouragement over the years kept me going. Kay has been a wise and insightful editor who has greatly improved my argument and prose. I also want to thank the team at Palgrave, who have guided this manuscript into final book form, especially my editors Sara Doskow, Farideh Koohi-Kamali, and Robyn Curtis; and Chris Robinson and Leighton Lustig, who have provided technical guidance in a prompt, patient, and professional manner. I wish to especially thank Deepa John and the Newgen team for their outstanding work in copyediting and proof-reading the manuscript. Many thanks also go to Jeff Drope and Stephan Leibfried for their helpful comments on an earlier draft of this book.

I also want to thank my employer, Marquette University. Teaching courses in American and comparative health policy at Marquette gave me the opportunity to think through the ideas that went into this book and for research assistants to help me complete it. Riggs Hickman, Joshua Hebda, Jillian Laumbacher, and Mashal Amjad all provided invaluable research assistance. Marquette University has also provided my family with comprehensive health insurance coverage that has made it possible for us to access high-quality health care when we need it. A special thanks goes to Steve McCauley for his commitment to securing such excellent health insurance for all Marquette University employees and their families.

God has blessed me with wonderful friends and family who have supported me on this project. My family, especially my mom, Marilyn Giaimo, provided the love and emotional support that are so vital to seeing through a project of this magnitude. I am also grateful for the support of others in my family—Mary Giaimo, Kathy Giaimo, Mark Giaimo, Paul Metzger, Gary Butler, Usma Khan, Eleanor Wend, Chris and Tammi Wend, and

Alice and David Wend. Thanks go to Nancy Bridich, Mary Custer, and Janet Cianciolo who brought good conversation, food, and a much-needed break at a key time during my writing. My friends Kathleen Stemper, Joanne Nelson, Anastasia Beznik-Frieseke, Jan Heinitz, Linda Manka, Diane Lieske, Deb Obermanns, Rhonda Plotkin, Ellen Anderson, and Dave Rynders have been wonderful supporting my writing of this book as well as providing me with much-needed breaks and fun to give my mind a rest. Thanks also go to Karen Hoffman for her encouragement. If I have inadvertently omitted anyone from this list, you know who you are and I thank you.

As a working parent, I have had enormous help from many other people in completing this book. Many thanks go to Lydia Lambert, Natalya Kahman, Miranda Quinn, Alex Nelson-Zirzow, Emily Hansen, and Marilyn Morris, who provided quality childcare for my son while I spent countless hours typing away on my computer. I am also grateful to Tammi, Laura, Paul, Jess, Becca, Taylor, and Tony, who have worked tirelessly with my son to help him reach his full potential. It made it easier for me to work on the book knowing that my son was in good hands with all of you.

There are others whom I do not know personally and whose artistry I could never possibly approach. But they have inspired me nonetheless. Nick Cave has noted that the writing process is hard work and is not often pretty. But his daily discipline and commitment to his craft has yielded some of the most amazing music and prose. Patti Smith has been a genuine role model to me. Even when she dropped out of public view and moved to Detroit to raise her family, she did not stop being creative. She kept at her art, while keeping her family at the forefront of her priorities. When she was ready to return to public life, she did so. And she shared with us her fantastic imagination in her music and books.

But my biggest gratitude lies with my son Sam and my spouse Henry. Sam's genuine joy for life is truly inspiring. He reminds me every day what really matters in this life. Henry has been a rock. He persuaded me to take on this book project and continued to push me to see it to its finish. He devoted countless days to parenting and running the household to give me the time I needed to write. Henry has also been an incisive editor who has helped sharpen my argument and prose. He has also been a wellspring of creative ideas. And without his love and support, I am certain that I would not have completed this book.

ABBREVIATIONS

AALL	American Association of Labor Legislation
AARP	American Association of Retired Persons (formerly spelled out)
ACO	Accountable care organization
AFL-CIO	American Federation of Labor-Congress of Industrial Organizations
AHA	American Hospital Association
AHIP	America's Health Insurance Plans
AIDS	Acquired immunodeficiency syndrome
AMA	American Medical Association
AMTA	Advanced Medical Technology Association
ANC	African National Congress (South Africa)
ART	Antiretroviral therapy
BMG	Bundesministerium für Gesundheit (Federal Health Ministry) (Germany)
BRICS	Brazil, Russia, India, China, and South Africa
CBO	Congressional Budget Office
CDU	Christian Democratic Union (Germany)
CHIP	Children's Health Insurance Program
CMS	Centers for Medicare and Medicaid Services
COSATU	Congress of South African Trade Unions
CSU	Christian Social Union (Germany)
DA	Democratic Alliance (South Africa)
DAL	Disability-adjusted life expecancy
DATA	Debt, AIDS, Trade, Africa
DHHS	Department of Health and Human Services (United States)
DKG	Deutsche Krankenhaus Gesellschaft (German Hospital Federation)
DMP	Disease management program
DOTS	Directly observed treatment, short course

DRG	Diagnosis related group
FDP	Free Democratic Party (Germany)
FJC	Federal Joint Committee (Germany)
GDP	Gross domestic product
GEAR	Growth, Employment, and Redistribution
GKV-SV	Gesetzliche Krankenversicherung Spitzenverband (Federal Association of Social Health Insurance Funds)
HAART	Highly active antiretroviral therapy
HCAN	Health Care for America Now
HIV/AIDS	Human immunodeficiency virus
HMO	Health maintenance organization
IDS	Integrated delivery system
ICC	Integrated care contract
IMF	International Monetary Fund
IPAB	Independent Payment Advisory Board
IQWiG	Institute for Quality and Efficiency in Health Care
KBV	Federal Association of Social Health Insurance Physicians
KV	Kassenärtzliche Vereinigung (Association of Social Health Insurance Physicians)
MCO	Managed care organization
MDRTB	Multiple drug resistant tuberculosis
MNC	Multinational corporation
NFIB	National Federation of Independent Business
NGO	Nongovernmental organization
NHI	National Health Insurance
NHS	National Health Service
NICE	National Institute for Health and Care Excellence
NLM	National liberation movement
NLRB	National Labor Relations Board
NP	National Party (South Africa)
OECD	Organization for Economic Cooperation and Development
OFA	Organizing for America
Patient CARE Act	Patient Choice, Affordability, Responsibility, and Empowerment Act
PCMH	Patient-centered medical home
PCORI	Patient-Centered Outcomes Research Institute
PEPFAR	President's Emergency Plan for AIDS Relief
PhRMA	Pharmaceutical Research and Manufacturers of America
PPACA	Patient Protection and Affordable Care Act
QALY	Quality-adjusted life year
SEIU	Service Employees International Union

SHI	Social health insurance
SME	Social market economy
SPD	Social Democratic Party (Germany)
TAC	Treatment Action Campaign
TB	Tuberculosis
TRIPS	Trade Related Aspects of Intellectual Property Rights
UNAIDS	Joint United Nations Program on HIV/AIDS
UNICEF	United Nations Children's Fund
WHO	World Health Organization
WTO	World Trade Organization

CHAPTER ONE

The Intersection of Health and Politics

Health care is vitally important to human life. Access to appropriate health care when needed can mean the difference between life, death, or permanent disability. The health care sector also constitutes a major portion of economic activity and employment. The public sector health care system in Britain is the largest employer in Europe. In the United States and Germany, health care comprises one-seventh of their economies. The importance of health care to human life and economic activity makes it a major concern of public policy.

Health care is also a matter of politics. Health care systems and health policies are the outcomes of political struggles over the role and power of the government and various health care stakeholders. These struggles also affect the balance among the key goals of any health care system, namely its ability to ensure equitable access to high quality care at a reasonable cost (to the individual and the country). These goals are not mutually exclusive, but nations must strike a balance among them. And that balance has become more difficult for the Western industrialized democracies. Unlike the era of welfare state expansion underwritten by robust economic growth between 1945 and 1973, these nations now face growing financial pressures associated with providing care for an aging population and the advances of expensive new technologies. Governments must meet these new challenges against a backdrop of slower economic growth and intensified global competition. The developing nations in the Global South share the same three health policy aims as those of the industrialized countries, but the challenges they confront are more formidable. They must combat the scourge of infectious diseases that afflict the poor while simultaneously constructing a comprehensive national health care infrastructure from a much lower financial base than the affluent Western industrialized nations.

This book explores health policy challenges in three nations – the United States, Germany, and South Africa—and how they are responding to such challenges. The United States and Germany belong to the exclusive club of rich nations of the West. South Africa is an emerging market economy that nevertheless confronts challenges common to developing nations of the Global South. A brief snapshot is illustrative of the challenges in each nation:

- The United States tops the world in health care having spent $8508 per person in 2011. Yet 50 million persons lacked health insurance in 2010, more than twice the number in 1980.[1] How can the nation ensure that everyone has access to good health care at an affordable price?

- Germany currently has one of the highest shares of senior citizens in the world. In 2010, 21 percent of its population was over the age of 65; by 2050, that share is expected to rise to 33 percent. At 1.36 children per woman, Germany also registered the fourth lowest birthrate according to the Organization for Economic Cooperation and Development (OECD) in 2009.[2] These demographic trends present a challenge to health policy. How can fewer workers finance their own health care needs and those of their elders in the future?

- South Africa has the highest prevalence in the world of people infected with human immunodeficiency virus/acquired immunodeficiency syndrome (HIV/AIDS), with over 19 percent of the population, or 6.3 million people, living with HIV in 2013.[3] The costs of caring for those with HIV place heavy financial and resource demands on the health care system, which must also address other infectious diseases as well as the growing burden of noncommunicable diseases like heart disease, stroke, and diabetes.[4] Since the advent of democratic politics and black majority rule, the country's under-resourced health care system, a legacy of centuries of neglect under white rule, has struggled to contain the AIDS epidemic. The government must address the scourge of AIDS and at the same time construct a health care infrastructure that addresses the other pressing health needs of all South Africans.

How are these countries responding to such challenges? The answer ultimately lies in politics. Each country's particular balance of health policy goals and policy choices reflect the distinctive politics and relative power of government policymakers and stakeholders in that country. The health care system in each of these nations has institutionalized rules and practices and a particular settlement among the state, health care providers, payers, and patients, about their respective roles, powers, and jurisdictions in health care. These settlements center on more concrete questions of financing, provision, and regulation of health care. The settlements also reflect core values that underpin the broader social and political life of each country and deal with fundamental questions of the boundary between public and private, the balance between individual freedom and responsibility and the collective good, and the extent of the market in social provision. But these settlements are now in a state of flux. Policy solutions to the substantial health care problems today are disrupting these long-standing agreements and threaten (or promise) to redefine the power, roles, and institutional arrangements within each health care system. Because the stakes are so high, the reform debates are marked by controversy and conflict in all three nations.

This chapter provides the basic framework of analysis for the subsequent case studies that follow. The first section, "Goals of Health Care Systems and Policies," elaborates the criteria used to evaluate a health care system's performance. The second section, "The Politics of Health Care Policy," presents the major challenges facing health policymakers and health care systems today, highlighting the main differences among industrialized and developing nations. The third section, "Contemporary Challenges in Health Policy," specifies the main political factors that shape health policy and health care systems. The final section, "Plan of the Book," provides a brief sketch of the health care and political systems and outlines the reform paths the three nations have taken.

At first glance, South Africa may not seem the best case to illustrate health policies and politics in a developing nation. As one of the emerging market economies, it is far from the poorest of the poor. Nevertheless, it is an appropriate case for the following reasons. South Africa joined the family of democracies with the introduction of universal adult suffrage and the end of minority white rule in 1994. The country has an independent judiciary (that has withstood attempts by the ruling party to politicize its decisions), a free press that is openly critical of the government (even if the government has sought to curb press freedom), and a vibrant civil society with an array of independent interest groups that vigilantly protect civil rights. South Africa is also a capitalist economy with a well-developed industrial base. Thus, using a similar systems approach, it is more easily comparable to the two other industrialized democracies considered in this book than a much poorer nation would be. At the same time, however, it shares important features of developing nations that brings into sharp relief the contrasting health policy challenges that the affluent Western industrialized nations do not face. In short, comparing South Africa to the United States and Germany allows us to glean insights by using a most different systems approach.[5] Although it is a middle-income country and the conditions of the poor have improved since 1994, South Africa still has high rates of poverty, even after factoring in the ameliorative effects of tax transfers and social spending. Using World Bank definitions of poverty, 16.5 percent of South Africans live in extreme poverty, that is, on less than $1.25 a day and 39 percent live in moderate poverty, on less than $2 a day.[6] Like other developing nations and in contrast to the United States and Germany, the South African government possesses far fewer financial resources available to them to meet the health care needs of their citizens.

And the health challenges it faces are daunting. Like other developing nations, the primary challenge for South Africa is to bring under control the scourge of infectious diseases that are tied to poverty and social exclusion. South Africa has the unfortunate distinction of being the country with the highest prevalence rate of HIV/AIDS in the world, and relatedly, one of the highest rates of tuberculosis (TB) infection.[7] These twin epidemics have placed an enormous burden on the overstretched and underfinanced public sector health care system. At the same time, as a middle-income country whose population is aging and adopting lifestyles more common in the West, South Africa must also face the growing burden of noncommunicable diseases. In other words, the country faces a dual challenge absent in industrialized nations and in the poorest developing nations. Finally, South Africa, like most nations in the Global South, has had to grapple with the entrenched legacies of imperialism. In South Africa, imperialism took the form of *apartheid*, the official system of segregation and political, social, and economic disempowerment of the black majority by the white minority.

The effects of imperialism and apartheid are deeply entrenched in the patterns of disease among South Africans as well as in the institutions that are expected to treat them. Racial inequality manifests itself in the distribution of the burden of illness, with black Africans suffering the brunt of infectious diseases such as HIV/AIDS and much worse health outcomes from noncommunicable diseases and incidents of violence than the white minority. Apartheid also created two separate and profoundly unequal health care systems in South Africa. While descendants of white European settlers have continued to enjoy private health care services on a par with the rich industrialized world, most nonwhites must seek care from a severely under-resourced public sector health care system or from traditional healers. The apartheid system, moreover, instilled a deep mistrust among the races that influenced the thinking and actions of key policymakers in the black majority government, with disastrous results for health policy.

Goals of Health Care Systems and Policies

The overarching aim of health care is to make people healthy and give them the best chance to live long, productive, and happy lives. But how and whether people are able to get such care depends on the health care system in their particular country. As noted, the primary goals are accessibility, affordability, and quality of care. We will also consider responsiveness to patients, although this could fall under the domain of access or quality.

Ensuring access to health care means having health insurance coverage, which eliminates or lessens the financial barriers to health care. But nonfinancial barriers to health care such as geography, may also be in play. Many rural areas or poor inner city neighborhoods face a shortage of doctors, nurses, and hospitals, so that even if one has insurance, a person might not be able to find a health care provider for timely care. The general debate over accessibility centers on the concept of equity. Those who view health care as a human right define equity as universal coverage, so that health care is available to everyone and based on need rather than the ability to pay. This formulation expresses the *solidarity* principle, which is realized through the mechanism of *risk pooling*. Risk pooling means that the healthier and wealthier subsidize the health care of the sicker and poorer, either through higher insurance premiums, contributions, or progressive income taxes. Otherwise, those who need health care the most will be unable to afford it. However, commercial for-profit insurers define equity in terms of *actuarial fairness*, or the idea that health insurance contributions or premiums should reflect the health care that one presently consumes or is expected to consume. This sort of equity is realized through the mechanism of *experience rated premiums*, which means that those who are younger and healthier pay lower premiums than those who are older or sicker.[8]

Health care must be affordable to both the individual who uses it, and to the broader society that may pay for all or part of it. While there is a broad pattern showing that richer nations devote more resources to health spending than poorer nations, cross-national data amply demonstrate that even the richer countries vary widely on how much they devote to health care expenditures, whether expressed as a percentage of gross domestic product or as per capita spending. They also differ on the extent to which government or private sources finance health care (see Figures 1.1 and 1.2). Understanding such differences requires an explanation rooted in politics. The definition of affordability is itself a political choice, not some absolute economic or scientific given.

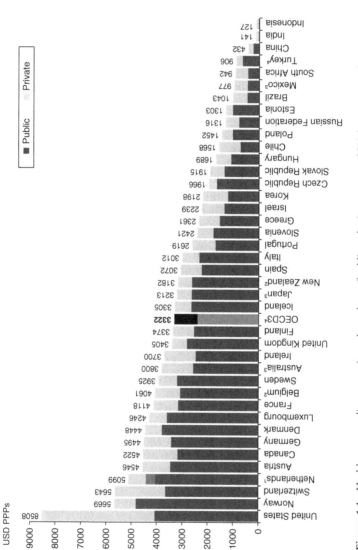

Figure 1.1 Health care spending per capita and as a share of public and private sources, 2011 (or nearest year).

1. In the Netherlands, it is not possible to clearly distinguish the public and private share related to investments.
2. Current health expenditure.
3. Data refers to 2010.
4. Data refers to 2008.

Source: Health at a Glance 2013 (OECD 2013).

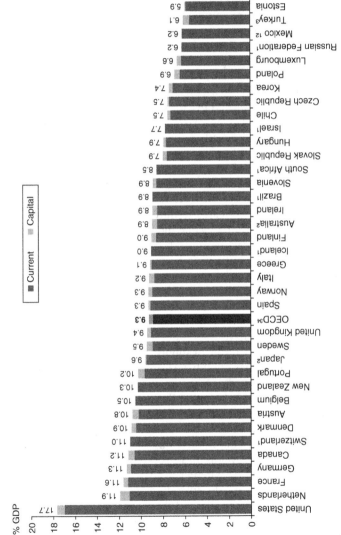

Figure 1.2 Health care spending as a percentage of GDP, 2011 (or nearest year).

1. Total expenditure only.
2. Data refers to 2010.
3. Data refers to 2008.

Source: Health at a Glance 2013 (OECD 2013)

Health care must not only be accessible and affordable, but it must also be of high quality. But like the other two goals of a health care system, quality can mean different things and can be difficult to measure. The OECD has compiled macro-level comparative indicators of quality, such as life expectancy and infant mortality rates among nations and subpopulations, which it uses to compare countries. But these are global measures lacking nuance and may mask significant disparities among subgroups of the population. For example, while most would agree that longevity is important, it fails to capture the quality of life that accompanies advancing age. Social scientists, particularly health economists, have devised new measures that incorporate such concerns. One such measure is the disability-adjusted life expectancy (DALE), which measures the number of years of good health the average person can expect to enjoy before developing a disability associated with aging. A nation's DALE is usually around seven years less than its life expectancy figure. Another is the quality adjusted life year (QALY), which calculates the additional years of life and the quality of those years gained through a particular medical intervention. Policymakers increasingly use QALYs to help them decide which treatments a nation should spend scarce resources on and which it should not. But because QALYs incorporate value judgments about quality, they raise difficult moral and political questions: For instance, who is to say six additional months of life for a patient with terminal cancer is not worth spending money on? Or what is the monetary value associated with each QALY above which a treatment is not worth funding? And is that monetary amount set so low as to exclude new drug therapies for cancer? As a result, how QALYs are used is subject to controversy and argument.[9]

Other measures of quality have their own limitations. Some of these define quality of care solely in terms of inputs, for example, the amount spent on health care, the number of high-technology interventions, or the number of doctors or hospital beds. Other measures define quality of care in terms of patient satisfaction and employ the now ubiquitous consumer survey following a hospital or doctor visit. But none of these measures tells us whether the particular health care intervention cured a patient's ailment or even improved her condition. Consequently, most industrialized countries are moving to develop measures that establish causal links between inputs and outputs (i.e., whether a given treatment produces a desired health outcome). Some are also introducing measures that evaluate treatments on both their clinical results and their costs. Such comparative effectiveness measures, as they are known, may compare two treatments that provide the same or similar outcomes but at varying costs.

On quality indicators, the United States provides a mixed picture. It leads the world in developing and diffusing many high-technology innovations, which are available to those with top-flight insurance. But if one is uninsured or has minimal coverage that includes high up-front out of pocket payments or excludes certain procedures, then she may not be able to access such innovations. The United States boasts lower rates of smoking but, at 36.5 percent, has the highest rate of adult obesity in the OECD. Both smoking and obesity are conditioned by racial and income inequality, with upper income whites having far lower rates than minorities. The US infant mortality is worse than all industrialized nations and even some developing nations. This global figure masks enormous disparities by class, with higher mortality rates among lower income women. But race is also a factor: African-American women experience double the infant mortality rate of white American women (11.6 percent to 5.2 percent, respectively).[10] Yet this is not a problem afflicting only poor African-Americans, since the infant mortality rate is higher for well-educated professional black women than for white women with only a high school education. After controlling for genetic differences, the findings suggest that broader social factors beyond income and education, such as racial discrimination, may be at work.[11] A final goal of a health care system its responsiveness to patients. Responsiveness can mean different things, however. It may be defined as good customer service or treating patients with dignity. It is usually measured by consumer satisfaction surveys asking patients about their satisfaction with the care they received, for example, how polite the doctor and office staff were, how long it took to get an appointment to a doctor or to receive elective surgery, and whether they have been able choose their insurer or health care provider, such as a doctor or hospital. As before, countries vary on these measures. One example is how long people wait to see a doctor or receive a particular treatment. In Britain, Canada, and Sweden, where the government is the sole payer for health care, wait lists for elective surgery are common, while in countries with multiple insurers, they are rare. The length and time of the wait list can constitute a measure of access or quality (of life) as well as the responsiveness of the health care system. In most countries, patients have their choice of a primary care doctor, although not of a specialist. Even in the United States, many insurers require patients to seek care from doctors and hospitals within a defined network or else pay higher out-of-pocket costs, and the poor and disabled reliant on government insurance (Medicaid) may experience long waits for treatment because the low reimbursement rates for providers mean that many of them refuse to treat patients with that coverage.

Policymakers must balance these different goals, yet they often find that the goals conflict with one another. Deciding the relative balance among these goals is a political process that necessarily entails broader conflicts about power, interests, and values. My focus will be on the first three goals because they are the ones most commonly used to evaluate health care system performance. But responsiveness will also figure in the analysis of different health care systems, especially patient choice of insurer or provider, as this has become a component of health care reforms in a number of nations, including the United States and Germany. We turn now to the politics that explain nations' policy choices in pursuit of these goals.

The Politics of Health Care Policy

To understand the health policies of any country, one must examine the interplay of the health care system with the broader politics of that nation. Public policies are the product of politics which, in turn, are the interplay of political system structures or institutions, the power of political parties and organized interests, and the play of ideas or values. Health care systems themselves reflect a nation's politics, and embody power arrangements among political parties and interest groups as well as dominant values about the role of government and private actors in health care provision and financing. At the same time, the design of a particular health care system may present policy problems of its own, and require solutions that may be unique to that system.[12] The temptation exists to look for single-cause explanations of policy choices and outcomes. But the real world is seldom so neat. Depending on what one is trying to explain, one factor may be more prominent than another. As the old adage goes, policymaking is a lot like sausage-making. Many different ingredients go into the mix, some of which we would perhaps not want to see. But since the task of this book is to understand health policy, we have to look at these ingredients.

An easy way to think about the key political ingredients that explain policy choices and outcomes is in terms of the "three I's"—political *institutions, interests,* and *ideas*—plus history, that is, past decisions and developments of a country's health care system that create policy legacies confronting current governments. A good place to begin is with political institutions. These set out the formal and informal rules of engagement and shape the tactics and strategies of interests and governments.

Institutions

The structures or institutions of any political system channel policy initiatives and conflicts among parties and interest groups, shaping policy outcomes by making it easier or more difficult to enact and implement particular policies. Political institutions may be the formal structures (such as the executive, legislature, and judiciary) and rules that specify the powers of different branches or levels of the political system as specified in a country's constitution, or informal rules, norms, or customs that have evolved over a long period of time but are widely accepted by the players in the political contest.[13]

Political systems can be classified by the extent to which they centralize decision-making. Most democracies in the world are *parliamentary systems*, and such systems tend to centralize decision-making in the executive. This is because parliamentary systems fuse the executive and legislative branches, binding them to a common electoral fate. Citizens do not directly elect the chief executive (prime minister); instead, they elect representatives to the national legislature (parliament). Usually, the party (or coalition of parties) that has the majority of seats in parliament forms the executive or *government*, consisting of the prime minister and cabinet. A minority government is also possible. In that situation, the cabinet lacks an outright majority in parliament and instead relies on the support of a number of parties that together comprise a majority in the legislature. Policy initiatives originate in the cabinet and attendant ministries and the ruling party or coalition in the legislature generally enacts the government's program. If it votes against a government bill or if a sufficient number of its members support a motion of no confidence, the resignation of the prime minister and cabinet, and fresh parliamentary elections will follow. Few members of parliament (MPs) are willing to take such an electoral risk, so party discipline and support of the government's program are the norm (but not the rule).

In a *separation of powers or presidential system*, by contrast, the legislative, executive, and judicial branches are roughly coequal and related to each other through a system of checks and balances. The legislative and executive branches are elected separately and may act independent of each other, employing the powers constitutionally assigned to each. The legislature can refuse to enact a president's bill and the president can veto a bill passed by the legislature or use other powers to act contrary to the majority will of the legislature. Each can act contrary to the other without facing the voters until their respective terms are up.

An independent judiciary also acts as a check on arbitrary government power. Many democracies grant the judicial branch the power to nullify laws enacted by the executive and legislature on the basis of their constitutionality. The high courts of the United States and Germany possess judicial review power, which serves, as a further check on government power.

Power can also be more or less centralized depending on the political system's vertical relations among different levels of government. Some democracies are *unitary systems*, whereby lower levels of government owe their existence and powers to the national government that creates them.

Such is especially the case in Great Britain, where the powers and existence of local and regional governments are set out by acts of Parliament in London. In *federal systems,* by contrast, subnational levels of government have policy jurisdictions distinct from the central government, as recognized in the nation's constitution; these subunits cannot be created or abolished at the whim of the national government. The central government in a unitary system thus possesses the capacity to formulate and implement policies at national level more easily than the national government in a federal system. Of course, political and policy conflicts between national and regional or local governments are features of both unitary and federal systems. And a central government with a preponderant decision-making responsibility (i.e., unitary system) may also be vulnerable to blame from citizens and opponents for local policy failures.[14] Yet federal systems often grant provincial or regional levels of government the power to veto or otherwise shape the implementation of policies enacted at the national level and may even bar national government intrusion into the areas of jurisdiction reserved for these lower units of government on constitutional grounds.

In general, the more dispersed and decentralized the decision-making process, and the more porous the political system is to interest group input, the greater the likelihood of either policy gridlock, or compromise solutions that can garner consensus from a number of different actors. A parliamentary system generally makes decision-making and formulation of policies easier than does a separation of powers system. The same is true for unitary as opposed to federal political systems. This is because parliamentary and unitary structures offer fewer points of access to the policy making process, and thus fewer veto points for opponents of a government bill (whether an opposition party, an interest group, or a branch of government) to block the forward movement of a policy initiative than do presidential and federal systems.[15]

Even within a particular branch of government, institutional arrangements can impede or facilitate policymaking. The US Congress, for example, is marked by a vast array of committees and subcommittees, often with overlapping jurisdiction. Such terrain is treacherous to navigate and many policy initiatives may never get out of committee for a vote by the full legislature. Bicameral legislatures often require the assent of both the upper and lower chambers, although in some cases only the assent of the lower house is required. Other polities provide voters and interest groups a potent say in policymaking through direct democracy initiatives like referenda or recall elections.

Likewise, the rules of the electoral system have a profound effect on the shape and fate of policy initiatives. Electoral systems that define the rules for winning seats in the legislature are a case in point. Electoral systems operating under *single-member districts* and *simple plurality rules* (first-past-the-post rules: i.e., the candidate with the most votes, as opposed to an absolute majority, wins the seat) encourage party systems consisting of two large parties capable of winning seats under such rules. This type of party system, in turn, fosters single-party government in which one party wins an absolute majority of legislative seats. Electoral systems based on *proportional representation* rules that accord parties seats according to the percentage of the popular vote they garner give small parties a fighting chance to win seats. Such rules for determining the winning of seats yield multiparty systems with several parties gaining representation in the legislature. In parliamentary elections, proportional representation usually yields coalition governments of two or more parties since no single party can normally muster an absolute majority of seats.

In short, the institutional terrain of a polity not only makes legislative enactment and implementation more or less likely but may also influence the political strategies that interest groups will pursue.[16] Polities with more centralized decision-making and fewer veto points have an easier time enacting and implementing radical policies than decentralized polities that allow a greater number of players entry to the policymaking process. In the latter situations, enactment and implementation of a policy usually require compromise and negotiations, and tend to be more watered-down solutions. These institutional considerations affect all policy decisions, including those related to health.

Interests

But institutions only tell part of the story of health policy. Political institutions channel policy proposals, and structure conflict and negotiations among political actors. The policy outcomes reflect which groups have power and which do not in this process. The key political actors are parties and interest groups, and policy proposals reflect their preferences and values.

Political Parties

The primary purpose of political parties is to serve as a vehicle for candidates to run for office and to aggregate and channel the demands of civil society into distinct policy platforms that candidates, if elected, will be expected to pursue in office. However, parties are quite distinct entities that institutionalize particular social identities and cleavages.[17] Historically, parties of the left (social democratic or socialist parties) have favored welfare state expansion and redistributive tax and spending policies that reflect the desires of their core working-class and lower-income constituencies.[18] Conservative parties of the right that have their origins in the aristocratic class of feudal times have generally viewed inequality of outcomes in economic and social domains as reflecting the natural hierarchical order of society. But there is a distinct difference in European and American conservatism that reflect their different historical trajectories in the development of capitalism and democracy. European conservatives are generally more tolerant of state intervention in society and the economy, stemming from the days of *noblesse oblige* (paternalism) whereby the feudal lords were obligated to look out for the welfare of their serfs. Christian Democratic parties in Europe express a different strand of conservatism. These parties originated in reaction to the social upheaval accompanying the Industrial Revolution, and the suffering it inflicted on the poor. Competing with socialist parties on the left for the allegiance of the working class, and adhering to official Catholic doctrine that gives preference to the poor, such parties have justified state regulation of the capitalist economy.[19] In the United States, however, where private entrepreneurs led industrialization and feudalism was confined to the slave economy of the South, conservatism has tended to mean both economic and political liberalism, that is, individual freedom and limited government.[20]

In much of Europe, liberal parties that champion more or less unlimited economic and political freedom of the individual tend to be smaller than the more dominant forces of conservatism or social democracy. European countries also have small but significant Green parties that support direct democracy, environmentalism, and human rights, as well as small parties of the Far Right that promote traditional social morality, nationalism, and anti-immigrant stances.[21] The type of party system produced by the electoral system influences the political formation of these political forces. Proportional representation election rules tend to encourage multiparty systems where smaller liberal or Green or Far Right forces can exist as independent parties. Simple plurality electoral rules tend to favor two larger parties that often absorb smaller challengers.

The particular configuration of parties in developing nations may differ from those found in the West. Some of the new democracies may have parties on the Left–Right spectrum found in Western industrialized democracies, but other types of parties may be more prominent. Such parties express the particular social and political identities and conflicts that are unique to each country's history. In countries that have recently emerged from colonial rule, parties of national liberation movements (NLM) that represent the indigenous majority may dominate politics and elections, not only at the dawn of democratic rule but even decades later. Parties representing a white settler minority will lack the voting strength to challenge the electoral dominance of the NLM party. Or the dominant party may be largely based on religion. In cases of overwhelming dominance of one party, single-rule will be the usual outcome of elections. In heterogeneous societies, a number of parties may court voters on the basis of ethnicity, region, language, or religion. Multiparty systems like these may yield a succession of unstable coalition governments.

As in other policy areas, different parties promote distinct health policies. Forces on the Left tend to favor health care available to all residents as a matter of right, financed by progressive income taxes, and with a large degree of government regulation if not direct provision of health care. This would approximate a National Health Service (NHS) model of health care finance and delivery. Left parties see such arrangements as the only way to assure equality of access to care without regard to ability to pay. Forces on the Right, particularly liberal parties, promote private market solutions to health care, under a liberal or predominantly "private health care system," in which individuals finance private insurance through premiums and obtain care from private providers. Such parties prefer only minimal government regulation in the belief that markets are self-regulating and that an overweening state stifles individual freedom of choice. Limited public health care programs are targeted to the truly needy, such as the elderly, children, or the disabled. Traditional conservative or Christian Democratic parties champion a social insurance model of national health insurance (SHI), which gives primacy to major groupings of societal actors in health care financing and administration of health care to unions, employers, and associations of private providers. Consistent with their mistrust of unbridled markets, their acceptance of social hierarchies, and the obligation to ensure social solidarity and provide for the vulnerable, these parties also routinely require the state to set the parameters of the health care system and provide oversight over its actors so that their behavior conforms to public goals.

Most developing nations lack a universal health care system. Instead, private insurers and providers cater to the wealthy minority or small middle class in formal sector employment in mostly urban areas. The vast majority of the population seeks care from traditional healers. Alternatively, they may seek medical treatment from a clinic run by a relief organization or a public health clinic that is most likely overwhelmed and underresourced.[22] A number of developing countries are constructing a system of universal health care coverage, but many are still rudimentary and do not reach the poorest.[23]

These are not the only health care systems found in the world; other models and hybrids of these certainly exist. But the general point bears repeating: the particular health care system crystallizes political settlements among different parties and health care stakeholders in each country. These stakeholders find their voice in the formation of interest groups.

Interest Groups

Interest groups seek to influence policy and policymakers. But they possess different types of resources that render them more or less powerful or influential. One set of resources is organizational. This includes the number of members a group has and the ability to call its members into action. It may also encompass centralization, that is, the decision-making authority of the leadership and its ability to discipline wayward or rebellious members. Money is obviously an important resource as well. This includes not only funds to mobilize members, but also money to channel to political campaigns or lobbyists to hire. A key resource is a group's organizational connections to a political party that is in government frequently and for long periods of time. The group–party linkages include an electoral base that votes for a particular party as well as overlapping membership among members of parliament or the executive branch of government with that of trade unions or business associations.[24]

In addition, the political system accords interest groups particular roles in policymaking which is a second major source of their power and influence. In the United States, the "pluralist" interest group system is highly fragmented with numerous groups vying with each other to bend the ear of policymakers. This fragmentation became more pronounced in the 1970s, with the explosion in the number of groups in Washington DC and state capitols, and the increasingly narrow focus of the concerns of such organizations, to the point that hyper-pluralism is a more accurate description of reality. In pluralist systems, interest groups lack an officially recognized role in policymaking or an official status whereby government leaders must consult them. Rather, they work to press their case from the outside, exerting pressure through lobbying and campaign donations.

In many European polities, by contrast, corporatist systems are the way that interest groups and the state interact with each other. Under corporatism, a limited number of associations representing the key sectors of the economy or a given policy arena possess de facto or legal right to serve as the official voice of that sector. So, for instance, there may be a single peak association that speaks for all trade unions, and a similar counterpart that represents the voice of firms in the political arena. The state accords these interest groups an official seat at the policymaking table, with government ministers or bureaucrats regularly consulting them on legislative or policy changes affecting their members or their sector either out of custom or by legal requirement. Not only do such groups claim a major role in making policies, but also the state often grants them exclusive administrative jurisdiction to implement policies in their sector. In exchange for such a privileged position, the group's leaders must possess the authority to ensure that the members can and will abide by agreements reached with the state.[25] Germany's social health insurance system illustrates such corporatist governance.

The main interest groups in the health policy arena are those representing providers and payers, and to a lesser extent, patients. Among health care providers, interest groups representing doctors and hospitals are key actors, but there are also groups that represent allied health professions. In addition, pharmaceutical companies and medical device manufacturers are powerful interests. The configuration of interests on the payer side depends on how health care is paid for. In health care systems financed by general revenues, private insurers play a marginal role, offering extras or supplemental services alongside the dominant government plan. In countries that finance health care through payroll taxes or premiums to insurers, then insurance associations are important players in health policy. Where health insurance is employment-based, then employers and labor unions also are players in the health policy arena. Finally, groups representing the interests of patients seek a voice in health policy. These may represent a particular age group or disease. Some are more powerful than others in voicing their concerns to policymakers or in mobilizing their members at election time. Generally speaking, those groups exclusively representing the poor tend to have fewer resources and less influence than those representing the middle classes or senior citizens.

Each country's health care system and political system gives entry to different stakeholders in policymaking and administration. Moreover, interest groups and political parties often align with one another to form potent alliances in health policy. In some cases, these alliances endure over a long period of time; in other situations, the partnerships are more fluid. Even long-standing pacts between parties and interest groups, and between interest groups themselves, can decay and disintegrate with time.[26]

Ideas and Ideologies

Policies are the expression of preferences or values of political actors. The dominant values or political culture of a society are widely shared beliefs about politics. People often unconsciously internalize these norms without deliberate reflection. Transmission of these values begins early, in the family or school, and continues through the mainstream media and other social institutions. In the United States, the dominant values are so pervasive that they infiltrate commercial advertising. Think of American car company ads that connect their trucks to images of the cowboy, that classic American icon that invokes values like independence, freedom, self-reliance, and grit.

Not all citizens or actors may subscribe to the dominant value system. They may have their own subcultures and corresponding practices and norms. But values become dominant, or hegemonic, when the vast majority of the population accepts them (consciously or not) and when all mainstream political parties feel compelled to invoke those values when making their arguments and policy recommendations. Heclo and Madsen captured this: "Hegemony need not consist of unanimous or even majority support: it consists of the fact that almost everyone, knowingly or unknowingly, dances to the tune of the leading player."[27] The dominant political culture also defines the acceptable parameters and types of political action. This includes the proper role and reach of the state, the market, the community or group, and the individual. The dominant political culture defines the limits of the possible when considering various policy alternatives.

Ideology is a more explicit and coherent set of values that provides its adherents a way to view and interpret the world. Ideology serves as a blueprint or guide for its adherents as they draw up policy options. Ideology values those proposals that fit within its parameters and discards those that do not. True believers will use ideology almost reflexively when deciding their position on a particular issue or policy alternative. Ideology also serves a retrospective purpose, as policymakers may reinterpret recent history of policy successes or failures through its lens.[28] Hegemonic ideologies are potent weapons that politicians, parties, and interest groups marshal in their efforts to frame a policy debate and to sway public opinion or voters to their side.[29]

Yet periodically these ideological frameworks are subject to challenges that call into question not only the details of existing policy and political settlements, but even the basic values underpinning them. This leads us to consider a final political factor, the effects of history and the nature of political and policy change.

Historical Policy Legacies

The past influences the present, but one must take care in specifying how it does so. Otherwise we fall into the trap of historical determinism, which views a path of development in mechanistic terms and ignores the influence of power. How to avoid simplistic explanations of this type? We must first bear in mind that the policy process does not proceed along a predetermined or linear path. Instead, it more often resembles a *feedback loop* in which policies decided on in an earlier period create new supportive or opposing constituencies, such as interest groups, parties, or voting blocs. In other words, "effect becomes cause," with policies creating politics.[30] Once a policy becomes settled and implemented over time, those who have a stake in the existing arrangement will resist radical attempts to alter that settlement at a later date and exert what political power they have to block changes they oppose. Far from being a mechanistic or pre-determined path, it is a recognition of the political forces and actors in play. If policymakers are to successfully enact changes that depart from the status quo, they will either have to bypass or negotiate with these constituencies. The porousness of the political institutions, their degree of openness to the input of interests, and the balance of party forces in power, will necessitate either negotiation or exclusion. There are plenty of examples in health care of policies creating new constituencies and new politics. One notable example is the rise of the American Association of Retired Persons (AARP) following the passage of Medicare, the govern-ment health insurance program for the elderly in the United States. This group is the foremost representative of senior citizens in health policy and a force that politicians ignore at their peril when they consider changes to that program.

Another way to think about policy continuity or change without fall-ing prey to crude determinism is a careful application of *path dependence*. This approach seeks to explain why policies persist for so long, even when their results may be suboptimal. The argument is that once a policy is enacted and implemented, and stakeholders adjust to it, a radical departure becomes less likely as time passes because those affected have invested so much in the current arrangement.[31]

But then how to explain instances of radical policy shifts? Some analysts point to a cataclysmic event, such as a war or economic depression, often external to the policy in question, that serves as a brief window of oppor-tunity that allows policymakers to create radical new policies. Such events lay bare the limits of the old ways of thinking and doing. For example, a critical election sweeps new political forces into power who then embark on a program of radical change. In situations such as this, a radical pro-posal that was once considered a fringe idea gains mainstream acceptance and is adopted as policy. Change of this type can be in the form of formal revision or outright displacement of an existing policy with something radically new.[32] Yet major policy change may also occur in less dramatic fashion as individual reformers or new policy communities define an issue as a policy problem and offer a specific solution. An idea gains traction not simply because of its inherent attractiveness but because key policymakers and groups coalesce in support of it.[33]

Fundamental policy change may also take place in less conspicuous ways. In some instances, a process of *layering* occurs, whereby new policies or institutions are grafted onto existing ones. Another avenue for change is *conversion*, whereby policies that were once created with a particular purpose in mind are harnessed to serve a new purpose. Such conversion may occur when new groups become beneficiaries of the policy and redirect it to new ends.[34] In both cases, a succession of seemingly minor policy changes or a redefinition of a policy to serve new ends can have far-reaching effects down the line that may go unnoticed at the time of their enactment or implementation. Finally, a subtle yet far-reaching policy change may be the result of *drift*. In this case, a policy is not modernized to address new social risks.[35]

Let us pause to summarize the argument. Policy proposals originate in parties, interest groups, research institutes, and even in the minds of individual policy wonks. The dominant political culture or ideology in a country sets the boundaries of what is politically acceptable for citizens and governments alike in their assessment of a particular policy option. Core political values also are tools that competing parties and interests invoke in framing the political debate and winning over the public. Formal or informal political institutions set the rules of political competition, channel the policy demands of society, and like values, shape calculations of political feasibility. Feedback loops, path dependencies, and legacies of previous policies constrain the realm of the possible. But institutions do not preordain policy outcomes. Cataclysmic events, such as wars or economic depressions, may sweep away these long-standing policies. Less visible processes of conversion, layering, and drift, can also fundamentally alter a program over time. All four political factors are in play and explain different facets of the processes underlying public policy. They help us understand why political actors choose or reject a particular policy, or why the policy may succeed or fail during the enactment and implementation stages of the policymaking process. With all this in mind, it is now time to turn to the contemporary challenges in health policy.

Contemporary Challenges in Health Policy

As health care policymakers face the ongoing tasks of reconciling the goals of health care—equitable access, affordability, quality, and, increasingly, responsiveness—new challenges have made their task harder in recent decades. The nature of new health policy challenges is qualitatively different for an industrialized country than for a developing nation, so we will examine each in turn.

Health Care Policy Challenges in Industrialized Nations

The richer industrialized nations face new demands on health care systems that drive up costs even as a shrinking financial base makes it more difficult to cover them. The difficulties are the result of technological innovations in health care, demographic developments, and structural changes in the nature of work.

First, the health sector employs and rewards technological innovation and scientific breakthroughs. New surgical techniques, drug therapies, and diagnostic tools enormously benefit the survival, prolongation, and quality of human life. But they are expensive.[36] Second, the aging of the population of industrialized nations, to varying degrees, creates new health care needs and exerts greater pressures on health care spending. People are living longer and birth rates are declining. Longevity, itself the product of better medical treatments and innovations in health care places new burdens on the health care systems of these countries. Improvements in public health (vaccinations, sanitation) have put death by infectious diseases at bay, but now chronic and acute noncommunicable diseases arising from affluence and old age afflict more people in Western nations. Heart disease, diabetes, high blood pressure, dementia, stroke, and cancer are now the leading causes of death. The cost of treating patients with these diseases, especially over a longer lifespan as life expectancy rises above 80 years, adds up. At the same time, declining birth rates mean that fewer people of working age will be shouldering the cost of their elders' health care in the future, be it through insurance contributions or taxation. The full impact of population aging on health care spending will play out over a generation, and will be most severe between 2010 and 2035 in most OECD nations, which is when the bulk of the postwar baby boom generation retires. Lifestyle changes in the rich countries of the world constitute another demographic pressure on their health care systems. As more people adopt a sedentary lifestyle and consume diets filled with fat and sugar, rates of obesity and related illnesses like heart disease and diabetes have soared across all age groups.[37]

Profound changes in the nature of work and employment constitute the third source of strain on health care systems. For the first three decades following World War II, Western countries enjoyed a period of unparalleled prosperity. Labor unions, which covered far more workers than they do now, negotiated good wages and benefits for those in full-time permanent employment. Salaried white-collar employment also expanded. The high value-added goods of manufacturing underwrote generous, family-supporting wages and welfare benefits, whether paid for as payroll contributions to social insurance or as general taxes, for the unionized working class.

In the past four decades, however, Western economies have undergone a gradual contraction of employment in manufacturing and a concomitant expansion of employment in services. Companies moving their manufacturing operations to lower-wage countries of the Global South have driven much of this. Some of it has come from labor-saving technical innovations within the industrialized West. In both cases, the result has meant slower wage growth, long-term structural unemployment among displaced factory workers, and the rise of subcontracting and part-time work, all of which spell more tenuous relationships between workers and employers. Together, these developments have reduced the revenue base (whether from tax revenues or payroll insurance contributions) for health care and other welfare state programs.[38] The rise of atypical employment has also frayed the link between insurance coverage and work. In many countries, job-based benefits like health insurance accrue only to full-time permanent employees.

An additional challenge, which I will discuss at greater length in chapter five, is coming to grips with the limits of the biomedical model of health care that dominates Western medicine. A clear body of evidence demonstrates that those with lower incomes have poorer health outcomes than those who are wealthy.[39] The question is why this is so and what health policy can do to change this. The biomedical model overlooks broader social forces that affect health outcomes and instead concentrates on microbiology, genetic inheritance, or individual lifestyle choices to explain physical illness. This understanding of disease ignores how individual choices and even genetics are shaped by broader social forces.

Under the contemporary biomedical model, the physician's attention is solely directed toward the individual patient who comes to the clinic. The medical intervention is reactive and seeks to cure the physical disease, or short of that, alleviate the patient's symptoms. Born in the scientific discoveries of the late nineteenth and twentieth centuries, the biomedical model esteems heroic medicine, life-saving interventions using complex technological procedures, done by specialist physicians. Far less glamorous are the more mundane treatments and consultations of primary care. We can see such different values in the greater social prestige and income of specialists, especially in the United States: the average income of a primary care physician in the United States is approximately $231,000 but for specialists, it is $397,000. Some specialties do even better: orthopedists earn almost double the latter figure.[40] Popular culture also reflects the higher worth society places on heroic, high-tech medicine; in the United States, shows like *ER* and *Grey's Anatomy* are common television fare.[41]

Yet a growing body of evidence points to a more complex interaction of the environment and biology in causing illness. Understanding health and disease in this way leads to a more holistic approach that focuses not simply on the individual patient but also on broader populations. It gives priority to prevention and primary care as a way to lessen the need for curative, high-tech medicine to treat conditions later on. It increasingly recognizes that coordination among medical practitioners and those in other fields, such as behavioral mental health and social services, is needed if an individual and her neighbors are to live in a state of good health. Good health not only requires access to medical care (including cutting-edge technology when appropriate), or information on eating right and exercising, but also giving people access to safe recreation and healthy foods in their neighborhoods so that they can exercise healthy choices. It also requires that health care policies work together with other social policies, such as education and training policies, and tax policies to alleviate if not prevent poverty by attacking a wide range of structural inequalities in society.[42]

Health Care Policy Challenges in Developing Nations

If the health problems of Western nations reflect an embarrassment of riches, the same cannot be said about the Global South where health policy challenges are far more formidable, for two main reasons: widespread poverty and the experience of Western imperialism, a legacy contributing to deep-seated economic problems and political instability decades after its formal dismantling.

Poverty

Poverty and inequality are particularly pernicious in the developing world. Poverty not only causes illness and disease, it also deprives governments of the financial resources to devise effective policy responses. Certainly, poverty and inequality contribute to ill health in the affluent Western countries. But in most of the Global South, poverty is qualitatively different from what it is in the West. The World Bank assigns countries into three classes of poverty: *extreme poverty*, which is defined as at least 25 percent of a nation's population living on less than $1.25 per day, a figure that is insufficient to meet the basic needs of daily life such as food, shelter, or health care. Above that is *moderate poverty*, which is at least 25 percent of the population living on less than $2 per day. At this level, people are just barely surviving; they have enough to assure the basic needs but nothing left to save or invest. The highest level is *relative poverty*, defined as a proportion of the population below one-half the median income of a country. A much greater proportion of the population in countries of the Global South must endure the grind of daily life under conditions of extreme or moderate poverty. By contrast, most of the poor in the affluent Western industrialized democracies are living in relative poverty, owing to social policies that lift people out of extreme or moderate poverty.[43]

The breadth and depth of poverty in developing nations has enormous implications for health and health policy. The causes of death vary by income, as Table 1.1 shows. Poverty also constrains government responses to illness. A poor country lacks the means to invest in broader public health interventions like sanitation or immunizations that would reduce preventable deaths in childhood. It also means that governments have too little tax revenue and most households have too little savings to pay for adequate health care. The public sector health care system that may exist

Table 1.1 Leading causes of death by country income group, 2012* (Deaths per 100,000 population)

Low-income countries	Upper-middle-income countries
Lower respiratory infections (91)	Stroke (126)
HIV/AIDS (65)	Ischemic heart disease (107)
Diarrheal diseases (53)	COPD (50)
Stroke (52)	Trachea, bronchus, lung cancers (31)
Ischemic heart disease (39)	Diabetes mellitus (23)
Malaria (35)	Lower respiratory infections (23)
Preterm birth complications (33)	Road injury (21)
Tuberculosis (31)	Hypertensive heart disease (20)
Birth asphyxia and birth trauma (29)	Liver cancer (18)
Protein energy malnutrition (27)	Stomach cancer (17)

Lower-middle-income countries	High-income countries
Ischemic heart disease (95)	Ischemic heart disease (158)
Stroke (78)	Stroke (95)
Lower respiratory infections (53)	Trachea, bronchus, lung cancers (49)
Chronic obstructive pulmonary disease (COPD)** (52)	Alzheimer disease and other dementias (42)
Diarrheal diseases (37)	COPD (31)
Preterm birth complications (28)	Lower respiratory infections (31)
HIV/AIDS (23)	Colon, rectum cancers (27)
Diabetes mellitus (22)	Diabetes mellitus (20)
Tuberculosis (21)	Hypertensive heart disease (20)
Cirrhosis of the liver (19)	Breast cancer (16)

*World Bank country income groups (using 2013 figures): Low-income countries = gross national income (GNI) per capita of $1045 or less; Middle income = more than $1045 but less than $12,746 GNI per capita; High income = $12,745 or more GNI per capita. Lower and upper-middle-income countries are divided at $4125 GNI per capita. Low- and middle-income countries are sometimes designated as developing countries.
**COPD = Emphysema.
Source: World Health Organization, "The Top Ten Causes of Death," Fact Sheet No. 310, updated May 2014, http://www.who.int/mediacentre/factsheets/fs310/en/); WHO, Health statistics and information systems; Definition of region groupings," http://www.who.int/healthinfo/global_burden_disease/definition_regions/en/; World Bank, "Updated Income Classifications," http://data.worldbank.org/news/2015-country-classifications.

is underfunded, understaffed, and overwhelmed. As a result, most of the population seldom if ever sees a medical doctor; if they do, there is a high likelihood that the practitioner is an aid worker working with a nongovernmental organization (NGO) that provides humanitarian relief, such as the Red Cross or Doctors Without Borders. Table 1.1 illustrates the differences in life expectancy around the globe depending on a nation's income.

The picture, however, is changing, particularly for lower middle-income countries. For these countries, industrialization and economic development have brought the benefits of higher incomes and better access to health care, at least for the middle and working classes who can obtain health insurance. Governments have devoted more spending on public health interventions including immunizations, sanitation, and electrification, all of which have begun to contain the spread of infectious diseases. Life expectancy has increased as deaths from infectious diseases decline. All of these are welcome developments. At the same time, however, economic modernization and urbanization have brought lifestyle and behavior changes such as growing tobacco use, the consumption of high-fat diets, and more sedentary routines. What all this means is that many lower middle-income countries face a double health care burden that their Western neighbors do not. The former continue to confront infectious diseases (in mostly poorer rural areas and urban slums), but increasingly face the burdens associated with the treatment of noncommunicable diseases. At the same time, they possess far fewer resources to devote to health care than the richer nations of the West, whose concerns are confined to the noncommunicable diseases of age and affluence.

The Legacies of Imperialism

Development experts, politicians, and pundits vigorously debate the causes of and solutions to poverty in the developing world. But the basic divide is clear. On one side are those who point to poor governance and weak political leadership in these countries following their independence from colonial rule. On the other side are those who blame the former imperial powers for the economic, political, and social ills of the developing world.[44] In a complex world, one can find truth in both accounts and both must be considered. Certainly, to omit the effects of history is to deny reality and prevent a fuller understanding of current conditions facing the different nations of the Global South. This does not mean that these countries are forever trapped in a history that they had little hand in making; politics involves human agency and collective choice. But it does require that we acknowledge the imprint of history, of the policy legacies that colonial rule bequeathed, that has contributed to contemporary challenges in health policy and politics.

So let us take stock of that history. The era of Western imperialism dates from the sixteenth to the twentieth centuries, when European and American powers created a global economic and political system that enriched their countries at the expense of the Global South. The imperial powers conquered the lands of the Global South and exploited their labor and natural resources for their own economic development, industrialization, and enrichment. That account is generally accepted today. But many scholars go further and argue that imperial domination continues today, albeit through indirect and less visible means. After surrendering their colonies in the latter half of the twentieth century, Western nations exerted their power to create the rules and institutions of the international economic system. Ostensibly based in free trade, the new economic order worked to maintain the dominance of the industrialized Western nations and their corporate allies who sought to retain their access to the natural resources, cheap labor, and hefty profits in the former colonies, even if it meant supporting undemocratic regimes there.[45] Western-based companies with operations in the Global South, international bankers, and economic development institutions had merely replaced direct rule by colonial administrators. Even nations that had not been formal colonies of the Western powers were subject to the toxic effects of geopolitical struggles (such as the Cold War) on their internal politics and policies.[46]

In the same vein, health care in the imperial era primarily furthered the interests and rule of the colonial powers. Colonial doctors initially treated the illnesses of conquering European militaries and later those of the white colonial administrators in cities and ports of these empires. Doctors also treated the illnesses of the indigenous labor force in the mines and plantations that were so important to the extraction of the colonies' natural resources for raw materials for the factories of Europe.[47] This history explains the location of many hospitals and clinics in urban areas where the white minority population continues to be concentrated today.

The profoundly unequal access to health care that originated in the colonial era persists today. The predominant health care model in developing nations consists of two distinct and unequal health care systems, one for the wealthy minority and one for the vast majority of the poor. The wealthy minority that can afford to pay for care through private insurance or directly out of pocket has access to a high quality system of private clinics and medical practitioners. These fortunate few are primarily the descendants of white colonial settlers, but also include the small but privileged cadre of ruling party members, civil servants, military officers, and the nascent middle class that has opened up to the indigenous population.[48] Everyone else, particularly the indigenous population, must seek care from the most rudimentary public sector health care system or, more likely, from traditional healers.

The legacy of inequality also translates into very different disease profiles, not only between rich and poor nations, but also between the white minority and the indigenous majority within the developing countries. As Table 1.1 indicates, in the industrialized countries, the leading causes of death reflect affluence and old age. The biggest killers are heart disease, diabetes, high blood pressure, dementia, stroke, and cancer. The leading causes of morbidity (living with an illness) are the same, as well as depression, anxiety, and obesity (which leads to heart disease, diabetes, and stroke). In developing nations, however, the major killers are infectious diseases like malaria, diarrhea, TB, and HIV/AIDS, and the victims are mostly young children or those of working age.[49] These are the diseases of poverty, and reflect insufficient investment in basic public health: foul water, sooty air, and cramped living quarters of the slums of the megacities (urban areas with more than 10 million people) facilitate the spread of such diseases. The costs associated with the construction of a public health infrastructure, as well as a health care system that can provide basic primary and preventive care as well as tertiary care like surgeries or drugs to combat infectious diseases, are beyond the reach of most private households and governments in these poor countries.

The scourge of infectious diseases is rooted in broader structural forces such as the global economic system and the inequality that has persisted following the end of formal imperialism. Labor migration patterns that are part of the web of global trade became transmission belts for infectious diseases. Local conflicts became bloodier as the West and Russia armed their proxies. Paul Farmer has termed this "structural violence" against the world's poor. By that he means "such suffering is structured by processes and forces that conspire—whether through routine, ritual, or more commonly, the hard surfaces of economics and politics—to constrain agency. For many, . . . choices both large and small are limited by racism, sexism, political violence, *and* grinding poverty."[50]

Simply put, poverty and inequality are hazardous to one's health, and this is especially so for those who reside in the developing world. The inequality between rich and poor nations as well as that between the rich and poor within the nations of the Global South make it far more likely that their people will contract an infectious disease (often one conquered long ago in the West by public health interventions), or endure illnesses arising from economic or political violence. Furthermore, they will lack the financial means to pay for treatment and therefore die a needless and preventable death at a younger age than someone in the West.[51] As Paul Farmer has succinctly stated, *"Thus do fundamentally social forces and processes come to be embodied as biological events"* (my emphasis).[52]

Imperialism has also left deep psychological scars in the former colonies that have undermined the trust and social cohesion necessary to the development and sustenance of healthy democracies. At the Berlin Conference in 1884, European powers divided up the African continent into their own respective areas for colonization. Much of Asia (and Latin America earlier) became territories reserved for the European and American powers. But the boundaries that these colonial masters set were artificial. In some cases, distinct ethnic groups or tribes, each with their own identity based in history, custom, language, or religion, were herded into a single colony. In other cases, the boundaries severed an ethnic group into two, leaving the majority of that group in one colony but also creating a minority population in a different colony. In Rwanda, South Africa, and Zimbabwe (formerly Southern Rhodesia), the white settlers constructed group identities on the basis of artificial racial categories, and used these categories to privilege one group over the other in a strategy of divide-and-rule. Once the colonial powers retreated after World War II, they left behind fractured countries with weak national identities and simmering resentments among the indigenous groups that erupted into horrific civil wars, as in Rwanda in the 1990s, or between the white minority and the indigenous majority groups, as in Zimbabwe in the 1960s and 1970s. Even in countries like South Africa, which escaped full-fledged civil war has, over a century of colonial oppression bred racial animosity and mistrust between white colonials and their descendants on the one hand, and the indigenous population on the other.

The ill will, resentment, and suspicion between the races have carried over into health policy. A vivid example is South Africa's response to HIV/AIDS over two decades. The system of racial segregation under white minority rule infected public attitudes and public policy toward AIDS even after the transition to democratic politics and black majority rule. Sharply delineated racial identities seeped into perceptions of disease risk and slowed the formulation of an effective national response to the epidemic, with tragic results.[53]

International Actors and Organizations

Poverty and inequality born of imperialism are not the only factors shaping the health care challenges and policy responses of the Global South. To a greater extent than the Western industrialized nations, actors and institutions at the international level impinge upon the domestic policies of the nations of the Global South. Their deep poverty has forced developing countries to rely on international development organizations and agencies, private multinational corporations and banks, and NGOs engaged in humanitarian aid and social and economic development work.

The key supranational institutions of the global economy are the International Monetary Fund (IMF), the World Bank (WB), and the World Trade Organization (WTO). The victorious western Allied powers agreed to establish the IMF and World Bank in 1944 and the WTO's predecessor, the General Agreement on Tariffs and Trade (GATT) in 1948 to stabilize the global economic and financial systems after World War II ended. These institutions were created to prevent another 1930s-style Great Depression that had undermined economies and fragile democracies and had culminated in World War II. Both industrialized and developing nations are members of these organizations, but in many cases these bodies serve as vehicles to advance the interests of the industrialized West at the expense of the Global South. These organizations not only give the Western powers inordinate influence on their governing boards, but have also inflicted great harm on nations receiving their help by imposing the dictates of a neoliberal strategy of "structural adjustment." Let us examine these bodies in greater detail.

The IMF is the lender of last resort to countries on the verge of bankruptcy whose governments no longer gain the confidence of private or foreign creditors and bondholders. To obtain a bailout from the IMF, the country in question must comply with the Fund's terms of structural adjustment. The IMF's diagnosis of structural adjustment rests on the conviction that excessive government meddling in a nation's economy and society is responsible for a nation's economic ills, and that the only lies in embracing free trade and the free market. The nation in question must undergo "shock therapy" involving measures to unleash free market forces and bring it back into the global free trade regime in rapid fashion. The specific policies of structural adjustment regimen remove trade barriers by eliminating import tariffs and quotas and encouraging foreign investment and ownership in domestic industries. It also compels the government to reduce its reach in the economy and society and balance its budget by privatizing state-owned enterprises, ending subsidies on basic foods and fuel because these distort market signals of supply and demand, and slashing public spending.

Less committed to structural adjustment than the IMF is the World Bank, a supranational bank financed by contributions from the governments of its member nations. It funds development projects, primarily physical infrastructure, but also education, health, and social services in poor nations. The WTO is an international body that sets the rules of trade and investment and adjudicates trade disputes among member nations. It, too, tends to promote structural adjustment and free trade, but does provide for some exceptions in specific cases. The WTO's rulings on intellectual property rights and patent protection have had a direct bearing on health care in all nations.

Critics of structural adjustment, both within the affected countries and in the broader international development community, argue that the bitter medicine of structural adjustment has toxic effects and that the cure is worse than the disease, if cure indeed there be. Privatization triggers layoffs in state enterprises, while the lifting of protectionist measures that had sheltered nascent domestic industries produces mass unemployment. Widespread poverty and hardship follow from mass unemployment, the ending of food and fuel subsidies, and deep cuts in social programs like education, health care, and income support. The social dislocation and misery in turn foster political unrest (such as strikes, demonstrations, or riots), often prompting a coup or revolution that installs a military government or dictator and spells the end of a fragile democracy.[54]

Several supranational organizations deal directly with health and welfare. The United Nations (UN) and its specific aid agencies, such as the United Nations Children's Fund (UNICEF) and the Joint United Nations Program on HIV/AIDS (UNAIDS), formulate health policies and assist nations and other actors in implementing them in developing nations. But the main body is the World Health Organization (WHO). Founded in 1948, it acts as a clearinghouse of information and statistics, creates reports, and makes policy recommendations on health policy topics for the world. It also provides technical assistance to policymakers and practitioners on the ground. The WHO does not directly fund projects, but it channels money from donor countries or organizations to developing nations. Relying on the international scientific community, health economists, as well as the input of delegates from member nations at world summits, the WHO, World Bank, and UNICEF exert significant influence over the health policies of developing nations.

The record of these organizations in combating disease and promoting health has been mixed. Even with the best intentions, they have sometimes recommended or implemented health policy interventions that have failed to meet their stated goals or have done little to improve the health of developing nations. Because officials at the highest levels of these organizations are far removed from the populations they serve, the policies they design do not always take into account local conditions and needs, as with the ill-fated WHO malaria eradication program between 1955 and 1969.[55] Sometimes the organizations adopt cost–benefit analyses that take resource constraints as a given, and in so doing devise interventions that are neither clinically effective nor cost effective. For example, the WHO recommendation for a short duration drug therapy for TB (directly observed treatment, short course, or DOTS) rather than a longer and more comprehensive (yet more expensive) drug regimen (DOTS-Plus) has allowed for the spread of multiple drug-resistant strains of the disease. The WHO has been slow to adopt the latter treatment into its guidelines of best practice.[56] Another example is the WHO's best practices for HIV/AIDS in poor nations. Initially the WHO recommended only preventive public health measures rather than expensive drug therapies that were common in Western countries, on the grounds that the drugs were not a cost-effective use of scarce resources. But renegade nations like Brazil bucked this advice and adopted free access to such drug therapies for all who needed it, along with prevention strategies for at-risk groups. Brazil's twin approach of prevention plus treatment led to sharp declines in AIDS mortality and prevalence rates, as drug treatment of those infected actually reduced transmission of the disease to their offspring or partners. The approach was also cost effective: with drugs suppressing the emergence of full-blown AIDS, the treatment also prevented opportunistic infections like TB from emerging in persons with compromised immune systems. This, in turn, saved money by reducing costly hospital admissions. It took Brazil's success—and the mobilization of AIDS activists globally—to convince the WHO to adopt prevention plus treatment as best practices for all nations.[57]

But there have also been notable successes. The WHO's campaign to eradicate smallpox is a stunning example.[58] Less dramatic but equally important actions to promote global health have come out of international meetings of national governments and aid organizations. One such example is the 1978 International Conference on Primary Care at Alma Ata, where delegates from 134 nations and 37 international organizations committed to achieving universal health care by 2000. Since Alma Alta, the WHO has continued to press nations to introduce health care systems that are centered in primary care and to address the social determinants of health. Perhaps the best known example of the WHO's advocacy is the Millennium Development Goals (MDGs). In 2002, UN member states adopted a declaration that committed them to pursue the improvement of human well-being through a range of health and social policy goals. At the centerpiece was the pledge to halve extreme poverty by 2015 and eliminate it by 2030, and the commitment of rich nations to spend 0.7 percent of their GDP on direct foreign aid. In 2010, the WHO published its report *Health System Financing: The Path to Universal Health Coverage*, which called on all nations to adopt policies to achieve universal health coverage. The WHO subsequently published documents outlining a framework and guidelines to realize this goal and UN member states adopted a resolution in 2012 that committed them to this project.[59] To be sure, these ambitious goals have not been fully realized, yet real progress has been made.[60] The WHO's efforts have focused minds and actions of governments, providing them and aid agencies with policy direction and technical assistance. These examples also highlight the limits of these supranational organizations to compel action by member states intent on preserving their national sovereignty. Lacking the authority to issue binding rules or the means to enforce them on recalcitrant nations does not render these organizations completely powerless. International organizations may exercise "soft power" of persuasion, admonishing nations to cooperate and take action or impose economic sanctions on renegades.[61] In some cases, the signatories may abide by the provisions of an international treaty even in the absence of enforcement mechanisms, as with the WHO's Framework Convention on Tobacco Control.[62]

Furthermore, in recent years intensified economic globalization has enhanced the influence of private economic actors on the domestic policies of developing nations, with both indirect and direct effects on health and health policy. Governments and firms in these nations must bear in mind the decisions of global financial creditors (private investment banks, currency and stock markets) and their willingness to extend credit to them. Multinational companies (MNCs) can decide to locate or shut down operations in developing nations. While most analysts consider these actors as falling under the realm of economic policy, their decisions at least indirectly influence the status of health in these nations. For example, a global company headquartered in a Western country may open a plant in a developing nation because the environmental and workplace safety standards may be weaker and the wage scales lower than in its home nation. While the plant creates jobs, it also puts the local population and workforce at risk for disability or death from industrial pollution (as in Bhopal, India) or workplace accidents or ill health and malnutrition because their earnings are too low to pull them out of poverty. Global food producers and tobacco companies that decide to pursue new markets in developing countries directly impact the health of these populations.[63]

In sum, governments in developing nations must often deal with international actors and rules on terms that are not of their making. The nations of the Global South still do not wield political power commensurate with their growing economic might. For example, the biggest emerging market economies (Brazil, Russia, India, China, and South Africa, or BRICS), wield only 10.3 percent of the votes on the governing board of the IMF, even though they comprise 24.5 percent of the world economy.[64] This is beginning to change, especially in the wake of the Great Recession of 2008. Whereas the economic crisis brought a number of Western industrialized nations to the brink of bankruptcy and required bailouts from the IMF and European Union, the effects of the downturn were far less severe in the Global South. Their relative economic vigor led them to claim a greater role in the management of the world economy. In 2009, the Group of Twenty (G20) officially displaced the more exclusive Group of Eight (G8) club of the eight richest industrialized nations as the main international forum for meetings of heads of state and central bank governors of the wealthiest economies.

Membership of the G20 includes the larger emerging market economies as well as the major Western powers. In a further effort to wrest greater control over their destinies and assert their autonomy from the West, the BRICS established their own economic development bank independent of the IMF and World Bank in 2014.[65] NGOs have become major actors in global health. Their sheer numbers have grown exponentially. In 1990, they numbered only 6000, but by 2000 there were over 26,000 such entities.[66] NGOs give organized expression to civil society in the health policies at international, national, and local levels of developing nations. NGOs engage in humanitarian work on the ground and seek to work with and strengthen civil society in developing countries or finance the work of such organizations. Some of the better-known organizations, such as Doctors without Borders, Oxfam, and the Red Cross, are headquartered in the West but operate worldwide. Other NGOs, such as the Bill and Melinda Gates Foundation, are philanthropist organizations that donate and channel large sums to health care research or finance the work of NGOs on the ground. NGOs have become increasingly active in advocacy and lobbying of government officials and international organizations on health policy issues that are of vital interest to developing nations, such as making sure drug therapies to treat infectious diseases like AIDS are affordable for those countries. Some of these groups have established networks with local NGOs to create transnational networks, such as DATA (Debt, AIDS, Trade, Africa) or the ONE Campaign, to put pressure on Western governments to make good on their financial commitments to meet the Millennium Development Challenge. Doctors without Borders and other NGOs have framed access to essential medicine in terms of human rights and pitted this against the profit-seeking behavior of global pharmaceutical companies. Such campaigns, particularly around AIDS therapies, have forced the industry to make their life-saving drugs affordable to the poorest nations. The Campaign for Essential Medicines spearheaded by Doctors without Borders is one such example. But NGOs have also forged innovative public–private partnerships instead of confrontational approaches to encourage the development of new treatments for the deadliest diseases afflicting the Global South. For-profit drug companies often shy away from research and development on medicines for poor countries because they fear that they will not see a return on their investment. But the Drugs for Neglected Diseases Initiative, which Doctors without Borders founded in 2003, coordinates the work of pharmaceutical companies, university researchers, and governments to develop essential medicines and has scored successes for drug therapies to treat malaria. In an effort to get essential medicines to the developing countries more quickly, international aid organizations have partnered with university researchers and drug companies to develop patent pools that allow for research on cheaper generic drugs before the patents expire while still allowing the patent holder to claim royalties.[67]

These difficulties have manifested themselves in one way or another in our three case studies. All three countries have sought, with varying degrees of success, to undertake reforms to address the challenges facing their health care systems.

Plan of the Book

Each of the case studies highlights some of the major challenges in health care today as well as the specific configuration of politics that shape their policy responses. Policymakers in the United States have begun repair a health care system with runaway costs that denied ever more millions of people access to care. A porous political system granting organized interests and political parties multiple points of entry to the policymaking process shaped the reform that emerged but ultimately did not prevent its passage. Still, the fragmented system offers political actors subsequent opportunities to halt or overturn reform at a later date. Successive German governments have had to confront the effects of an aging population on the financial sustainability of the health care system while promoting greater coordination of health care delivery. Coalition politics and federalism have entailed difficult negotiations with a range of stakeholders and parties, producing compromise solutions. In South Africa's young democracy, governments face the arduous task of institution building in their construction of a durable health care system that assures equitable access to all. But the burden of history weighs heavily here. Deep poverty and cleavages based on racial lines, the legacies of the country's colonial past, have often hampered effective policy responses. In addition to these internal political factors, international forces have impinged upon South African health policy, complicating the government's policy response. To a greater degree than in the United States and Germany, international actors have influenced the policy choices of the South African government. The international development community has been an important source of assistance— financial, technical, and coalition building. But at the same time, the rules of the global economy have limited the maneuver room of South African policymakers and their economic strategy has sometimes conflicted with the health needs of the population.

The book addresses these case studies of health policy and politics as follows. Chapter Two examines the politics of health care policy and reform in the United States. Chapter Three covers similar ground for Germany. Chapter Four sets out the South African case. The conclusion chapter draws together lessons for health policy from these three case studies.

CHAPTER TWO

The United States: An Ambivalent Journey toward Universal Coverage

The United States remains the only industrialized nation that does not provide universal health insurance. The passage of the Patient Protection and Affordable Care Act (PPACA) of 2010 brings the country closer to its peers, but in its own fashion. This is a far more limited role for government in health care than the health care models in other industrialized nations. Canada, for example, relies on a tax-financed single government insurance plan in each province. The single-payer insurance model, however, allows for primarily private providers. In the national health service of Britain and Sweden, the government's role is even more extensive, financing health care from a single government insurance program and providing health care services from public clinics and hospitals. By contrast, American policymakers have taken steps to fill in coverage gaps through a dualistic model of private employment-based insurance and public insurance programs for those outside the labor market, namely, the elderly, poor, disabled, and the military. Germany's statutory national health insurance based in employer and individual mandates perhaps comes closest to the United States.

The PPACA builds upon this dualistic structure by mandating individuals to carry insurance obtained through employment or on the individual market while greatly enlarging the reach of public insurance to extend to the working poor. If fully implemented, the law will cover millions of people who had been left behind. The law also plants the seeds for major long-term institutional change in the way that health care services are provided to address high costs and uneven quality of care. For these reasons, the law stands as a transformative piece of legislation in the history of American health care policy. Though ambitious in scope, the law nevertheless reflects the historical legacies of past choices in health policy and the political institutions, interests, and ideas that such choices encompassed. But it also signals a new alignment of forces that successfully advocated and mobilized for major change.

It would be a stretch to call health care arrangements in the United States a system because that would imply a coherence and coordination that is all too often lacking. This health care system is a product of a political system that makes radical sweeping reforms infrequent, though not impossible. A system of fragmented political institutions that disperses power, multiple interest groups that work to sabotage change, political values that render the public suspicious of government intervention, and past policy legacies that constrain subsequent policy choices have thwarted ambitious initiatives of policymakers most of the time. Even so, there have been a few periods when policymakers have instituted major reform. The PPACA of 2010 is one such example.

This chapter describes the US patchwork health care system and the political dynamics that have underpinned efforts to reform it. The first section "A Private–Public Patchwork Health Care System in the United States" describes the main features of health care financing and provision in the United States. The second section "A Polity that Disperses Power" describes the political forces that disperse power in the United States and make a national consensus on health care reform difficult to achieve. The structures of the political system, the configuration of health care stakeholders, and an ideology that is suspicious of government intervention has time and again obstructed efforts to introduce national health insurance. The dual system of private and public coverage thus emerged by default rather than by conscious design. The third section "Bringing Stakeholders Back In: The PPACA of 2010" analyzes the latest effort at reform, the PPACA, giving special attention to the politics surrounding its enactment and implementation. The fourth section analyzes Republican Party alternatives to the Democrats' Affordable Care Act. The last section considers two possible futures for health policy in the United States.

A Private–Public Patchwork Health Care System in the United States

Health Care Financing

Voluntary Employment-Based Insurance

The majority of working-age Americans and their dependents obtains health insurance through the private market, and especially through their place of employment as a fringe benefit. Indeed, the availability of health insurance through employment is often a decisive factor in choosing where to work. Health insurers are private, and increasingly, for-profit entities. Public government insurance programs extend to many, though not all, of those outside the labor market: senior citizens aged 65 and older have Medicare; low-income families and the disabled obtain coverage through Medicaid; while members of the armed forces and their families are covered under government programs associated through the Veterans Administration (VA). This dual system of primarily private coverage alongside government programs for certain eligible categories of the population evolved in a haphazard fashion rather than through some conscious grand design. Private insurance based in employment dates from the early twentieth century, while government programs designed to ameliorate the health hazards of those outside the labor force followed several decades later.

In the early twentieth century, health insurance was mostly an individual affair. Health insurance originated in funeral benefits that commercial insurers offered members of the working class. Individual policies offering limited health benefits were tailored to each individual policyholder and insurance agents collected premiums on a weekly basis. As such, it was a costly enterprise with low profit margins, thus deterring most insurance companies from entering the market.

Employment-based health insurance first gained a toehold during the Great Depression of the 1930s. The economic crisis ushered in mass unemployment and put the incomes of health care providers at risk as individuals could no longer afford their individual health insurance policies or their medical bills owed to providers. To counter this, providers set up their own nonprofit insurance companies to offer group insurance to employers at a low prepaid monthly premium, thus ushering in "the Blues." State hospital associations created Blue Cross insurance plans to cover hospital bills while state medical societies followed with Blue Shield plans to cover doctors' fees. The Blues made health insurance more widely affordable and available by employing *risk-pooling* mechanisms. First, they offered *group insurance* to employers, which placed a large number of healthier people along with sicker people across a larger group rather than insuring each individual by means of a separate insurance policy. This practice not only cut down on administrative costs but it also spread the cost of insurance among healthy and sick people. Second, the Blues calculated insurance premiums by using *community rating* in which the same premium would apply to all members of the insurance pool regardless of their individual health status, and would also apply to all employer groups in a defined geographical region. Community rating made health insurance affordable to sicker and older members of a group because they would be paying less than their actual health care costs, while healthier and younger members paid more than their health status would indicate. The Blues also typically offered *first-dollar coverage*, that is, full coverage of medical and hospital bills with no out-of-pocket payments by patients at the time of medical treatment rather than requiring patients to pay their bills in full and then seek reimbursement from their insurer, which was the practice of indemnity insurance. The Blues were also nonprofit entities whose surpluses went back into the operations of the company rather than as profits to shareholders. Acknowledging their public service in making insurance affordable to many, the government granted the Blues tax-exempt status as nonprofit entities serving the broader community.

Voluntary employment-based insurance became firmly entrenched during and after World War II, again with the help of government policies.[1] In 1939, the Internal Revenue Service (IRS) ruled that employers could deduct the cost of fringe benefits from their taxable income as a business expense rather than as a portion of employee income subject to income tax. This ruling not only gave a huge tax break to employers who provided health insurance to their workers but also to employees since their fringe benefits would not be considered part of their taxable income. Another significant ruling came in 1942, from the National War Labor Board, whose remit was to prevent inflation and industrial strikes in an environment of tight labor markets during World War II. To prevent inflationary wage settlements, the board froze wages but permitted employers to boost fringe benefits to attract and retain workers in short supply. This ruling provided a further impetus for employers to offer health insurance and other fringe benefits in lieu of wage increases. Following the war, labor unions faced a threatening political environment with a Republican-controlled Congress enacting legislation restricting unions and refusing to pass a national health insurance bill. In response to such hostile government action, the two umbrella organizations of the labor movement, the American Federation of Labor (AFL) and the Congress of Industrial Organizations (CIO), decided that unions would have to seek income security for their members via collective bargaining on fringe benefits, like pensions and health insurance, as well as wages. Though employers contended that fringe benefits were the exclusive prerogative of the management, the National Labor Relations Board (NLRB) disagreed. In its 1948 *Inland Steel* decision, the NLRB ruled that fringe benefits were a condition of employment subject to collective bargaining, thus paving the way for labor unions to negotiate for health insurance benefits on behalf of their members.

The private insurance landscape altered significantly with the entry of for-profit commercial insurers beginning in the 1950s. The rapid expansion of employment-based insurance in the postwar period demonstrated to commercial insurers that health insurance could be profitable venture. The commercial insurers entered the market and went head-to-head with the dominant nonprofit Blue Cross–Blue Shield plans by using medical underwriting practices, pursuing *experience rating*, and an array of coverage exclusions as a strategy to gain market share. Instead of community rating offered by the Blues, which spread the costs of health care evenly to all employers and individuals in a region by charging the same premium, commercial insurers used experience rating to tie insurance premiums to the health status and expected or actual use of health care by an individual or a firm's employees. In this way, commercial insurers could win market share by offering lower premiums to firms with healthier workers whose lower health care costs made them more profitable to insure than sick people. To cover losses and enhance profits, commercial insurers also inserted exclusion waivers into policies that listed specific medical conditions that would not be covered. The most insidious instrument was the *preexisting medical condition* clause that allowed insurers to deny coverage of any condition that had existed in the year prior to a person's enrollment in the health plan, regardless of whether the person knew that the condition existed or had not sought treatment for it. Such clauses also permitted an insurer to cancel an individual or employer's health plan once the preexisting condition was discovered. These kinds of underwriting practices pervaded the individual and small business insurance markets.[2]

Commercial insurers' use of experience rating and exclusion clauses proved successful in winning market share at the expense of the Blues, whose community-rated premiums were higher for firms with healthy employees. But such *cream skimming (risk selection)* practices segmented the market into healthier and sicker communities and placed health insurance out of reach for the weakest market players. Thus, insurers charged women higher rates than men for the coverage in the individual insurance market because of the associated costs of pregnancy (even if they were not pregnant), or else excluded pregnancy from coverage altogether. Those who were sicker face prohibitively high premiums based on their poor health or were deemed uninsurable and denied coverage altogether.

Small businesses, too, faced distinct disadvantages in obtaining affordable insurance for their employees than do larger firms. Unlike large employers, small businesses have fewer healthier employees to spread the costs of health care of a few sicker employees. Many small firms were also charged experience-rated premiums for each employee, a burden that large companies did not bear. Small businesses also shouldered much higher administrative costs for insurance coverage than large companies: such administrative costs typically gobbled up 33 to 37 percent of the cost of medical claims for small firms but only 5 to 11 percent for large firms.[3] More significantly, small firms lacked market clout that comes with size to negotiate better premiums from insurers. Indeed, many large employers have been able to take the ultimate exit option by self-funding (also known as self-insuring), that is, setting aside money to pay for the health care costs for their employees alone and hiring a company to administer the plan. This allows employers to extricate themselves from a risk pool of sicker individuals and small businesses, and escape state mandates to cover particular medical services. Self-funded plans have grown from covering 44 percent of the workforce in 1999 to 60 percent in 2011.[4] But it is not an option for small employers because they lack enough healthy employees to offset the costs of even a few sicker workers.

Premiums and coverage reflected the differential treatment of large and small employers in the health insurance market. In 2011, only 48 percent of firms with three to nine employees offered insurance but nearly all larger firms with more than 100 workers did so. Small businesses typically faced annual premium increases of 30 percent per year in the twenty-first century compared to large firms whose rate increases were 10 percent or less. Those who worked for small businesses typically had to pay higher deductibles and other cost sharing than those working for large employers.[5]

The success of commercial insurers in gaining market share was a game-changer by the 1990s. To stay competitive, many nonprofit insurers abandoned community rating and switched to experience rating. The latter became the dominant tool for calculating premiums in the individual and small group insurance markets. Facing criticism and possible legislative action by state governments for such action, Blue Cross–Blue Shield plans converted from nonprofit to for-profit entities in the 1990s. All of the above changes made insurance increasingly difficult to access for individuals and small businesses.

Government Insurance Programs[6]

Employment-based insurance spread rapidly in the 1950s and became a common feature of collective bargaining between unions and management, particularly in the manufacturing sector, the biggest sector of employment at the time, and the public sector. Blue Cross and Blue Shield plans were the dominant insurers in this market. Even so, not everyone was covered by employer-sponsored insurance, particularly, retirees, children, and the disabled who were not in the labor market and thus cut off from this source of health insurance. In response, policymakers in Washington created two government insurance programs, Medicare and Medicaid, to cover those deemed deserving of government help in 1965. Since then, policymakers have expanded the scope of the programs to cover more services and people.

Medicare is government health insurance that covers all Americans aged 65 and older. The program, financed and administered by the federal government, covers senior citizens, disabled individuals who receive Social Security disability income, and patients receiving kidney dialysis treatments. Medicare Parts A and B were enacted in 1965. Medicare Part

A covers hospitalization, some home care, and skilled nursing home care for a limited duration. All seniors are automatically enrolled in the program when they turn 65. Medicare Part B covers physician and outpatient medical expenses. Technically a voluntary program, virtually all seniors choose to enroll in it. Under Medicare Parts A and B, seniors have full choice of physicians and hospitals and the federal government directly reimburses providers for their services.

Medicare does not cover all services, however. It excludes skilled long-term care, and, until 2003, did not cover prescription drugs. Many seniors had to either pay for their medications out of their own pocket or take out supplemental insurance plans to cover such expenses. The Medicare Modernization Act of 2003 promoted private health plans and introduced drug benefits. Part C is the Medicare Advantage Program that allows seniors to enroll in private health plans that contract with the federal government to provide health services to enrollees. Such plans typically restrict members to a specific network of doctors and hospitals in exchange for additional benefits and lower out-of-pocket costs for their members. The legislation also created a prescription drug benefit under Medicare Part D, giving private insurers the sole authority to provide drug coverage plans to seniors and barring the government from negotiating drug prices with pharmaceutical companies. The program is popular, with nearly 60 percent of seniors opting for prescription drug coverage.

Medicare has done much to expand access to health care for senior citizens. Nevertheless, the program has gaps in coverage and requires significant cost sharing from recipients. Payroll taxes provide the bulk of Medicare Part A financing, but seniors also pay an annual deductible and a co-payment for hospitalization beyond 60 days. Part B Medicare is financed by federal income and general tax revenues but also by monthly premiums by enrollees. Medicare reimburses doctors only up to 80 percent of an approved amount for their services. Consequently, many seniors have supplemental insurance (Medigap policies) to pay the 20 percent balance, or pay the amount themselves, unless the provider accepts government payment as payment in full. Medicare Part C and D receive federal tax revenues for the bulk of their financing. Yet the drug coverage saddled seniors with out of pocket costs up to almost $5000 annually. In 2010, a typical Part D plan charged an enrollee a $30 average monthly premium, $300 deductible, and paid 75 percent of drug expenses up to $2,830. The patient paid the 25 percent share. Above that, an enrollee entered the "doughnut hole," in which insurance coverage stopped until the person had paid $4,550 out of pocket (minus the premium). For catastrophic drug expenses above that amount, insurance paid 95 percent of the costs with the patient being responsible for the 5 percent remainder.

Despite these shortcomings, the Medicare program is popular and carries with it significant legitimacy. Most Americans recognize that senior citizens, who tend to be sicker and needing medical treatment with advancing age, require health insurance. Furthermore, Medicare epitomizes the model of *social insurance*, which is government insurance provided on a universal basis (in this case, to nearly all seniors aged 65 and above, regardless of income), and financed largely by contributions (as premiums or payroll taxes) from the beneficiaries themselves.[7] This contributory aspect makes Medicare akin to an insurance program and seniors believe that with their contributions, they have "earned" or are "entitled to" their benefits (hence, the term, entitlement program). Social insurance programs such as Medicare also garner broader political support because their universal nature makes them a middle class program. Seniors, moreover, tend to vote in elections in higher numbers than their younger cohorts, so they are a force that politicians must reckon with.

Medicaid, enacted in 1965, is health insurance for low-income families with dependent children, the disabled, and low-income pregnant women. In 1997, the federal government enacted the Children's Health Insurance Program (CHIP), which extended Medicaid to children in low-income households with earnings up to 200 percent of the federal poverty line or $39,580 for a family of three in 2014. Adults without dependent children were explicitly barred from Medicaid. Though Medicaid and Medicare were enacted as part of the ambitious Great Society legislation, the two programs contain stark distinctions. Unlike Medicare, which is financed and administered by the federal government, Medicaid and CHIP are jointly financed and administered by the federal government and the states. The federal government pays roughly half of a state's Medicaid costs, but this share varies by each state's income. Hence, the federal government shoulders 50 percent of Medicaid costs for 15 states but 74 percent for poorer states like Mississippi. The federal government also increases its contribution to states' Medicaid programs during recessions as more Americans lose their jobs and insurance and then turn to Medicaid for coverage. Within federal guidelines, state governments enjoy significant freedom to determine who is eligible for Medicaid and which services are covered. States may apply for waivers to the federal government to experiment with more efficient ways of providing health care services to their Medicaid population, so long as these are budget neutral. Under such waivers, however, states may reduce eligibility and benefits.[8]

Finally, because it is *social assistance* rather than social insurance with earned benefits, Medicaid carries a stigma and differentiates between the "deserving" and "undeserving" poor through means tests and eligibility rules. Not all poor people are covered: childless adults are expected to provide for themselves in the labor market. Recipients must also pass a means test of their assets and income, which carries with it the stigma of charity.

Since most who pay income taxes earn too much to qualify for Medicaid, the program can fuel resentment among low-wage workers whose earnings exceed the income limit yet who are uninsured. Though the popular perception of a Medicaid recipient is a low-income household headed by a minority single mother, most Medicaid recipients are white, and the bulk of Medicaid spending goes to formerly middle-class senior citizens in need of long-term care who must spend down their assets to meet the income eligibility requirement.

The other group of the population that receives government insurance and health care is the military and their dependents, which the federal government finances and provides. Active members of the military and veterans receive health care directly from VA hospitals. Military families receive health insurance through the government.

The patchwork quilt of health care financing has frayed with the passage of time, leaving an increasing number of Americans uninsured. Between the Great Depression and the 1970s, insurance coverage expanded, thanks to employment-based insurance and the introduction of Medicare and Medicaid in 1965. Still, not everyone was covered. Insurance coverage peaked in 1976 but since then the trend has gone into reverse. In 1980, 25 million Americans were uninsured; by 2009, the depth of the Great Recession, 51 million lacked coverage.[9] That same year, 49 percent of the American population received insurance from work, 5 percent from individual private insurance, and 19 percent from Medicare and Medicaid combined.[10]

The major reason for the rising numbers of uninsured has been the erosion of employment-based coverage. Small businesses in particular have found it difficult to obtain affordable coverage. Roughly half of small firms with fewer than 10 employees offered insurance in the 1990s, and only 47 percent of them offered it in 2009, the trough year of the Great Recession.[11] Unlike large employers, small businesses face experience rated premiums and lack the size to negotiate manageable premium increases with insurers. Yet broader changes in the American economy have also left their mark. With deindustrialization, high-paying manufacturing jobs with union-negotiated wages and fringe benefits like health insurance have disappeared. For the unskilled, employment opportunities are confined to low-wage service sector jobs that lack health insurance and other fringe benefits. Even when an employer in this sector offers health insurance, many workers forego it because their wages are too low to afford their share of the premium and other out of pocket costs associated with the health plan. Finally, medical inflation has been far higher than inflation in the general economy. Facing rising health insurance premiums, firms have either dropped coverage or shifted a greater share of the premium and other cost sharing to employees.

The Provision of Health Care

A mix of private and public providers comprise the American health care delivery system. The system is plagued by fragmented, uncoordinated care that overemphasizes high technology procedures and acute care, all of which make health care costly and the quality uncertain. Hospital ownership is varied, with 58.4 percent nonprofits, 20.3 percent owned by state or local governments, and 21.3 percent for-profit private entities.[12]

For most of the twentieth century, the dominant model of physician practice took place in individual or small-group settings. Doctors freely chose their specialty and patient mix and faced virtually no oversight of their clinical decisions by payers or their medical peers. Health care providers have been paid primarily on a *fee-for-service* basis, which pays a provider for each item of service. This reimbursement system rewards high volumes of services and technical procedures rather than counseling and coordinating care. This form of reimbursement and the crushing burden of medical school debt that students incur in the United States have led to a distribution of doctors favoring specialists over primary care. Indeed, two-thirds of physicians are specialists, whereas only one-third are primary care practitioners. The trend toward specialization has become more pronounced since the 1980s as incomes of primary care doctors have lagged further far behind those of specialists. A family practitioner typically earns $186,000 per year, while a radiologist earns as much as $400,000; and while primary care physicians in the 1980s earned 75 percent of that of the average specialist, by the late 1990s they earned only 50 percent.[13]

Government and private insurers have largely accommodated and encouraged the model of the autonomy of the solo practitioner, with its preference for acute care, excessive specialization, and nearly complete freedom of individual doctors to set their fees and to determine which treatments to provide. The 1946 Hill-Burton Act committed federal money to the construction of hospitals that, quite naturally, led to the growth of acute care settings to the detriment of ambulatory care settings. The Medicare program has been an important source of medical education, paying for medical residency programs only in hospital settings. Both of these federal policies have favored hospital over ambulatory settings for care. State governments have taken the same approach, enacting laws that ceded to state and local chapters of medical societies the authority to collectively regulate their own by controlling licensing, and disciplining procedures of individual practitioners. In practical terms, this meant little or no discipline or oversight of either clinical decisions of individual practitioners or their choice of specialization. Furthermore, state laws enacted in the early twentieth century essentially granted physicians a monopoly over health care by outlawing alternative providers.[14]

And private insurers and government have long rewarded specialty care with higher fees than primary care services. The Medicare program initially allowed physicians to set their own fees on a "usual, customary and reasonable" fee-for-service basis and reimbursed hospitals fee-for-service plus 2 percent basis to account for their investment in capital and high-tech equipment.[15]

While most physicians remain in private practice, the terms of their work have changed significantly since the 1990s. More doctors are part of multispecialty group practices that refer patients to specific hospitals. Such integrated delivery systems (IDSs) bind together physicians and clinics, hospitals, pharmacies, and home care and other related services as a single package that contracts with large for-profit insurers to treat their members. Physicians may be salaried employees of the provider network, or may bind together as an independent network to contract with insurers on a fee-for-service reimbursement arrangement, but their freedom to set their own charges has been circumscribed by fee schedules negotiated by insurers or government.[16]

Government payers have taken the lead in cost containment beginning in the 1980s. The first big change came in 1983 when Medicare switched from fee-for-service reimbursement of hospitals to prospective payment on the basis of diagnosis related groups (DRGs). DRGs pay hospitals a fixed average amount calculated in advance that reflects the cost of treating a particular diagnosis. Later in the decade, Medicare took action to curb physician costs, introducing a binding fee schedule intended to narrow the gap between fees of primary care and specialist physicians.

Government efforts to bring coordination to this system through planning have been short-lived. One example was the National Health Planning and Resource Development Act of 1974 that required states to create certificate-of-need programs and planning agencies to approve or deny the construction of new hospitals or the addition of new high-tech wings in such entities. President Ronald Reagan, expressing a preference for market competition to allocate health care resources, abolished the certificate-of-need programs in 1982. What followed was a pattern of deprivation and duplication as hospitals in inner cities serving many poor uninsured or Medicaid patients closed their doors and abandoned their populations. The same hospital chains then opened new facilities in higher income and privately insured suburban areas. In many instances, this led to the siting of identical facilities only a few miles apart that needlessly duplicated the services provided by existing hospitals but without lower prices expected under a competitive market model.[17]

In short, the American health care system was broken. It left millions uninsured who either went without care or waited until their conditions were advanced and more costly to treat in hospital emergency rooms. Providers' market power allowed them to charge high prices to payers than their peers in other countries, while fee-for-service reimbursement rewarded high volumes of specialty care. High administrative costs and uncoordinated care also plagued the system. Taken together, the health care system erected formidable barriers to access to affordable quality care. Not surprisingly, this emphasis on high-tech, acute care interventions taking place in hospital settings corresponded to an insufficient attention to primary care, preventive care, and public health. In 2009, only 3 percent of US spending was devoted to public health.[18]

A Polity that Disperses Power

The design of the American polity—its political institutions, interest group universe, and dominant political culture—fragments government authority and undermines purposive, coordinated action by policymakers. Multiple and competing centers of power vie for influence, often work at cross-purposes, and yield incremental policy changes that reflect compromise and sometimes incoherence. This is the political reality that must be grasped if one is to make sense of health policy in the United States.

Fragmented Political Institutions

The American political system disperses decision-making authority and create numerous veto points at which a minority can block action on a bill.[19] Under federalism, the states possess exclusive powers, but also jointly finance and administer many programs with the federal government. Separation of powers creates a relationship of checks and balances among the executive, legislative, and judicial branches of government, allowing each branch to check the other and at the same time requiring cooperation among them for laws to be valid. For a bill to become law, both the Senate and House of Representatives in Congress, and the president, must agree. A president can veto a bill passed by Congress and Congress can override the presidential veto but only by a two-thirds majority vote in both houses. Such disagreements are all the more common under periods of divided government, when different parties control the executive and legislative branches. Even when the president and Congress agree to pass a law, the federal courts may wield their power of judicial review to void a law on the grounds that it violates the Constitution. In that case, Congress and president must pass a new law.

Party discipline, which might serve as the binding factor to counteract centrifugal institutions, is lacking in the American polity and stands in stark contrast to a parliamentary system. In a parliamentary system, the prime minister and cabinet are drawn from the party or parties winning the majority of seats following legislative elections. A vote of no confidence by the legislature can remove the prime minister but requires fresh legislative elections. The threat of all legislators losing their seats fosters party discipline in a parliamentary system. In America's presidential system, by contrast, the separate election of the president and congress makes party discipline less pressing. Members of Congress are elected to promote their state or district interests as much as their party platform. Moreover, members of Congress who refuse to toe the party line may claim that they are representing the interests of their constituents who elected them. The designation of "maverick" may be a badge of honor rather than one of opprobrium.[20]

The design and rules of the US Congress give substantial power to the legislature and further fragment decision-making authority. First, unlike parliamentary systems, where bills originate in the executive branch, the Constitution designates Congress as the source of legislation. Second, the Constitution's provisions for bicameralism require that both the House and Senate must pass identical legislation before it can be forwarded to the President for consideration. The committee system within Congress also allows for multiple points of decision-making.[21] A bill may languish in committee and never reach the floor of the House or Senate for debate. Senators have an additional weapon in the filibuster, which requires a supermajority of 60 senators to cut off debate and force a vote on the bill by the entire chamber. The filibuster applies to all bills save budget items. Many bills die because a minority of 40 senators deploys or merely threatens to invoke the filibuster weapon.[22]

Interest Group Hyperpluralism

In addition to parties, key actors in health policymaking are interest groups. Their political influence has grown in tandem with the attenuation of the power of party leaders in politics. Separation of powers has historically made it difficult for party leaders to rally members around a professed party line. Intentional reforms of political parties in the twentieth century have weakened parties even further. During the early decades of that century, the Progressives, a reform movement that aimed to clean up the corruption in politics by curbing the power of party bosses and big business, secured the passage of laws in several states that removed candidate selection and policy decisions from party leaders working behind smoke-filled back rooms and into the hands of ordinary citizens. Such mechanisms of direct democracy included (1) direct primaries that allowed voters to directly select candidates for elections, (2) the creation of nonpartisan offices in city government, (3) recall elections that allowed voters to remove officials for malfeasance, and (4) initiatives and referenda that placed policy questions on the ballot for voters to decide directly. The Watergate scandal that engulfed President Richard Nixon unveiled a host of irregularities and dirty tricks during the 1972 campaign that led to the passage of laws intended to reform campaign financing. Though the aim of such legislation was to set limits to and require disclosure of the sources of donations to political parties, it weakened parties and party leaders in selecting candidates and effectively ceded that role to interest groups.

Interest groups also spend money, and lots of it. Since the campaign finance reform laws of the 1970s, organized interests have replaced political parties as the chief source of campaign financing through political action committees (PACs). While large organizations like corporations and labor unions had already created their own PACs in the 1940s to channel campaign donations, the 1970s laws encouraged a proliferation of such organizations. By 2009, 4,618 PACs were registered with the Federal Election Commission (FEC), the government agency that oversees them.[23] And, thanks to the Supreme Court decision in the *Citizens United* case in 2010, corporations have been freed from campaign spending restrictions on the grounds of free speech. Groups and individuals may also donate money to "issue advocacy" groups that are ostensibly not affiliated with a particular candidate. In reality, the line separating PACS and candidates is not so clear. Moreover, unlike contributions to PACs and election campaigns, interest groups face no limits on their donations to issue advocacy groups.[24] Critics worry that the inordinate influence of interest group money in financing elections has corroded the democratic process and fueled public cynicism with politics.

Besides money, interest groups seek to influence policymaking in a number of other ways. Most obviously, they lobby members of Congress and the executive branch. But they may also use less direct means, such as orchestrating public campaigns to mobilize their members or running political ads in key congressional districts to rile up voters. With the latter tactic, groups hope that the candidate will take a favorable position to curry voters' favor or avoid their wrath at the ballot box. Starting in the 1960s, broader social changes muscled their way into the insular world of interest group politics. That world had extended to only a handful of associations representing the economic interests of business and labor, operating in closed-door meetings with congressional committee leaders and the cabinet. But new groups promoting particular causes like civil rights, feminism, peace, and environmentalism, proliferated. At the same time, economic and professional interests splintered into smaller associations representing more specific constituencies. By 2011, there were 12,220 registered lobbyists in the nation's capital.[25]

Contemporary politicians now confront an interest group terrain best described as hyperpluralism. Not only does this involve a far greater number of interest groups, but also these associations are narrower in scope than their predecessors. Such hyperpluralism makes it difficult for interest groups and their contacts in Congress or the executive branch to forge durable alliances on policy initiatives. Interest group power is more often than not negative power, as groups are too numerous and fragmented to take positive action than they are to block a policy initiative.[26]

Not all groups are equal in this hyperpluralistic universe, least of all in the health policy arena. For much of the twentieth century, the most influential alliance in health policy was that uniting business, insurers, and doctors in their opposition to national health insurance.[27] The key interest groups in the health policy arena have been those representing providers, chiefly, the American Medical Association (AMA) for doctors, the American Hospital Association (AHA), the trade association for large pharmaceutical companies (Pharmaceutical Research and Manufacturers of America, PhRMA), America's Health Insurance Plans (AHIP) representing the insurance industry, and employers and unions (American Federation of Labor–Congress of Industrial Organizations, AFL-CIO). Unlike providers, employers lack a single peak association to speak for them and the political power of labor has waned with the decline in union membership since the 1980s. The American Association of Retired Persons (AARP), which represents senior citizens, achieved prominence after the passage of Medicare. By contrast, the most vulnerable segments of the population—the poor and disabled—possess fewer resources upon which to draw for the representation of their constituents' interests in the political and policy arenas.

Nevertheless, the power and influence of interest groups may change over time. Seemingly impregnable alliances may unravel and new coalitions may arise to take their place. Such alternations in interest group politics happen for a number of reasons. New groups entering the health policy arena may challenge existing coalitions. Coalitions may change in response to new challenges in the broader economy or within the health care system itself. Groups may redefine their interests, their policy preferences, and their partnerships. Changes in the partisan composition in Congress and executive branch and in the ideological outlook within the Democratic and Republican parties may furnish openings for interest groups to forge new alliances with policymakers.

A Political Culture Promoting Limited Government and Free Markets

Dominant values concerning the proper reach of government and private actors infiltrate debates over health policy. The translation of such values on politics is not always direct, however. Rather, politicians and interest groups deploy values as a weapon, invoking them to frame the public debate over health policy to shape public opinion in their favor.

The dominant political culture in the United States blends political and market liberalism, that is, a mistrust of government power and an almost unquestioning trust in the beneficence of the market. This suspicion of an overweening government dates to the Founding Fathers whose distrust of the centralized, arbitrary power of the British monarchy prompted their design of a political structure that separates and fragments government power. The reification of the private market followed much later with the Industrial Revolution following the Civil War, when private entrepreneurs rather than an assertive government bureaucracy took the lead in transforming America from an agrarian nation to an industrial power. The government's role largely supported this path of economic development, through the waging of wars with Native Americans to settle the frontier. The captains of industry propagated the gospel of the free market, and their message became fused with long held ideas of political freedom.[28]

Even so, these dominant values concerning the appropriate role and balance between government and individual, and public and private are not static but have been subject to challenges from reformist politicians and social movements from below, as in the New Deal and Great Society social reform eras of the 1930s and 1960s, respectively. Those championing communitarian values have faced powerful advocates of free enterprise and individual freedom, and both periods of social activism were followed by periods of conservative-led rollbacks. The reason for this state of affairs lies in the specific historical development of the United States in which the business community's economic and political power saw no serious challenges from the state or other classes. Successive waves of immigration and the existence of African-American slavery divided working-class identity by ethnicity and race. Early suffrage for white males severed the link between economic and political democracy that had been the rallying cry of social democratic parties in Europe. Through the nineteenth century, the possibility of moving westward offered a safety valve for working-class disaffection with the abysmal working and living conditions associated with industrialization. Outside of the South, the United States did not have a feudal past and an aristocracy bound by a code of *noblesse oblige* that specified their duties and obligations to safeguard the welfare of their agricultural laborers. As a result, American conservatism differs from the European variant. It champions economic and political freedom rather than accepting an activist government to foster social peace and interclass harmony or to promote the welfare of the lower orders.[29] This libertarian brand of conservatism, which the New Deal and Great Society had threatened, has become politically ascendant again since the election of

President Ronald Reagan in 1980. It has continued to find a home in the neoliberal wing of the Republican Party since then.[30]

The two major parties have tended to identify with these different value orientations and interests. Even though both parties are broad catch-all parties that seek to attract the electoral center ground, Republicans have generally been allied with business interests and the values of private enterprise and limited government, whereas Democrats have promoted the interests of unionized working class, minorities, and the poor in redistributive programs aimed at reducing inequality.

Policy Legacies

Finally, past policy decisions have shaped subsequent health policy battles. A "policy feedback loop" is set in motion as policies enacted and implemented at one point in time generate new politics.[31] A new program creates new arrangements that affected stakeholders learn to live with. A new law encourages society to form new interest groups with a stake in its survival. This dynamic has been at work in the history of national health insurance efforts in the United States spanning the last hundred years. The growth of employment-based private insurance created formidable constituencies in favor of the status quo. The spread of employment-based insurance and the creation of Medicare and Medicaid subsequently muted calls for government national health insurance from workers and labor unions.

Even so, there are limits to policy legacies. Different conditions in later periods may drive a wedge between former allies and forge new partnerships advocating major policy change. A brief window of opportunity may open up, allowing reformers to significantly modify or even jettison past practices.

Political Forces Blocking National Health Insurance

The battles over national health insurance in the twentieth century illustrate the interplay of political system institutions, interest groups, ideology, and policy legacies in shaping policy outcomes. Together, these forces combined to yield policies that initially sharply limited the government's role in health care financing and provision and instead gave primacy to private actors and solutions. This was true even in the public Medicare and Medicaid programs.

The 1910s marked the first major effort to introduce national health insurance. Informed by the country's federal political structure, the American Association of Labor Legislation (AALL), a group of reformist academics and labor union leaders, used states as laboratories of social policy innovation. They unsuccessfully sought to get universal coverage laws passed in key states, which would then serve as a model for a national insurance program. However, their model of universal coverage, based on Germany's national health insurance program, was ill timed given that the United States was fighting Germany in World War I. The anti-communist Red Scare in the wake of the Bolshevik Revolution in Russia also provided ammunition for opponents to portray the AALL's reform idea as a socialist threat to free enterprise and democracy. Employers seeking to safeguard their prerogative to decide the terms of work, private insurers fearing national health insurance as the entering wedge of government in their business, and the AMA arguing against any outside intrusion in the doctor–patient relationship were opposed to the scheme.

A cross-party alliance straddled separation of powers and teamed up with key health care stakeholders to thwart subsequent efforts to introduce national health insurance, even when Democrats controlled the White House and both houses of Congress. President Franklin Roosevelt discovered this in 1935. He included national health insurance as a component of his Social Security Act for statutory pensions and industrial accident insurance. But conservative southern Democrats feared that the bill would empower African-Americans and threaten the power structure of white supremacy in the South. As chairmen of key congressional committees with the power to bottle up the legislation, Southern Democrats allied with congressional Republicans who advanced the interests of a powerful alliance of employers, private insurers, and the AMA opposed to national health insurance. In the face of likely defeat, Roosevelt dropped the national health insurance proposal. He also made additional concessions to Southern Democrats, excluding domestic servants and agricultural laborers (who were largely African-American in the South) from Social Security, to ensure enactment of pensions and accident insurance.

President Harry Truman resurrected national health insurance in 1949, but his plan faced the same opponents, as did his predecessor's. The alliance of conservative Southern Democrats and pro-business Republicans in Congress possessed a majority to defeat Truman's proposal, as did the business community, insurers, and the AMA. Masking doctors' economic concerns over incomes and professional autonomy, the AMA mounted a public campaign depicting national health insurance as a socialized medicine. This proved a very effective message with the public in the Cold War era of fervent anti-communism.[32]

With policymakers unable and unwilling to enact national health insurance, the United States headed down the road of voluntary, private insurance in the workplace. In the industrial economy following World War II, millions of workers and their dependents enjoyed comprehensive health insurance coverage negotiated by their unions and employers. Such arrangements satisfied firms seeking to attract and retain scarce workers while giving the unions substantial legitimacy and membership. Yet those outside the labor market remained uninsured as they had before. This group comprised nonunion workers, the elderly, poor (mostly female-headed) families with children, and the disabled. Policymakers turned their efforts to helping these groups and succeeded with the passage of Medicare and Medicaid in 1965.

The reasons for this legislative success had as much to do with the modest scope of the programs as with an environment ripe for government action. First, Medicare and Medicaid drove a wedge among the usual forces arrayed against national health insurance. Private insurers had long shunned elders, the disabled, and the poor because they were not profitable clients. Employers had no interest in these groups since they were not in the labor force. This left the AMA as the main group opposed to Medicare and Medicaid. Bereft of their powerful business and insurance allies, the AMA alone could not defeat the legislation, even if it did secure some prize concessions from policymakers in the final bill. By contrast, the forces in favor of reform were broad. Groups advocating for senior citizens supported Medicare, as did organized labor as a way to relieve unions of the burden of negotiating health insurance for retirees. State governments realized that Medicaid promised an injection of federal funds for their cash-strapped health care programs for the disabled and poor. Finally, the message of socialized medicine fell flat in the face of the public discourse on the reality of poverty in a land of prosperity, and the broadly shared belief that vulnerable groups deserved government help.

The composition of Congress also changed decisively following the assassination of President Kennedy. The watershed election of 1964 brought an influx of northern Democrats from urban areas who were favorably disposed to an activist government role in social policy. Their numbers swamped those of conservative southern Democrats and decimated the Republican membership in Congress. President Lyndon Johnson relied on huge Democratic majorities in both houses of Congress to enact his ambitious Great Society social policy agenda, which included Medicare and Medicaid.

In addition to cementing party unity in Congress, Johnson also made key concessions to health care stakeholders to make sure that his legislation would pass. Far from threatening the existence or profits of private providers and insurers, Medicare and Medicaid enhanced them. Private insurers were awarded major responsibility for claims processing and administration of both Medicare and Medicaid. Doctors and hospitals' participation was voluntary. The coverage of seniors represented a new income stream for doctors and hospitals, even if Medicare and Medicaid paid less than private insurance. Moreover, the legilsation retained fee-for-service payment of providers and allowed physicians to dictate fees locally, at least for the first two decades of Medicare's existence. State governments also did well under Medicaid, receiving federal dollars for their health care programs for the poor and disabled as well as preserving their role in defining eligibility, benefits, and reimbursement rates for providers.[33]

Following the passage of Medicare and Medicaid, demands for national health insurance receded to the background. But the problems of rising costs and the rising uninsured did not. Between 1987 and 1993, employment-based insurance premiums climbed by 90 percent. US employers came to view this trend as an unsustainable assault on their profits and survival. In the brave new world of globalization, manufacturing giants like General Motors now faced stiffer competition from overseas competitors enjoying the advantage of lower labor costs. Even on their home turf, firms offering health insurance had to shoulder higher labor costs, which put them at a competitive disadvantage against rivals who did not. In 1989 Chrysler's CEO Lee Iacocca took the unheard-of step of publicly calling on the government to enact national health insurance.[34] The logic was that if all firms were forced to offer insurance to their workforce, it would level the competitive playing field. This new reality, in turn, drove a wedge in the coalition that had long opposed national health insurance, as employers began to resent the profits of health care providers and insurers at their expense. Working Americans voiced growing unease over rising health care costs and declining access to insurance as the recession of the early 1990s drove up the number of jobless and uninsured, while those who remained employed found themselves shouldering higher premiums and other forms of cost-sharing. Opinion polls showed that Americans were deeply worried about losing their workplace health insurance, with majorities agreeing that the health care system needed to be "totally rebuilt" and in favor of the federal government guaranteeing universal coverage.[35]

By the early 1990s, national health insurance was again on the political agenda. Democratic President Bill Clinton came into office in 1992 by promising major health care reform. Yet he believed that national health insurance that built on the existing system of employment-based insurance would inoculate himself and his party against charges of socialized medicine. The "New Democrat" wing of the Democratic Party, which Clinton epitomized, sought to forge a new electoral coalition uniting the middle class, working class, and the poor. By employing public and private solutions to health care, the Democrats would rid themselves of their "tax and spend" image and would overcome wedge issues, such as social welfare, that had divided their electoral base on racial and class lines.[36]

Clinton's national health insurance plan, which he dubbed Health Security, reflected this effort to span this wide electoral and interest group divide. It would build on existing employment-based private insurance but would achieve universal coverage by mandating all employers to offer coverage to their workforce. Insurance would be financed primarily by payroll taxes but also excise taxes. Small businesses would receive federal tax credits to make such coverage affordable.

The Clinton plan contained several innovations intended to realize the twin goals of universal access and cost containment in health care. Foremost among these was managed competition, which involved government regulation of the insurance market to ensure universal access to care, and competition and choice among health plans to encourage cost containment. The idea for managed competition came from Stanford health economist Alain Enthoven, who first proposed such a scheme in 1980 and refined it in subsequent journal articles.[37] Managed competition under Health Security would require all employers to offer their workers at least three plans that would differ in terms of cost-sharing, premiums, and choice of providers. The reformers expected that employees would choose the lower cost plans, thus bringing down health care costs. At the same time, managed competition would set new regulations on insurers to bar them from competing by simply selecting healthier, more profitable customers. They would no longer be allowed to shun only the sick through coverage denials, preexisting condition exclusions, and experience-rated premiums. Instead, insurers would be required to offer a comprehensive basic benefits package to all applicants, and charge community-rated premiums, i.e., levying the same rate for all in a region rather than differentiating by a person's medical condition, to spread health risks more evenly across the population and make insurance more affordable for the sicker. As an additional safeguard, plans with healthier members would have to make risk-adjusted payments to plans with sicker members. Responsibility for administration of the health care system would be split between the federal and state governments. State governments would create and administer the individual and small-group insurance markets (or delegate this job to a nonprofit entity). To appease large firms, employers with at least five thousand employees could opt out of the state exchanges and instead assume their own financial risk for insuring their members, which many already did as self-insured plans. At the national level, Congress would set and update the basic benefits package. A National Insurance Board with members appointed by the president would have the authority to regulate alliances and health plans. If competition failed to deliver health care cost containment the board could cap premium increases to the rate of inflation.

Clinton publicly launched his health care reform plan in a speech to Congress and the American people on September 22, 1993. Opinion polls shortly following the speech showed that most Americans were supportive of Health Security. Yet hopes for its passage were dashed in the ensuing year. The president's proposal never made it to a floor vote in Congress despite Democrat majorities in both houses of Congress. By August 1994, health care reform was dead. In the congressional midterm elections, the

Democrats lost control of both houses of Congress to the Republicans, a political event not seen since 1952.

This spectacular turn of events owed to the mobilization of an anti-reform coalition led chiefly by health insurers and employers allied with congressional Republicans. The strategy that President Clinton chose to undertake health care reform also had to bear its share of the blame for this outcome. The president failed to work with the realities of the political terrain, discounting the obstacles posed by separation of powers, party indiscipline, and the extreme pluralism of the interest group universe. Moreover, the spirit of bipartisanship that had marked the 1960s had become a poisoned environment of polarization. And, in the face of Democratic disarray, Republicans marshaled an extraordinary degree of unity in their quest to defeat Health Security. Republicans viewed the battle in strategic terms, as a way to usher in a new Republican majority in Congress. But they also viewed it in ideological terms, invoking key symbols in American political culture by portraying the reform as socialized medicine and big government run amok.

The president created a special task force in early 1993 to draw up health care reform, but its proceedings alienated potential allies. The task force worked behind closed doors, shutting out key Democrats in Congress who had had years of experience in health policy. Feeling snubbed by the president, Democratic and Republican members of Congress produced their own competing versions of health care reform so that as many as seven bills were being considered by Congress in 1994. The task force was equally insensitive to the need to win over important health care stakeholders, such as associations representing employers and insurers. It formally consulted these stakeholders in hearings but did not engage them in genuine negotiations and the resultant give-and-take that would have accompanied such a process. As a result, these groups went public with their grievances and the administration responded with a campaign to demonize the insurance industry. In short, Clinton's strategy was the polar opposite of President Johnson's co-optation of key interest groups and congressional leaders that had been so essential to the enactment of Medicare and Medicaid.

To be sure, the interest group terrain made it much harder for Clinton to forge a pro-reform coalition. Over eleven hundred interest groups had a stake in the outcome of health care reform, which made the forging of a broad coalition in support of reform difficult.[38] Employers, who lacked a single association to aggregate their demands in the political arena, demonstrated the power of interest groups to block reform. Infighting among the different business associations and the loss of members to rival organizations led large employers to pull their support for Clinton's health care reform. This left the field open to groups firmly committed to defeat

Health Security, particularly the small business federation (National Federation of Independent Business, NFIB) and the association representing smaller insurers, who waged a public campaign that involved direct lobbying, media advertising, and grassroots mobilization in key congressional districts. In contrast, the forces favoring national health insurance, such as the AARP and organized labor, expressed only tepid support and failed to mobilize their members on a scale to match their opponents. Also notable was the phenomenon of "reverse lobbying" by Republican congressional leaders who pressured business associations such as the Chamber of Commerce to take a neutral stance on health care reform or else risk the loss of congressional action on other legislation that business held dear.[39] The AMA, a major player in previous health care reform debates, proved strikingly impotent in this one. Its weakness arose from the loss of members to rival organizations over the years as well as its exclusion from negotiating the content of Health Security.[40]

Finally, some of the design features of Health Security proved difficult to sell to the American public. Foes of the Clinton plan won the battle for public opinion by portraying the legislation as a government leviathan that would stifle patients' choice of doctor and kill off small businesses. Opinion polls reflected the effectiveness of this campaign: while 59 percent of poll respondents had expressed support for Health Security right after Clinton's September 1993 speech, it had dropped to 42 percent by summer 1994.[41]

Employers Go it Alone: The Managed Care Revolution and Subsequent Backlash

Following the government immobility on health care reform, employers pursued a go-it-alone strategy to control their own health care outlays. In essence, they used competitive forces and managed care but with none of the rules to safeguard the sick that Health Security would have provided. Instead, employers herded their workers into managed care plans that controlled costs by means of preauthorizing (often denying) expensive high-tech procedures and referrals to specialists, and by putting physicians at financial risk for the health of their patients via capitated payments. Some of the goals of managed care were laudable, such as an emphasis on coordinated care through primary care doctors and efforts to move away from the perverse more-is-better incentives of fee-for-service reimbursement. Other practices, however, were less benign and even harmful to patient care. These included financial bonuses to physician reviewers who met a targeted level of treatment denials, paying bonuses to groups of doctors for staying within a preset financial target, and basing medical treatment denials on the absence of agreed-upon clinical practice guidelines based in scientific research. Whereas fee-for-service reimbursement had encouraged physicians to perform more procedures and more expensive ones, the managed care revolution contained equally perverse incentives but in the opposite direction, tempting insurers and providers to reduce access to care even if it was medically necessary. In the absence of good information on clinical effectiveness a regulatory framework that protected patients from unwarranted denials of care and that assured universal coverage, competition became a sledgehammer to pulverize the weakest market players, especially small firms and sicker patients. At the same time, the utilization review processes adopted by insurers spawned a gargantuan private sector bureaucracy of medical reviewers and claims processors.

Managed care without proper regulation allowed insurers and employers to trim health care costs for a few years in the mid-1990s, but at the expense of inciting a popular backlash. Managed care horror stories abounded.[42] Facing rising employee dissatisfaction with insurance, employers retreated and offered health plans with more choices of doctors and only discounted fee-for-service physician reimbursement. Such accommodation came at a cost, however, as the upward trend in health insurance premiums resumed. Between 1999 and 2012, premiums for an individual employee more than doubled from $2,196 to $5,615, while premiums for family coverage nearly tripled from $5,791 to $15,745.[43] These figures only refer to premiums. But workers increasingly shouldered a greater proportion of overall health insurance costs, in the form of rising premiums, coinsurance, copayments, and deductibles. High-deductible health plans became more common especially among smaller firms. The total cost of health insurance for a typical family of four, which included not only premiums but also the cost-sharing arrangements just described, jumped from $9,235 in 2002 to $23,215 in 2014. Of this, employers covered an average of 58 percent of the cost, or $13,520, with employees picking up 42 percent, or $9,695.[44] The national figures were no better. In 2011, the United States topped all nations in health care spending at 17.7 percent of gross domestic product and $8,508 per capita; by contrast, the OECD average was 9.3 percent and $3,322.[45]

Managed care had also done nothing to staunch the rising tide of uninsured. This is not surprising, since employers were focused on controlling their labor costs, not solving the general problem of the uninsured. Even the long economic boom of the 1990s did not solve the problem either. Even as labor force participation rates soared, the number of uninsured continued to climb. In 1995, 40.6 million, or 15.4 percent of the nonelderly population, lacked insurance. By 2007, the year before the Great Recession hit, the uninsured had swelled to 47 million, or 17 percent, of the population under age 65.[46]

Bringing Stakeholders Back In: The PPACA of 2010[47]

Economic Crisis and an Unsustainable Health Care Model

The Great Recession that hit in 2008 ushered in an era of economic insecurity not seen in the United States (or Europe) since the Great Depression of the 1930s. The root cause lay in the reckless lending and trading practices of investment banks in the US real estate market. When the housing bubble burst, it brought the rest of the economy to the brink. Unemployment, which had stood at only 4.4 percent in 2007, rose quickly to peak at 10 percent in October 2009.[48] To avert a complete breakdown of the international financial system and a major economic depression, national governments in the United States and Europe had to intervene with massive taxpayer bailouts of the banks. In the United States, government bailouts also extended to the car industry, which faced steeply falling demand and the near bankruptcy of General Motors and Chrysler. Such government intervention in the economy had not been seen since the Great Depression and World War II (1939–1945).

Naturally, the turbulent economy had major repercussions in health care because most working-age Americans and their dependents received health insurance from their workplace. Mass unemployment drove up the numbers of uninsured. Each 1 percent increase in unemployment translated into one million Americans losing their health insurance coverage. The US Census Bureau estimated that 50 million people, or 16.3 percent of Americans under age 65, were uninsured at the depth of the recession in 2010.[49] Yet government programs like Medicaid and CHIP for the poor and near poor were unable to cover all of these uninsured people.[50] The state and federal governments fund these programs jointly, but the states were facing huge budget gaps owing to the recession-induced fall in tax revenues plus greater demand for these health care programs and unemployment benefits. Furthermore, state governments did not have much maneuver room; unlike the federal government, nearly all state constitutions require their governments to balance their budgets annually. This foreclosed the option of deficit spending. Other than a few states like California, most governors did not want to raise taxes to pay for additional state outlays. Lastly, the Medicaid and State CHIP coverage rules excluded certain people by design: they covered poor families with children but left out low-income childless adults. The health care safety net was stretched so tightly that it was fraying in many places.

The political terrain had also shifted, with Democrats recapturing the White House after eight years of Republican rule. Democratic President Barack Obama soundly beat his Republican rival Senator John McCain in the November 2008 election, and Democrats also secured comfortable majorities in both houses of Congress. Obama had placed health care reform at the front and center of his campaign, and the election results indicated that he had a mandate for action. Even so, the economic crisis and federal deficit that Obama had inherited from the previous administration at first glance seemed an inauspicious environment in which to undertake any major health care reform. Paradoxically, however, the desperate economy provided an opening for a health care overhaul. The federal government had already intervened in the economy with its bailout of the banks and the car industry. If the banks, which were responsible for the mess, could receive billions of dollars of government aid, should not the millions of ordinary Americans experiencing unemployment and loss of their health insurance obtain a helping hand from the government? With this argument, Obama and his advisers turned vice into virtue and transformed the economic crisis into a window of opportunity to move forward a plan for health care for all.

The question was what kind of reform would the Democrats pursue? Reform had to address the growing number of uninsured and bring runaway health care costs under control without sacrificing quality of care. Left-wing Democrats and their trade union allies initially pushed for a single-payer government health plan for all, but then settled for a more modest "public option," or government plan that would compete with private insurers. For conservative Democrats and key health care interest groups, even the public option was too much. What was needed was a compromise that would satisfy enough Democrats and the health care industry. Table 2.1 summarizes the main provisions of the law that passed.

Content of PPACA

Expanding Access to Insurance

The compromise solution that Democrats finally agreed on built on the dualistic framework of health care financing. The Affordable Care Act retained employment-based private insurance for most Americans (since they already had it) while making it more affordable to them via income-based tax credits. In addition, it expanded Medicaid to cover all individuals, even adults without children, with incomes at or below 138 percent of the federal poverty limit.

Many of the provisions centered on shoring up employment-based insurance by imposing new rules on insurers, and designing insurance markets that fostered fair competition based on price and innovation rather than simply cream skimming the healthiest and most profitable customers. An online marketplace, or exchange, for health insurance for individuals and small businesses would operate in each state. The exchanges

Table 2.1 Main Provisions of the PPACA of 2010

Health care financing reforms: expand access to affordable insurance	*Health care delivery system reforms to improve quality and efficiency*

1. Medicaid expansion
   –expanded to all low-income adults below 138% of the poverty line
   –Federal funding for Medicaid expansion 100% for first 3 years; 90% after that
   NOTE: Medicaid expansion optional, so not all states participating.
	1. New forms of coordinated care
	   –Patient-centered medical homes
	   –Accountable care organizations

2. Online insurance marketplaces (exchanges) small businesses and individuals in each state:
   –promote competition and choice of health plan
   –subsidized premiums
	2. Payment reform
	   –bundled payments instead of fee-for-service
	   –pay for performance (rewarding good health outcomes)
	   –Independent Payment Advisory Board for Medicare

3. Insurance reforms
   –ban on preexisting conditions exclusions
   –insurers must accept all applicants
   –adult children covered under parents up to age 26
   –modified community rating for premiums
   –essential benefits package
	3. Promoting evidence-based medicine
	   –Patient-Centered Outcomes Research Institute to disseminate best practices
	
	4. Electronic medical records
	
	5. Investing in primary care workforce and community health clinics

Source: Author.

would put into practice the theory of managed competition: insurers in the exchanges would compete on price of premium and associated cost sharing, but not on health risks. A transparent easy-to-compare format, much like the site Travelocity for airfares, would make it easy for consumers to shop for the plan that fit their needs. Individuals and small firms would be able to choose among tiered health plans, each offering an essential minimum benefits package. But plans could differ on price, the degree of choice of provider offered, and extra benefits. A classification system ranked plans by medal category. Platinum plans offered the greatest choice of providers and would cover 90 percent of average health care costs, but would also be the most expensive in terms of premiums and cost sharing. Gold, silver, and bronze plans were the next categories, covering 80, 70, and 60 percent of the average costs of the plan, respectively. Patients would shoulder higher cost sharing in each successive tier.

New insurance reforms would prohibit some of the most odious discrimination by insurers that had made coverage unattainable for the sickest individuals and small firms. Thus, all insurers, whether inside or outside the exchanges, would no longer be able to exclude people from coverage through preexisting conditions clauses, exclusion of specified illnesses, or experience-rated premiums. Instead, they would have to accept all applicants, would not be able to drop coverage based on health status, and would have to charge modified community-rated premiums that would vary only by age, family size, region, and whether a person smoked tobacco. Modified community rating was the means to pool risks and thereby make insurance more affordable to those who were the sickest. Under modified community rating, all in a region pay the same premium beyond those factors noted above. The healthier cross-subsidize the sicker by paying higher premiums than they would if their rates were based solely on their good health. Likewise, sicker persons pay lower premiums under community rating than they would if they were charged rates that reflected their health status. If insurers still attracted sicker members, they would receive risk-adjusted payments from those insurers that had a healthier membership. This provision would offset insurers' subtler attempts at cream skimming, through targeted advertising to healthier people, as well as compensate them for having the misfortune of attracting a sicker membership.

Finally, new insurers inside and outside the exchanges were required to provide an essential benefits package encompassing medically necessary ambulatory care, emergency and hospital services, laboratory services, prescription drugs, prevention and wellness services, maternity and newborn care, pediatric care, (including vision and dental care), mental health and substance abuse services, rehabilitative and habilitative services, and chronic disease management. The inclusion of a minimum essential benefits package would prevent insurers from cream skimming healthier patients by offering them barebones coverage, and would allow the insurance market to function properly by making it easier for consumers to compare health plans on the basis of price rather than complicated differences in what they covered. In addition, the coverage of preventive services without patient cost sharing sought to reorient the health care system away from its emphasis on treating patients only after they became ill. However, individuals under age 30 could choose a plan with a very high deductible, but the plan would still provide the basic benefits package. Policymakers hoped that this provision would encourage younger, healthier people to sign up for insurance and thereby cross-subsidize the health care costs of sicker persons who would be more likely to enroll.

The Affordable Care Act exchanges were similar to the Clinton plan alliances, and both plans rested on managed competition. But Obama and his team did not have to rely on a theoretical model of managed competition as Clinton had, but could draw on the real-world example of the

Massachusetts Health Plan. Enacted by a Democratic-controlled legislature and Republican governor Mitt Romney in 2006,[51] the Massachusetts Health Plan introduced near-universal coverage of state residents through employment-based private insurers. It outlawed insurers' practices that discriminated against the sick. The state created an online exchange where small businesses and individuals in the state could shop around for coverage from competing private insurers. The state mandated all individuals to carry insurance, but subsidized premiums to make it affordable and expanded Medicaid for the poorest.

The Affordable Care Act contained similar provisions. Chief among these was the individual mandate requiring nearly all Americans to have health insurance, with a tax penalty levied against those who refused to comply. That penalty was phased in with a negligible rate of $95 in 2014 but rising to $695 for individuals (up to $2,085 for a family) or 2.5 percent of household income, whichever was higher, by 2017. However, requiring people to buy insurance that was not affordable was neither fair nor politically sound. Hence, the law paired the individual mandate with the offer of premium tax credits for those with incomes between 100 and 400 percent of the federal poverty level. The size of the premium subsidies would decrease the higher the household income and would be pegged to the second-least expensive silver plan in the exchange. The subsidies would limit premiums to 2 percent of income for low-income households and to 9.5 percent for those with higher incomes. PPACA also set a ceiling on annual out-of-pocket costs (deductibles, coinsurance, co-payments, and services not covered by the health plan), but also provided subsidies for such cost sharing for those with incomes below 250 percent of the poverty line. PPACA's framers hoped that the subsidies would make insurance afordabel for millions of Americans. Yet the annual cost-sharing ceilings ($6,600 for individual coverage and $13,200 for family coverage in 2015) still represented considerable financial outlays for many Americans. PPACA fell short of achieving universal coverage, by certain segments of the population from the insurance mandate: those for whom insurance premiums would exceed 8 percent of their income, those with religious objections to carrying insurance, Native Americans, and undocumented immigrants.

PPACA departed from the Clinton plan on the question of mandates. Unlike the Clinton plan, which had mandated all employers to offer insurance, the Affordable Care Act put the responsibility for carrying insurance on individuals and medium to large employers. Under the play-or-pay scheme, firms with more than 50 full-time employees that refused to provide insurance and had employees obtaining coverage on the individual insurance exchange would pay a financial penalty of $2,000 per full-time employee, over and above the first 30 full-time workers. At the same time, PPACA exempted firms with fewer than 50 full-time employees from the requirement to offer insurance, but also offered tax credits for small businesses that chose to do so.

Interestingly, the idea of an individual mandate originated with moderate Senate Republicans led by John Chafee in the early 1990s. Most Republicans, however, favor subsidized individual coverage to promote personal choice but reject mandates as infringing on individual freedom. In the 2008 presidential campaign, John McCain advocated tax-subsidized individual insurance without an individual mandate, for the same reasons. Obama was initially cool toward the individual mandate, but his advisers subsequently convinced him that it was critical to the survival of insurance markets. Without it, only sicker people would sign up for subsidized insurance. Insurers would then have to hike premiums for everyone to cover their health care costs or else go bankrupt.

Covering millions more Americans through subsidized insurance and an expanded Medicaid program would cost money, and that would come from a number of sources. First, the health care industry, including pharmaceutical companies, commercial insurers, medical device companies, hospitals, and even tanning salons, would be subjected to new taxes. Second, Medicare taxes would increase from 2.4 percent to 3.9 percent for those with higher incomes (individuals earning $200,000 per year or families making above $250,000 per year). Notably, the tax on wealthier Americans would apply not just to their wages and salaries but also to their nonwage income and assets. Third, Americans enjoying generous health benefits would have to contribute: Beginning in 2018, a 40 percent premium surcharge would apply to so-called Cadillac insurance plans that totaled $27,500 or more for family coverage or $10,000 per year for individual coverage. Health economists justified the surcharge as a way to discourage superfluous coverage, though policyholders of such generous plans may have disagreed. Fourth, Medicare reimbursements to doctors and hospitals would decrease, though primary care physicians would see a two-year boost in Medicaid reimbursements while hospitals would be spared the reimbursement cuts for the first ten years. Fifth, private insurers who offered Medicare Advantage Plans, which are prepaid plans that provide seniors with supplemental benefits in exchange for limiting their choice of doctors and hospitals, would see their payments clawed back. The Obama administration justified this cut on the grounds that the federal government had been overpaying these plans by 17 percent, when they were attracting healthier and more profitable enrollees than those in traditional fee-for-service Medicare. Finally, most insured Americans would pay some portion of the cost of their health insurance, in the form of premiums or cost-sharing fees at the point of service, though there would be annual caps on such payments as noted above. As President Obama repeatedly stated, everyone would "have some skin in the game."

The nonpartisan Congressional Budget Office (CBO) estimated that the new law when fully implemented would extend health insurance coverage to nearly 30 million persons and cost $938 billion over the first decade. But the CBO also calculated big savings, to the tune of $143 billion in federal budget deficit reduction in the first decade and $1.2 trillion over the second decade.[52] Notably, the CBO exercised caution in its estimates, counting only the new tax revenues and the reimbursement cuts to providers. It did not try to estimate possible savings from reform of the health care delivery system since these innovations were largely untested pilot programs. It is these delivery system reforms to which we now turn.

Reforming the Health Care Delivery System

PPACA did not stop at expanding access to affordable insurance, however. It also sought to reform the provision of health care to slow the growth of health care spending and improve quality and health outcomes. Though perhaps not as bold and certainly less publicized than the reform of insurance markets, the new law funded innovations in a number of areas of provider reimbursement and delivery of health care. The intent was to shift the American health care system away from its overspecialization and fragmentation of care and reorient it toward more population-based, coordinated care with primary care at the center. By emphasizing health promotion and wellness rather than treating advanced diseases with expensive high-technology procedures, the hope was that health outcomes would improve and would slow the rise in health care spending over the long term.

One simple measure in this regard has been to mandate coverage of preventive services and screenings without any patient cost sharing. This change is part of the new essential health benefits package and applies not only to private insurers but also to Medicare and Medicaid. In addition, the PPACA finances a number of pilot programs on the ground to develop new forms of coordinated care and innovations in the payment of providers. Some, like patient centered medical homes, are health care organizations with a primary care team of doctors and allied health professionals like nurses and physician's assistants, who coordinate the entire spectrum of patient care. Another innovation comes in the form of Accountable Care Organizations (ACOs), in which health systems integrate care of those with chronic illnesses across primary and specialty care providers, and accept new forms of reimbursement to do so. ACOs deploy different types of payment reforms but all of them seek to reward doctors for achieving good health outcomes rather than simply encouraging them to provide a greater volume of more expensive procedures, which fee-for-service tends to do. Many of the innovations in provider reimbursement fall under the rubric of "bundled payments," which can range from capitation or a flat fee per episode of care or per diagnosis. Some ACOs participate in "shared savings," whereby a medical group can retain a portion of the savings that accrue from reducing avoidable emergency room use or hospitalizations while at the same time meeting good health outcomes. Other ACOs offer physicians shared savings but also shared risk in the form of financial penalties if they exceed spending targets. Some ACOs offer physicians additional payments or bonuses ("pay for performance") for meeting health outcome targets such as lower cholesterol or blood sugar levels, or increased preventive screenings and immunizations among their patient population. Still others mix capitation with additional payments for specified services. Through these varied mechanisms, the hope is that providers will be financially rewarded for providing the right kind of care (especially primary, preventive, and coordinated care) rather than being encouraged to skimp on necessary care as might be the case under a rigid capitation system.

Significant potential exists for system-wide diffusion of such innovations in care and provider payment. PPACA created the Center for Medicare and Medicaid Innovation to establish ACOs and promote advances in quality and delivery in government insurance programs. Many private insurers are partnering with provider networks to introduce similar innovations.[53]

The drive to coordinate care would be impossible without improved communication among health care providers. Accordingly, the PPACA provides financing to medical practices and hospitals to adopt electronic medical records. This should reduce medical errors and duplication of tests and services and costs associated with paper records and allow providers in geographically different settings to communicate effectively about patient care.

Weaning the American health care system off its excessive specialization also requires training more primary care providers. The law not only funds the training of more primary care doctors but also physicians' assistants, nurses, and nurse practitioners whose training is shorter and incomes are lower than physicians. PPACA also funds scholarships and loan reduction programs for those who enter careers in primary care, public health, and agree to locate in underserved areas. Medical school curricula are also now offering residents training in preventive and public health. The government also pledged an $11 billion increase in funding for community health centers that provide primary and preventive care and public health services to a broad population that is often uninsured or on Medicaid.

The law finances a number of measures to reconcile both cost and clinical effectiveness and safeguard quality from a single-minded drive to cut costs. The pay for performance measures discussed above are one such example. But a more controversial provision is the creation of the Independent Payment Advisory Board (IPAB) for the Medicare program. This body, comprised of major health care interests (providers, insurers, and patients) as well as health care experts appointed by the president and Congress, reviews annual Medicare expenditures and suggests quality improvements as well as ways to lower health spending to meet a predetermined target linked to inflation in the health sector and the broader economy. The law expressly prohibits IPAB from recommending cuts in benefits or eligibility or increases in premiums. Instead, it can only recommend cuts in provider reimbursements or new innovations in care. If Congress fails to respond to IPAB with measures that have the equivalent effect, the board's recommendations become automatically binding. IPAB was designed to bring medical expertise to Medicare program decisions while insulating the board from the pressures of health care industry lobbyists and members of Congress. However, critics contend that IPAB is undemocratic because it transfers congressional authority over Medicare spending decisions to an unelected board (never mind that Congress must give assent to IPAB's appointees). IPAB's critics also warn that its spending targets are too austere. Yet IPAB has not had to issue any recommendations thus far, since Medicare spending has remained below the predetermined target.[54]

PPACA also funds comparative effectiveness research, which compares different treatments for their clinical efficacy. The main instrument to promote this is the Patient Care Outcomes Research Institute (PCORI) at national level, whose job is to finance and disseminate medical outcomes research on best practices that can be used to develop scientifically-based clinical guidelines. [55]

Both IPAB and the PCORI represent cautious first steps by the US government to encourage system-wide improvements in the direction of providing treatments that work, based on the scientific evidence. To the extent that this drive eliminates treatments that are not clinically effective, it could also save the health care system money. Still, lawmakers have tread carefully. IPAB's remit extends only to Medicare, not the entire health care system. And as noted above, it cannot recommend cuts in eligibility or benefits. Congress may also overturn its recommendations if it enacts measures having the equivalent magnitude on program costs. PCORI's remit is also to evaluating treatments on clinical, not cost-effectiveness grounds.[56] Further, while PCORI is charged with making knowledge about evidence-based therapies widely available to health care providers, insurers and patients, the law explicitly forbids PCORI's findings from being construed as guidelines or mandates or to be used to deny benefits or coverage. Instead, the hope is that by making information on clinical effectiveness widely available, providers and insurers will voluntarily incorporate best practices in their treatment decisions. Decisions on coverage beyond the PPACA's mandated essential benefits package remains up to individual insurers to decide at a decentralized level in the United States. The law also leaves it to the states, not the federal government, to determine which specific services are to be included in the essential benefits package.

Why Reform Passed: Health Care Politics

Why did health care reform pass in 2010 when it resembled much of the failed Clinton plan two decades earlier? There was no single overriding factor but rather a few key developments that converged. Chief among these was the policy learning among Democrats from the failed Clinton effort. This entailed a reckoning of the powerful health care interest groups, the political system's numerous veto points, and party indiscipline that had wrecked reform nearly twenty years earlier. Obama and Democratic leaders in Congress fashioned a strategy that aimed to bring key interest groups into genuine negotiations early on, and made key concessions when necessary, to gain their support of reform. In addition, Democratic leaders in Congress also took care to centralize and coordinate the work of congressional committees to come up with a single bill in each chamber and preempt wavering partisans with critical deals when necessary to keep the legislation on track. The ground war of interest group mobilization was also more balanced than it had been in 1994. Key interest groups defected from previous anti-reform coalitions as a result of Obama's concessions to them, which made reform advocates' task easier. The war of ideas also played out differently than in 1994. Then, foes of health care reform masterfully shaped public opinion by depicting the Clinton plan as "big government" and "socialized medicine." In 2008, however, the federal government had embarked on a massive bailout of the banking and automobile sectors with a trillion dollars of taxpayer money during the Great Recession. Such government intervention in the American economy was to a degree unmatched since the 1930s Great Depression. The case for federal government inaction to address the health care crisis in the face of postwar record-high unemployment and the unraveling of job-based health insurance, was far less compelling in the 2008 than in 1994. In short, the dire economic conditions in 2008 made the case for government intervention in health care more convincing. Democrats and their allies also invoked key values normally associated with the Right, such as individual responsibility and reward for hard work, to make their case, while effectively using stories of personal hardship that resonated with advocates of reform. Finally, like the earlier Clinton effort, PPACA did not fundamentally break with the familiarity of private employment-based insurance. Rather, it explicitly sought to shore up that system and extend the existing Medicaid program to fill in the gaps.

Partisan Politics

President Obama had initially sought a bipartisan approach to health care reform, particularly in the Senate. The Senate Finance Committee chairman, Max Baucus, assembled a small committee of Democratic and Republican members to seek a compromise on reform in the summer of 2009. That effort failed, however, with the two parties far apart on the role of government in health care. In both the House and Senate, not a single Republican voted for the final health care reform bill.

The real struggle to enact health care reform lay within the Democratic Party itself. Although Democrats proved more unified than their predecessors during the presidency of Bill Clinton, party leaders still had to offer key concessions and compromises to keep wavering Democrats on board and to contain the number of defectors. Democratic leaders therefore decided to unify the different committee bills into a single piece of legislation for consideration in each chamber. Such action focused Democratic minds on one bill rather than on several competing versions of reform that had exerted such a centrifugal effect on party unity during 1993 and 1994. In a further departure from the Clinton strategy, Obama decided to give Congress the lead in drafting health care reform legislation and was content to publicly outline his broad goals for reform. This deference did much to forge a partisan bond able to traverse the institutional divide of separation of powers.

The most important concession that Obama made to ensure party unity was to drop a "public option" from the final version of health care reform. The public option would have created a government health plan along the lines of Medicare to compete alongside private insurers on the exchanges. Even though as a presidential candidate in 2008 Obama had called for a public option, as president he announced that he could live without it, as long as health care reform still met his basic conditions of fairness and affordability. This about-face was done as the politics of necessity to keep both powerful health care stakeholders and wavering Democrats on board. House Democrats, who enjoyed a comfortable majority and whose Speaker was among the liberal wing of the party, had the votes (just barely, as it turned out) to include a watered-down version of the public option in their reform bill. Senate Democrats were more conservative and their majority much smaller than in the House. Were the public option included in the Senate bill, the defection of even a few moderate Democratic senators would have been enough to kill the legislation in the event of a Republican-led filibuster. Ending filibuster required a supermajority of 60 senators, which the Democrats did not have. In order to keep health care reform on track, Obama announced his willingness to drop the public option from the final bill. Accordingly, the bill that made it out of the Senate did not have this feature.

Democrats inserted two provisions to appease those who had lost their cherished public option. One was a provision allowing for nonprofit health care cooperatives to offer insurance on the state exchanges. The nonprofit nature of cooperatives was intended to appease those who had wanted a government insurance program to be able to compete against for-profit insurers on the exchanges. Cooperatives would also be eligible for federal loans to offset formidable start-up costs associated with entering a market dominated by large for-profit insurers. At the same time, cooperatives faced a number of restrictions on their business activities meant to assuage the fears of the insurance industry that feared new competitor.[57] The second concession was to allow a federal multistate insurance plan to be offered on each state exchange.

Broader issues beyond immediate health policy also found their way into the final legislation. The unresolved issue of immigration reform, specifically, the question of amnesty for undocumented immigrants, was an issue that divided both Democrats and Republicans internally. To bridge the intraparty divide and ensure that Democrats did not appear soft on immigration, PPACA bars undocumented immigrants from purchasing insurance on the exchanges or receiving subsidies for insurance. Another compromise bridged the divide between social conservatives and progressive Democrats on abortion and contraception. In the end, Democrats agreed to follow restrictions on federal funding of abortions that already existed in the Medicaid program. Hence, PPACA limits taxpayer subsidies for insurance to cover abortions only when the mother's life is in danger or if the pregnancy is the result of rape or incest. States may go further to bar insurers both inside and outside the exchanges from covering abortions. In addition, PPACA exempts religious organizations from the requirement that employers offer contraception coverage to their workforce. Instead, employees can access this benefit directly from insurers.[58]

Cutting Deals With Health Care Interest Groups

Not only did Obama give Congress a leading role in the project of health care reform, he also differed from Clinton in bringing key interest groups to the negotiating table early on. Obama hoped to forge a consensus on the content of reform that could withstand the onslaught from opponents that was certain to follow during the long and tortuous legislative process. The strategy of stakeholder inclusion consisted of two parts. The first was bringing interest groups to the table as genuine negotiating partners. The second was the mobilization of a new reform coalition interest group coalition that brought together previous foes.

Winning over powerful health care interests was not simply the administration's purview. Rather, Obama relied on key politicians and interest group leaders as well. Senator Edward "Ted" Kennedy (D-MA; in office 1962–2009), a longtime advocate of universal health coverage who was suffering from terminal brain cancer, held closed-door talks with major health care stakeholders, many of whom had bitterly opposed the Clinton plan, to see if he could build a consensus on a new health care reform effort that would expand access to insurance and control costs. Health insurers and providers recognized the large potential market among the uninsured, while employers wanted some relief from their skyrocketing labor costs.[59] In May 2009, Obama announced the outlines of a breakthrough with major health care stakeholders. In a letter addressed to the president, the interest groups pledged to work together to slow the rate of health care inflation by 1.5 percent in the decade from 2010 through 2019. The list of participants at the announcement was a who's-who of the medical industrial complex: the AMA; the AHA; the Pharmaceutical Research and Manufacturers of America (PhRMA); the Advanced Medical Technology Association, which represented medical device manufacturers; America's Health Insurance Plans (AHIP) representing health insurance companies large and small; and the Service Employees' International Union (SEIU). Published in *The New York Times* on May 11, 2009, the letter noted, in part:

> We are committed to taking action in public–private partnership to create a more stable and sustainable health care system that will achieve billions in savings through:
>
> - Implementing proposals in all sectors of the health care system, focusing on administrative simplification, standardization, and transparency that supports effective markets;
> - Reducing over-use and under-use of health care by aligning quality and efficiency incentives among providers across the continuum of care so that physicians, hospitals, and other health care providers are encouraged and enabled to work together towards the highest standards of quality and efficiency;

- Encouraging coordinated care, both in the public and private sectors, and adherence to evidence-based best practices and therapies that reduce hospitalization, manage chronic disease more efficiently and effectively, and implement proven clinical prevention strategies; and,
- Reducing the cost of doing business by addressing cost drivers in each sector and through common sense improvements in care delivery models, health information technology, workforce deployment and development, and regulatory reforms.

None of the groups specified what exactly they would do to reach this ambitious goal, but all of them pledged to work with the president and each other to get there. All realized, however, that they would have to accept some responsibility for financing the expansion of coverage to the uninsured. It was in their self-interest to do so, as fewer uninsured translated into more certain incomes for providers and new markets for insurers.[60]

Key to bringing about this deal was the SEIU, whose leaders Dennis Rivera and Andy Stern viewed health care reform as vital to preserving union jobs.[61] SEIU president Stern also explained the need to bring employers on board and drive a wedge between the traditional foes of health care reform:

> If the business community, the pharmaceutical industry and Wal-Mart all opposed health care reform, this bill would be dead…What keeps it alive is that conservatives are isolated from their traditional business base. The business community appreciates that our country needs to do something about health care.[62]

The Obama administration and its Democratic allies in Congress offered key concessions to providers, insurers, and employers to prevent a repetition of their obstruction that had been so damaging to the fate of Health Security in 1994. One by one, their associations cut deals with the administration. The pharmaceutical industry was the first to move. PhRMA agreed to close the gap in Medicare Part D drug coverage insurance (the so-called donut hole) by granting discounts of 50 percent for name-brand drugs and promising to spend $150 million in ads supportive of health care reform. In return, Obama agreed to keep many of the Medicare Part D provisions that would maintain the hefty profit margins of the industry. Under the PPACA, the Medicare program would not be able to negotiate drug prices with manufacturers or reimport cheaper prescription medicines from abroad.

Other provider groups followed the pharmaceutical industry's lead, making concessions in exchange for new revenues that would follow on the heels of expanding coverage to millions of uninsured patients. Obama's expressed willingness to drop the public option also made them more willing to deal. The AMA publicly came out in favor of the House version of reform on the eve of that chamber's vote, even though it contained a watered-down public option provision. The American Hospital Association (AHA) acquiesced to cuts in government Medicare reimbursements of $155 billion over ten years to finance the expansion of coverage to the uninsured, since fewer uninsured would reduce the burden of uncompensated charity care that their members had to bear. The AHA also successfully negotiated a ten-year delay in the introduction of such cuts.

Obama's decision to jettison the public option was crucial to neutralizing the health insurance lobby, whose chief representative was the America's Health Insurance Plans (AHIP).[63] Private insurers loathed the specter of a public option because it threatened their profit margins and perhaps even their survival. Indeed, AHIP complained that the public option would enjoy unfair advantages in the marketplace (such as size and lower administrative costs) and would essentially drive private insurers out of business. Obama's decision to drop the public option, however, came with a price: insurers had to accept a host of new regulations prohibiting their practices that had allowed them to cream skim the healthy and shun the sick. Hence, the new regulations required insurance companies to accept all applicants and charge modified community-rated premiums instead of rates based on an applicant's health risk. At the same time, both the president and insurers agreed on the need for the individual mandate. Without it, adverse selection would be the likely outcome, as sicker individuals who had been denied coverage or priced out of the health insurance market would now rush to sign up for subsidized coverage. Without healthier people enrolling and offsetting these bad risks, the profits and even survival of insurers would be threatened. By requiring everybody to carry health insurance, the individual mandate would ensure the risk pooling necessary to the proper functioning of insurance markets. Having healthier people in the pool would keep average premiums lower and entail lower taxpayer outlays for premium subsidies than otherwise. The provision for risk-adjusted payments among insurers was an additional corrective to unintended cream skimming as a result of enrollment choices, or to deliberate efforts by insurers to attract healthier subscribers through subtle tactics (like targeted ads depicting healthier people) in order to gain a competitive advantage.

The Obama administration also made a number of key concessions to employers to mute their opposition to reform. Chief among these was the exemption of small businesses from the play-or-pay provisions, as well as the offer of tax credits to small businesses that voluntarily chose to provide coverage. Despite these allowances, organizations representing small business, such as the NFIB and US Chamber of Commerce, ran negative ads against the law. In the end, however, Obama's accommodations to employers' concerns made business opposition to reform less convincing, and, in fact, many large employers (and even small ones) supported PPACA.[64]

The second prong of the interest group strategy was the mobilization of supporters of reform in a highly coordinated and effective way. This was in effect a continuation of the mobilization of the electorate that had swept Obama into office in 2008. The leading groups in this issue-based campaign centering on health care reform were Health Care for America Now (HCAN), Organizing for America (OFA), and MoveOn. These groups coordinated their work and that of others favoring reform, such as associations representing segments of the medical profession as well as nurses and other allied health professions, labor unions, and consumer groups. HCAN and OFA organized rallies, circulated Internet petitions, and garnered online contributions to finance this issue campaign. These tactics sustained ordinary citizens' support for health care reform and targeted congressional Democrats in vulnerable districts whose votes for the PPACA were not assured.

Such mobilization of grassroots supporters succeeded. Proponents of reform would not let differences of opinion destroy health care reform efforts as they had in the past. Though some groups such as MoveOn and the AFL-CIO initially pushed hard for the public option, when President Obama made it clear that he would not sacrifice the entire reform project for the preservation of this one idea, they acquiesced. And, they continued to rally their members to support reform and to pressure congressional Democrats to do the same. Their efforts paid off, with Congress enacting the PPACA in March 2010.

The War of Ideas: The Role of Government

Though the pro-reform coalition faced opposition from small businesses and even a last-ditch stand by insurers, the main challenge came from the Tea Party. The Tea Party was neither an organized interest group nor a new political party. Rather, it was a conservative backlash among mostly white, relatively affluent Americans, many of them Republicans, in reaction to that party's fiscal profligacy and bank bailouts under President George W. Bush. Tea Partiers generally abhorred big government, including the Democrats' health care reform plans. They held particular disdain for the individual mandate, which they viewed as government intrusion on an individual's freedom to go uninsured. While many Tea Party adherents formed spontaneously among grassroots citizens, the movement was also supported financially and otherwise by powerful conservative elites, such as former Republican representative Dick Armey's FreedomWorks and the conservative industrialist Koch brothers.[65]

Tea Partiers engaged in a number of actions to try to stop health care reform. In summer 2009, they disrupted town hall meetings that Democrats had organized to explain and build public support for Obama's reform plans. Tea Partiers' shouted down speakers and garnered widespread media coverage in the process. In addition to such direct action, the Tea Party movement sought to reorient the Republican Party by running conservative candidates in Republican primaries for Congress and the presidency. Rather than form a breakaway third party, which is nearly impossible under the simple plurality rules of the electoral system, the Tea Party movement infiltrated the Republican Party to steer it back to its true small-government roots. Though failing to block the passage of the PPACA, Tea Party candidates did well enough to help the Republicans regain control of the House of Representatives in the 2010 midterm elections and the Senate in the 2014 midterm elections. However, they fell short of their aim to retake the White House in the 2012 elections.

To counter Tea Party foes, pro-reform groups mined other cherished American values to frame the debate on their terms. Pro-reform groups and Democrats invoked norms of individual responsibility to carry insurance and pointed to the subsidies to help make it affordable. They argued that a person's decision to forego insurance was simply shirking responsibility, shifting the cost of one's care when one became sick to taxpayers or those with private insurance. They also made the case for health care reform by invoking fairness, and illustrated their case with numerous personal stories of those who had fallen on hard times beyond their control. The typical story was that of a hard-working person who was self-employed or working for a small business but could not find affordable coverage due to insurers' decisions to deny them coverage because of their preexisting medical condition. Or, unemployment in the Great Recession meant loss of one's insurance. Such accounts were all too common and were an affront to fairness and the basic tenets of the American Dream, which held that hard work and personable responsibility would be rewarded, not punished. Pro-reform groups also countered opponents' distaste for government intervention by citing the trillion dollars in taxpayer money that Republican President George W. Bush had marshaled to bail out the big banks that bore substantial blame for the financial crisis and Great Recession of 2008. If the government could reward irresponsible financial institutions for their actions in the Great Recession, all the more should it help out ordinary hard-working Americans losing their jobs and health insurance as a result.

The Limits of Path Dependence and
the Fate of the Public Option

Path dependence was clearly in play in this episode of health care reform. PPACA borrowed from earlier theories and actual deployment of managed competition and built upon the existing structure of Medicaid and private employment-based insurance. Democrats also learned from the mistakes made by the Clinton team in 1994. Nevertheless, the fate of the public option demonstrated the limits of path dependence in explaining health policy choices.

The architects of the public option argued that it followed past precedent by building on the popular Medicare program for seniors, and by stopping well short of a universal single-payer government plan would have been acceptable to private insurers. Moreover, the public option was fiscally responsible: by retaining employer-provided insurance, tax revenues would not have been the only source of health insurance financing as they would have under a single-payer option. Keeping employer contributions in the mix would have therefore put less strain on the federal budget that already faced enormous deficits. The champions of the public option also envisioned it as a way to bridge the differences between the progressive wing of the Democratic Party, which wanted the single-payer option, and the conservative wing, which advocated smaller government and deficit reduction. Finally, advocates of the public option made a case on cost containment grounds: The public option, like the Medicare program, would have enjoyed the economies of scale and the market power to negotiate lower reimbursement rates with providers and hopefully would force private insurers to do the same to stay competitive.[66]

Yet the attempt to promote the public option as a less radical reform that built on past programs failed to appease powerful stakeholders. First, the fiscally conservative "Blue Dog" wing of the Democratic Party in Congress could not countenance such an expansion of government outlays, given the existence of enormous budget deficits. Private insurers vociferously opposed the public option on the grounds that it put their very existence in jeopardy. There was also the unstated concern that a government competitor would spell lower profits for private insurers. Providers, such as the AMA and AHA, feared that the public option would spell lower reimbursements, not just from the government plan but also from all insurers trying to stay competitive. Their fears were not groundless since Medicare and Medicaid have historically used their market clout to negotiate lower reimbursement rates with provider than more fragmented private insurers. Finally, there was uncertainty over what the public option would mean for American health care over the long term. Some liberal Democrats openly expressed their hope that the public option was the first step toward a single-payer government insurance plan for all Americans, while conservative Democrats and Republicans feared the same fate. In the end, the plan did not have enough votes to pass the Democratic-held Senate, and President Obama took a pragmatic path and declared his willingness to jettison the proposal to ensure passage of health care reform in that chamber.

Implementing PPACA: Technical and Political Hurdles

If the process of enacting health care reform was tortuous and fraught with uncertainty, the same has been true of the subsequent implementation of PPACA. Opponents of PPACA, with Republicans leading the charge, have pursued a number of strategies to derail the law. These have encompassed attempts by Congress to defund the law, challenging the constitutionality of PPACA in court, and presenting alternative legislation. Yet the Democrats must also take some share of responsibility for the law's rocky implementation.

Obama Administration Missteps and Deliberate Delays

Some of the setbacks in getting PPACA up and running rested squarely with Obama administration blunders. The first and most visible was the botched launch of the online marketplaces for insurance for individuals and small businesses. The reform law required each state to set up its own online marketplace; for those that refused, the federal government would either work with the state governments to do so or would set it up alone. In many cases, partisan politics and the associated ideological divide over the role of government shaped the decisions of state government on whether to create their own marketplace. As of July 2015, 16 states and the District of Columbia had created their own marketplaces or had accepted federal government financial assistance to implement their own innovations. Most of these state governments were under Democratic Party control. The remaining 34 states, where Republicans dominated legislatures or held the governorships, declined to do so, leaving the task solely to the federal Department of Health and Human Services (DHHS) to construct and administer these "federally facilitated marketplaces."[67]

It became apparent that the federal government was not ready for a task of this scale and scope and in a short time frame allowing two years. Aggravating the situation, DHHS officials had delegated the construction of the healthcare.gov website for the federally facilitated marketplaces to multiple contractors who proved incapable of coordinating their operations and software with one another. Ignoring contractor warnings that the website was not ready, DHHS launched the federal website for the individual insurance market on January 1, 2014, with disastrous results. The website crashed repeatedly in its first weeks, and there were concerns with software incompatibility and data protection. This poor start frustrated Obama's supporters and offered ample ammunition to his foes, who charged that the PPACA was "big government" run amok. In response, the Obama administration extended the enrollment deadline on the online marketplace by three months and ironed out the technical difficulties so that by April 1, 2014, approximately seven million had enrolled. While this figure fell short of initial projections, enrollment surged in the latter months as DHHS corrected the problems with the website.[68]

The Obama administration backpedaled on other provisions of the law in hopes of heading off an electoral backlash in the 2014 midterm congressional elections. Of particular concern was the potential loss of the Democrats' slender majority in the Senate. The first retreat centered on the comprehensiveness of benefits offered by individual insurance plans. Under PPACA, all new insurance plans offered inside or outside the online marketplaces were required to provide an essential benefits package. Though the intention was to prevent underinsurance and cream skimming, it conflicted with the President's publicly stated pledge that people who already had insurance and liked their coverage could keep it. Insurers sent out letters warning individual policyholders that they would be dropped from existing coverage and required to choose a more comprehensive plan, prompting complaints and confusion from those affected. Criticisms ranged from charges that President Obama had lied to the people, big government was intruding into individuals' freedom to choose coverage, to worries that the minimum benefits requirement forced people to take out more insurance than they needed. In response to the criticism, Obama announced that those who held individual policies that fell short of the essential benefits requirements would be allowed to keep them for a year and after that be required to upgrade to a more comprehensive plan.

The Obama administration also delayed the implementation of key provisions of the employer mandate, first delaying the start date a year to 2015, then extending it to 2016 for firms with 50 to 99 workers. Much of the delay owed to the technical difficulties associated with implementing the mandate, such as how to count full-time employees. But some of the decision to delay was also in response to complaints from businesses. Medium-sized firms were the clear beneficiaries of these postponements, since PPACA from the beginning exempted small businesses with fewer than 50 workers from the mandate, while nearly all large companies already provided insurance to their employees.[69]

In other instances, the administration abandoned some of the law's provisions that it deemed prohibitively costly. Such was the fate of the voluntary long-term care insurance scheme for community-based care known as the CLASS Act, which had been part of the PPACA. This long-term care program would have relied on payroll tax financing. But because participation would have been voluntary, the program would have likely attracted sicker enrollees, leading to funding difficulties that would have necessitated substantial government subsidies to keep it solvent. As a result, the Obama administration and congressional Democrats quietly decided to not fund it.[70]

The Politics of the Medicaid Expansion

The most substantial modification to PPACA came not from the Obama administration but from the Supreme Court. In *NFIB vs Sibelius* in June 2012, the high court ruled on the constitutionality of two major provisions of the reform law. On the first question of whether the individual mandate was constitutional, a five-to-four majority agreed, but for unexpected reasons. Instead of basing its decision on the authority that the US Constitution gave to Congress to regulate interstate commerce, the majority held that the tax penalty for not complying with the mandate, fell under the jurisdiction of Congress to levy taxes.

On the second question of the constitutionality of the Medicaid expansion, the court handed PPACA's architects a defeat. Under the reform law, the federal government pledged to cover 100 percent of the cost of the Medicaid expansion through 2017 and then 90 percent thereafter, with the states shouldering the 10 percent remainder. If states refused to expand Medicaid, they would lose not only the promised expansion funding but also the entire share of federal funding for their existing Medicaid program. This was a substantial amount of money since the federal government's share of Medicaid financing ranged from 50 percent for wealthier states up to 73.4 percent for poorer states.[71] In the Supreme Court's decision, some of the progressives joined forces with conservatives to rule that the financial consequences for states that refused to expand Medicaid amounted to coercion and thus was an unconstitutional infringement on states' rights. By ruling this way, the Supreme Court had essentially rendered the Medicaid expansion optional.[72]

The ruling has allowed for substantial variation among the states on whether to expand their Medicaid programs. As of July 2015, 30 states plus the District of Columbia had accepted federal funding and extended Medicaid to all childless adults and families with household incomes at or below 138 percent of the federal poverty line, one state was considering it, and 19 states had declined to do so. The federal government has left the door open for these states to change their mind and accept the federal expansion money later on. Of the 30 states that have expanded Medicaid, six of them have introduced some provisions that depart from the PPACA provisions. These departures include some cost sharing requirements for higher income recipients, some benefits exclusions, and incentives to encourage patients to adopt healthy lifestyles. Arkansas and Iowa are using federal money for premium assistance to enroll adults eligible for the Medicaid expansion in private health plans approved by their online marketplaces for private insurance. But all six states have had to meet federal safeguards in order to qualify for the waivers and funding, The safeguards, for example, prohibit states from imposing work requirements in exchange for Medicaid coverage or levying cost-sharing provisions on those with incomes below the federal poverty line.[73]

More important, the high court's decision to make Medicaid expansion optional has opened up a yawning coverage gap of 3.7 million persons that PPACA's architects did not intend. Medicaid has historically covered children in low-income families, but states have the authority to determine eligibility levels for parents. And many states set income eligibility limits for parents to levels well below the poverty line. In Texas, for example, the eligibility limit is only 19 percent of the poverty line while in Alabama it is a meager 16 percent. Such stringent eligibility requirements, coupled with Medicaid's exclusion of childless adults from coverage, meant that the government program only reached 30 percent of low-income adults in the United States in 2012, before the PPACA's Medicaid expansion went into effect.[74]

PPACA was supposed to vastly expand coverage in two ways, first, by expanding Medicaid to nearly all low-income persons—even adults without children—with incomes up to 138 percent of the poverty line, and second, by providing subsidized insurance on the exchanges to those with incomes between 100 and 400 percent of the poverty line. In nearly all of the states that have chosen not to expand Medicaid, 3.7 million residents living below the poverty line fall into a coverage gap: they earn too much to qualify for their state's current Medicaid program but not enough to qualify for premium subsidies on the exchanges that start at 100 percent of the poverty line. In those states not expanding Medicaid, the median eligibility limit for parents to qualify for such coverage is only 46 percent of the poverty line. For those with such low incomes, affordable insurance is simply out of reach: unsubsidized premiums on the exchanges may cost as much as 25 to 50 percent of their income. This does not include additional out-of-pocket medical costs they may incur.[75]

The reasons for the unwillingness of some states to embark on the Medicaid expansion varied. Some were out of revealed partisan and ideological considerations while others were more pragmatic in nature. Most of the states declining the federal dollars were led by Republican governors or legislatures or both, who either resented the expansion of federal authority into the domain of the states, opposed such a sweeping initiative from a Democratic president and congress, or both. Policymakers in some states did not trust the federal government to keep its promise to pay 90 percent of the Medicaid expansion costs in the future and feared being saddled with a burdensome unfunded mandate. Still other states with large uninsured populations, such as Texas, reckoned that even with the federal government shouldering 90 percent of the Medicaid expansion, the 10 percent share paid by state taxpayers would still be prohibitively expensive.[76]

In short, the fate of the Medicaid expansion bears the imprint of several important political factors. The fragmented institutional structure of the American political system was clearly in play. The Supreme Court's decision striking down the original Medicaid expansion demonstrated the checks and balances provided by separation of powers, while the states' varying decisions on whether to accept federal Medicaid expansion money was a clear expression of federalism. Partisanship was also an important factor, since Republican governors and legislatures led all of the states that declined the federal Medicaid dollars, while all states led by Democrats accepted the federal funds. Ideological aversion to big government and the intrusion of Washington into their domain also played a role in the decisions of many states to decline the money. Even so, in some cases pragmatism overcame ideological and partisan concerns, with Republican-led states such as New Jersey, Ohio, and Utah eventually opting to accept the federal expansion dollars.

Republican Alternatives

Unable to block the passage of PPACA, the Republican Party in Congress has sought to defund, repeal, and replace the Democrats' health care reform law. Republicans and their allies have also continued to use the courts as an avenue to block the implementation of PPACA. These varied tactics have centered on a broad argument that with PPACA the federal government has overstepped its authority and that President Obama in particular has asserted executive power to implement the law in ways that violate the Constitution.

In the House of Representatives, for example, the Tea Party wing of the Republican Party refused to authorize spending for the law, thus precipitating a partial federal government shutdown in October 2013.[77] That effort, however, was a monumental failure and a public relations disaster, for the party, and convinced Republican leaders to pursue their opposition through less dramatic means. Health care industry groups, too, have repeatedly sought to renege on their deal with the Obama administration to reverse the taxes they agreed to in order to pay for insurance expansion. In some cases they have secured delays in implementation but not outright reversal of these provisions.[78]

The reality of divided government has thus far made it impossible for Republicans to repeal the PPACA, even after capturing the Senate and expanding their grip on the House following the 2014 midterm elections. President Obama has repreatedly refused to dismantle key elements of his signature legislation. Republicans might yet prevail if they win the presidency and retain control of Congress in 2016. Even then, they may find it infeasible eradicate all of the Affordable Care Act. In the meantime, Republicans have begun to proffer bills that would retain popular provisions of PPACA, while repealing elements that they dislike and replacing them with their own alternatives that would get rid of the various mandates in the Democrats' law, drastically cut government spending, and shift the balance of responsibility toward individuals for their choices and financing of health insurance and actual medical care.

Paul Ryan's Paths to Health Care Reform

Medicare Reform

Representative Paul Ryan is arguably the most powerful and visible opponent to President Obama on the matter of health care reform. He has risen rapidly through the party ranks, first as chairman of the House Budget Committee, then heading the powerful House Ways and Means Committee, as well as serving as the Republican vice-presidential candidate in 2012, and is currently Speaker of the House. As the party's foremost thinker on social and economic policy, Ryan has authored detailed proposals for health care reform that center on competition, private insurance, and sharply reduced federal outlays on government health programs in the quest to reduce the nation's budget deficits and debt. He first set out his reform proposals in his *A Roadmap for America's Future* in 2008, but his Republican colleagues at the time found the document too radical and distanced themselves from it. Ryan reiterated his core ideas in *A Roadmap for America's Future, Version 2.0* in January 2010. By then, his ideas had become more palatable to his Republican colleagues, particularly as the Tea Party wing of the party gained seats in Congress. Many of his proposals have found their way into the proposed Patient CARE Act discussed below. Ryan has also modified some of the most controversial provisions in successive *Path to Prosperity* documents, which present the Republican-dominated House Budget proposals. In the intervening years, moreover, Tea Party activists have shifted the Republican Party further to the right in its ideological and policy orientation. For both reasons, Ryan's proposals have become the mainstream canon in the Republican Party.[79]

Ryan's Medicare reform proposals have garnered the most attention. His Medicare plan borrows some of the innovations found in PPACA. He calls for an online Medicare insurance marketplace with government and private plans competing on price. This essentially introduces into Medicare the managed competition provisions and insurance regulations already in place for small businesses and individuals under PPACA. Similarly, Ryan would prohibit insurers from discriminating against seniors with health conditions through experience-rated premiums or plan exclusions, and require them to offer an essential benefits package, again borrowing PPACA protections in the insurance marketplaces for small business and individuals into Medicare.

However, to meet his stated goals of fiscal responsibility, specifically, reducing the size of the federal debt and ensuring the long-term solvency of Medicare, Ryan's plan envisions radical structural change to the Medicare program. Chiefly, Ryan proposes to transform the financing of Medicare from a defined-benefit plan, in which government spending meets the health care costs of seniors by either raising taxes or cutting reimbursements to providers, to a defined-contribution plan in which the government's share of Medicare financing would be fixed and seniors themselves would make up the difference. Such fiscal responsibility would be achieved by "premium support," more commonly known as a voucher. The federal government would give each senior a fixed amount in advance, who would then use that money to select his or her own health coverage on an online Medicare marketplace. Seniors could choose a government Medicare plan consisting of fee-for-service reimbursement and free choice of provider as currently, or a health plan offered by private insurers. To prevent cream skimming, all plans would have to offer an identical basic benefits package (though they could offer additional benefits), charge community-rated premiums rather than experience-rated premiums based on a person's health status, and accept all applicants regardless health status. The premium support from the federal government would reflect the second cheapest plan available on the exchange, but the voucher would be more for sicker and poorer seniors and less for wealthier seniors. Senior citizens, who chose a more expensive plan or incurred additional cost-sharing expenses at the time of health care services, would be responsible for these amounts above the voucher.[80]

Ryan would also repeal PPACA's Independent Payment Advisory Board (IPAB) that oversees Medicare spending on the grounds that faceless, unelected bureaucrats will ration health care to seniors. Under this scenario, IPAB will recommend such deep cuts in provider reimbursements to meet the law's Medicare expenditure target that providers will flee the

Medicare program in droves, making it increasingly difficult for seniors to find doctors and hospitals willing to treat them. Even though PPACA prohibits IPAB from recommending cuts in benefits or eligibility or increases in premiums or cost-sharing, Ryan insists that IPAB will indeed recommend deep reimbursement cuts that will constitute de facto rationing.[81] As an alternative, Ryan would require Congress, rather than an appointed board, to decide on the magnitude of reimbursement cuts.

To avert a possible political backlash from senior citizens, Ryan's Medicare proposals would be phased in over time and would not apply to current retirees. The premium support would only affect those turning 65 in 2024. Ryan's plan would also gradually raise the retirement age from 65 to 67 years.

Ryan's proposals have garnered praise from conservatives and worry from progressives. The Heritage Foundation, the conservative research institute that earlier proposed a voucher for Medicare, lauded Ryan's proposals because it would "put Medicare on a budget."[82] But progressives as well as some health economists have expressed concern that Ryan's specific design of premium support would burden seniors with a rising share of health care costs over time. This is because under current law, all Medicare beneficiaries receive the same essential benefits for the same premium and deductible (unless they opt for private Medicare Advantage plans that cover more cost-sharing in exchange for obtaining care within a closed network of providers). Under Ryan's plan, premiums and cost-sharing could vary by health plan on the exchange, which would be consistent with a managed competition model premised on price competition. The sticking point is Ryan's formula to adjust premium support over time. Ryan's formula would allow premium support to increase in line with growth of US gross domestic product plus 0.5 percent. This formula would be quite effective in slowing the growth of Medicare spending because the government's premium support would be tied to economic indicators rather than medical spending. Historically, average Medicare spending per beneficiary, as well as medical price inflation more generally, has risen faster than the rate of economic growth. In other words, Ryan's premium support may not keep up with the actual health care costs of the Medicare program. In that case, seniors would shoulder an increasing burden of program costs in the form of higher premiums or cost sharing to keep the same level of benefits that they had enjoyed in the past.[83]

By contrast, the Medicare spending target that guides IPAB is a blended formula of the average rate of inflation in the broader economy and in the health sector. By taking into account medical inflation, PPACA's target is less stringent than Ryan's. Indeed, IPAB did not recommend any spending cuts for Medicare in 2015 because the program's spending was well below the stated target.[84] This suggests that Ryan's prediction of draconian spending cuts and rationing may be exaggerated.

Critics of Ryan's plan also question whether managed competition would actually be more cost effective than the current Medicare plan. Price competition among a number of health insurers could conceivably hold the line on premium and cost-sharing increases. But Medicare has historically outperformed private insurers in terms of lower provider reimbursement and overall costs. This is chiefly because Medicare functions as a single-payer insurance plan, which gives the government the market clout to negotiate lower reimbursements with providers. Medicare also has lower administrative costs than private insurers (3% vs. 14%, respectively). As a result, between 1969 and 2009, Medicare spending per beneficiary grew by 400 percent while private insurance premiums increased by over 700 percent. So, while a Medicare exchange could give seniors a greater variety of health plans to choose from, it may not be as cost effective as the current Medicare single-payer system. And the savings from managed competition may come through narrower provider networks than the traditional Medicare plan, or through higher premiums and cost sharing borne by seniors.[85] A further concern with Ryan's managed competition proposal is that the traditional fee-for-service Medicare plan, with its free choice of provider, might disproportionately attract those with the most serious health conditions. Such adverse selection would drive up premiums in the traditional plan and could force healthier seniors to exit for cheaper options. This "death spiral" of rising premiums and exit of healthier members could eventually lead to its demise.

Finally, leaving Congress in charge of restraining the growth of Medicare spending may not deliver the hoped-for savings. The membership of IPAB, which includes scientific and economic research expertise alongside representatives of insurers, providers, and patients, is designed to insulate spending decisions from direct lobbying by powerful health care interest groups and encourage more reasoned discussion and debate informed by scientific evidence. At the very least, it may improve the chances of consensual solutions through the mechanisms of inclusion and negotiation. Ryan's plan leaves it to Congress to make the difficult spending cuts to Medicare, and it is not clear that the legislature has the backbone to stand up to health care industry money and lobbying. Were Congress to fall short, Medicare spending could overshoot Ryan's target and undermine his projected reduction in the federal deficit and debt.

Medicaid Reform

Ryan has also outlined big plans to reform Medicaid. Again, the stated purpose of his reform is to reduce federal spending on Medicaid and give states more flexibility and responsibility for their own program. First off,

Ryan would repeal PPACA's Medicaid expansion to persons with incomes below 138 percent of the poverty line and allow states the freedom to set income eligibility limits for the program, as they do now. But Ryan would radically reconfigure the financing of Medicaid by converting the federal government's share of funding to a block grant for each state. This funding scheme would entail far less federal money than under current law. Currently, the federal government's contribution to Medicaid is set to meet the health care costs of the program in each state. The federal share takes account of not only health spending for beneficiaries but also economic conditions, rising during recessions when unemployment and the Medicaid rolls increase, then falling back during periods of economic growth. Under Ryan's block grant formula, however, increases in the federal share would be linked to the general inflation rate plus 1 percent, along with the state's population growth. It would not adjust for the economic cycle or for the actual health care spending for Medicaid in a given state. To compensate for this loss of federal money, Ryan promises that states would receive greater latitude to redesign their Medicaid programs, including allowing recipients to enroll in private plans. States would also receive more discretion to decide range of covered benefits, eligibility requirements, delivery of services, and reimbursement of providers.[86]

Ryan's proposal clearly would reduce federal spending on both Medicaid and Medicare, as the nonpartisan CBO study attests. Indeed, Ryan's 2012 House Budget called for a reduction in federal spending on Medicaid and CHIP from 2 percent of GDP in 2011 to 1 percent in 2050.[87] He would reduce Medicaid spending by $1.7 trillion, or 38 percent, between 2013 and 2022 alone. While the congressman believes that the states would use their new freedom to innovate to keep costs and benefits steady, critics fear that cuts in federal Medicaid outlays deficit would simply shift a greater share of program costs to the states, providers, or the poor.[88] Even if states were able to achieve some savings through program innovations, they would not be enough to make up for such draconian cuts to federal funding outlined in Ryan's plan. In that case, state governments would be faced with unpalatable choices to either raise taxes, cut reimbursement rates to providers (which are already only 60 percent of private insurance), or cut benefits and eligibility. Indeed, a study by the Urban Institute estimated that the 2012 Ryan plan requires states to reduce their Medicaid enrollment by 31 to 37 million persons over the decade to make up for the drop in federal spending.[89]

The Patient CARE Act[90]

Congressional Republicans have repeatedly vowed to "repeal and replace" PPACA. But other than Paul Ryan, the party had done little to articulate a replacement, until the Patient Choice, Affordability, Responsibility, and Empowerment (CARE) Act proposed in January 2014. And even this proposal borrows many of Congressman Ryan's ideas for individual and employer-based insurance.[91] The CARE Act leaves Medicare reform for another day, but does propose to overhaul Medicaid. The Medicaid provisions for the most part mirror those of Paul Ryan outlined above, calling for the repeal of PPACA's Medicaid expansion and introducing block grants to states to fund the federal portion of Medicaid. Other "patient-centered" provisions under CARE encourage Medicaid beneficiaries to assume more responsibility for their health care by giving them the option of enrolling in private health plans, and choosing high-deductible coverage paired with a health savings account (HSA), partially funded by government, to cover some of the costs they might incur at the time of medical care. Whether Medicaid beneficiaries with low incomes would have the means to pay for health care costs beyond the government contribution to their HSA is unclear.

The CARE Act also proposes major changes in employment-based and individual insurance for those under 65. The Republicans would retain popular provisions of PPACA, such as coverage for adult dependent children until age 26, barring lifetime limits on insurance, require insurers to accept all applicants regardless of health status, and levy modified community rating. The CARE Act would also continue with insurance premium subsidies, but only up to 300 percent of the poverty line rather than PPACA's 400 percent ceiling, and would be adjusted only to the general inflation rate plus 1 percent.

Yet the CARE Act would also break with PPACA in important respects. It would repeal the individual and employer mandates in PPACA, the taxes on the health care industry, and caps on out-of-pocket expenses for individual and family coverage. It would also permit insurers to set premiums for older enrollees five times higher than for younger ones, compared to the three-to-one ratio under PPACA. And, while no longer requiring individuals to carry insurance, the CARE Act contains a continuous coverage provision. While this prohibits anything other than community-rated premiums for those who maintain their insurance coverage, insurers would be able to levy experience-rated premiums on those who let their coverage lapse. This prospect might provide sufficient incentive for people to retain their insurance, especially since experience-rated premiums for those with medical conditions could be very expensive. But it does not consider the reasons for letting one's coverage lapse, such as loss of job-based insurance through unemployment or divorce. In such instances, some people may not have the financial resources to maintain their prior insurance coverage. However, for those unfortunate persons with preexisting medical conditions who find themselves unable to purchase a regular health insurance policy, the CARE Act would allow them to enroll in a high-risk pool in their state. The government would subsidize these pools, but the CARE Act did not specify the amount or relative share of federal and state taxpayer contributions. Historically, high-risk pools in the 35 states that operated them suffered from low enrollment due to high premiums and cost-sharing, even with state taxpayer funding. Because such pools segregate the sickest individuals and do not allow for risk-pooling with healthier individuals, premiums do not cover the health care costs of those in the pool and thus require tax subsidies. But making premiums affordable would require much higher tax subsidy than has been the case in the past. Indeed, a 2008 CBO study estimated that a national high-risk pool would cost $16 billion or more over a decade.[92]

Finally, the CARE Act would reduce the tax subsidy on employment-based insurance. Under current law, employers can deduct their share of premiums as a business expense and the amount does not count as taxable income for their workers. To encourage employers to continue to offer coverage, the CARE Act would still permit them to claim the tax deduction. But employees would only be able to claim up to 65 percent of the cost of an average health plan. While the constriction of the tax deduction for workers would certainly make more government funding available for other subsidies under the CARE Act, it would come as a shock to many accustomed to having the entire employer premium not count as taxable income, who would likely view it as a tax on their income.[93] In short, the CARE Act, would provide government-financed premium subsidies, but these may not keep pace with actual health care costs as they would under PPACA. The CARE Act may also lead to far fewer Americans being covered by health insurance, especially older individuals facing higher rates and those who may, for example, lose their jobs and their insurance and be subject to higher experience-rated premiums.[94]

In sum, the two political parties offer distinctly different visions of health care reform and the country's future. Republican proposals would slow the rate of increase in federal outlays for Medicare, substantially cut federal spending on the Medicaid program for the poor, and repeal or reduce federal subsidies for insurance for those not covered by Medicare or Medicaid. Yet the party's budget axe would not fall evenly, targeting social and health programs, holding the level of spending on other programs to far below that since World War II, while sparing defense from automatic cuts. Ryan's budget would also alter the tax code to sharply reduce tax rates on the wealthiest Americans and corporations while promising to close tax loopholes.[95] Even then, Ryan's austerity to attain the prize of fiscal responsibility would be a war of attrition: under his plan the federal budget deficit would not disappear until 2050.[96] In the larger scheme of things, then, both Republican and Democrat visions for health care reform are part of a more fundamental struggle over the proper role of government in the American economy and society, and whether the burden of economic adjustment should be borne equitably by all or disproportionately by the most vulnerable.

Two Possible Futures

So, what do we make of all this activity around health care reform in the past few years? And where is US health policy heading? Looking at PPACA, the evidence shows that the law has begun to meet some of its goals, but not all. The future of the Democrats' health care law, and the direction of health policy more generally, will be determined by political factors. An important Supreme Court decision on PPACA in June 2015 (discussed below) has settled some uncertainties. But the presidential and congressional elections in 2016 will also leave an imprint on the law's future course. Yet whatever the outcome of these highly charged political events, PPACA has shifted the terms of debate over health policy for both parties in important ways. This may be one of its chief legacies in the longer term.

The Affordable Care Act and Republican
Alternatives Compared

Assessing health care reform a year since the most important provisions of PPACA have been implemented reveals that the law has had a dramatic impact in some areas of health care system performance but less so in other areas.[97] PPACA has played a big part in reducing the number of uninsured. Between October 2013 and June 2015, almost ten million people had signed up for coverage on the exchanges. During the same period, Medicaid and CHIP added 13.6 million members.[98] This is in stark contrast to the end of 2013, the period just prior to the enrollment period under PPACA. At that time, 16.2 percent of the population under age 65 lacked health insurance. By the end of 2014, that number had fallen to 12.1 percent, and preliminary data from the first quarter of 2015 showed the rate had declined further to 10.7 percent. An improved job market since the depth of the Great Recession has contributed to the rising number of workers with employment-based insurance.[99] But an improved employment picture is not the only reason for the decline in the uninsured. Indeed, the growth in insurance coverage since 2013 was the greatest among Hispanics, Blacks, and households with incomes of less than $36,000.[100] They were more likely than other groups to be working in jobs that did not offer insurance, even before the recession. In other words, the Affordable Care Act has helped those who needed it most. Moreover, for those who enrolled on the exchanges in the first year, 85 percent were able to access premium subsidies making insurance more affordable. Still, despite nearly 24 million people getting insurance through PPACA, millions of Americans still lack coverage. This is due to the optional nature of the Medicaid expansion and less than hoped for enrollment in the exchanges in the first year, as well as PPACA's exemptions of certain sectors of the population (those in the Medicaid coverage gap and undocumented immigrants) from the individual mandate.[101]

Costs of US health care spending have slowed in the last two years. For example, premiums for employment-based and individual coverage on and off the exchanges rose by only 3 percent between 2013 and 2014, the lowest rate of increase since the mid-1990s. How much of this is due directly to the Affordable Care Act or to other factors like demographic change and the transition of older Americans onto Medicare is hard to disentangle.

PPACA's impact on the quality of health care is indeterminate and too early to judge. After all, many of these experiments in reimbursement and delivery system reforms are pilot projects whose effects may take a decade to fully assess. Yet the federal government has signaled its willingness to move forward with such demonstrations: in July 2015, the Centers for Medicare and Medicaid Services announced that it would introduce bundled payments for hip and knee replacements in 75 metropolitan areas. Significantly, the 750 hospitals in this project would be required to participate.[102] The success of payment and delivery reforms will hinge on their design. The experiments must be able to specify and measure health outcomes. There is also concern of the extent to which providers can and should be held accountable for patient outcomes. Some diseases are caused not simply by patient behavior, but also by broader social and environmental determinants such as poverty, lack of good healthy alternatives available, and violent neighborhoods that induce chronic stress. Programs must take incorporate risk-adjusted measures to account for these factors. Studies of ACOs yielded mixed results thus far. Early evaluations of some ACOs have found improvements in the quality of care, as measured by reductions in preventable hospital admissions and emergency room use. Other ACOs, however, have achieved little or no cost savings perhaps because they rely on fee-for-service reimbursement, which as we have seen, tends to reward physicians for higher volumes of more complex and costly procedures.[103] Recent evaluations of patient-centered medical homes have likewise documented mixed results but some positive indicators. A number of medical homes have registered improvements in costs, quality of care, access, and patient satisfaction as well as reductions in preventable emergency room and inpatient care. But challenges remain, particularly in devising payment systems that adequately reflect the higher costs of caring for those with multiple chronic diseases and that reimburse primary care teams for performing vital yet time-consuming tasks such as office visit consultations and management of patients' medications and referrals to other providers.[104]

Despite these unknowns, clear differences separate PPACA from Republican alternatives. In general, Republican proposals would do a better job than PPACA at cutting federal spending on health care, as the nonpartisan CBO has concluded. But holding the line on federal outlays for health care would depend on shifting the burden of financing to the insured themselves, through higher cost sharing via the "patient-centered reforms" touted by Ryan and his colleagues. These include setting stringent premium support or, vouchers for Medicare, reducing or eliminating premium subsidies for individual and small group insurance, and treating employment-based insurance as taxable income. The Medicaid block grants would also assure the federal government of reduced health care spending on that program, but would most surely shift any shortfall to state taxpayers, providers, and the poor. Republicans' belief that health savings accounts paired with high-deductible health plans will empower individuals in the market is also a leap of faith. Aside from favoring the healthier and wealthier, it is hard to see how an individual armed with his or her account will have the market clout to negotiate lower prices with formidable entities like large hospitals or integrated provider networks. These plans will also leave more people uninsured than under PPACA, due to the much heavier burden of health care financing that individuals or states will have to assume.

For those with lower incomes or severe health conditions, the likelihood of remaining uninsured is greater under the Republican alternatives than under PPACA. The Affordable Care Act provides stronger risk-pooling arrangements and spreads the burden of health care financing to include those with greater ability to pay, such as high-income earners and the health care industry. But the CARE Act has harsh consequences for those who are less healthy and who lose their health insurance coverage. They will either face experience-rated premiums based on their medical condition, or be shunted into a state high-risk pool. Neither of these options may guarantee affordable premiums and cost sharing. In the end, the Democrats' approach offers more equitable burden sharing for both health care financing and larger federal deficit reduction than do the Republican alternatives.

Further Politics

The possibility that some or all of the Republican offerings may become law remains to be seen. Following the 2014 midterm congressional elections. Republicans strengthened their grip on the House of Representatives and also retook control of the Senate by a 54 to 46 seat margin. Despite this setback, President Obama and congressional Democrats have stood firm in the face of Republican efforts to repeal any part of his signature health care reform law. Any attempt to repeal PPACA would require the votes of 60 senators to defeat likely Democrat attempts at a filibuster. But the Republicans are six votes short of this hurdle. In the current toxic partisan environment, compromise between the two parties on this issue is little more than a pipe dream. Paul Ryan has become a dominant figure in the Republican Party, having secured the chairmanship of the powerful House Ways and Means Committee following the 2014 elections. As chair of this committee, Ryan enhanced his influence over the party's policies. This is because the Ways and Means Committee has the final say in the House on the spending for all federal programs, including health care. In October 2015, Ryan became Speaker of the House, being seen by his colleagues as the only one who could bring discipline and direction to a fractious Republican caucus. Ryan has signaled his party's priority to replace the Affordable Care Act, but has acknowledged that this will be a long game: "We need to articulate a different vision for health care. I do believe Obamacare is going to collapse under its own weight for lots of reasons...so I think we need to be prepared for what to replace it with...And I know we won't pass a repeal and a [new] law with this president."[105] Should the Republicans hold their majorities in Congress and capture the presidency in 2016, their promise to repeal and replace PPACA with their own alternative vision may well become reality.

Before that date, however, PPACA had to overcome another major legal hurdle in 2015. In the *King v. Burwell* case, conservative groups challenged the legality of the premium subsidies in the federal government-run exchanges operating in 34 states (16 states plus the District of Columbia had set up their own exchanges). The Obama administration, the Internal Revenue Service, and PPACA's supporters held that the intent of the law was to make premium subsidies available on the exchanges in all 50 states. But the conservative plaintiffs maintained that the wording of the law limited premium subsidies only to "an exchange established by the state."[106] Had the Supreme Court agreed with the plaintiffs, it is estimated that between 7 and 9.5 million people who had already enrolled or planned to do so in health plans on the 34 federally facilitated exchanges would have been ineligible for premium subsidies. Without premium subsidies, insurance would have been unaffordable for many, giving them little choice but to forego insurance.[107] Certainly, the 34 states could have subsequently chosen to set up their own exchanges so that their citizens with incomes between 100 and 400 percent of the poverty line would gain access to premium subsidies. But Republicans who previously rejected PPACA lead many of these states, and it was unclear how many of these would have reversed their stance had the Supreme Court ruled in favor of the challengers.

A Supreme Court decision declaring premium subsidies illegal in these exchanges could have had far-reaching consequences, setting in play a death spiral that would have destroyed the Affordable Care Act. This is because the law mandates individuals to carry insurance but also pair this requirement with subsidies to make coverage affordable. Recall that the individual mandate was put in place to ensure that healthier people would enroll and offset the health care costs of those who are sicker. Community-rated premiums would reflect the average cost of insurance coverage for both the healthy and the sick. However, unable to obtain premium subsidies in the 34 states, many of the healthier among the middle and working classes might have decided to forego coverage and pay the tax penalty, leaving only the sickest on the exchanges. Insurers would have had to hike premiums to retain profitability or solvency, prompting even more people to drop coverage. The ensuing death spiral would have made insurance unaffordable except for the wealthy. Under this scenario, the Affordable Care Act's key elements to expand insurance would have unraveled, and it is difficult to see how the law would have survived in its current form.[108] As it turned out, the Supreme Court accepted the logic of the Obama administration. In its decision in June 2015, by a six to three majority, the court held that the subsidies extended to all 50 states.[109]

Even so, electoral politics could make PPACA's future uncertain. Should Democrats hold onto the White House or retake one or more chambers of Congress in 2016, the law should survive. But if Republicans capture the presidency and hold onto Congress in 2016, all bets are off. A Republican president and Congress could yet succeed in repealing or simply defunding budgetary parts of PPACA by simple majority vote in both houses. Or a few wavering Democrats could defect from their own party's filibuster attempt.[110] Even without a supermajority of 60 senators, Republicans could thwart a Democratic filibuster to defend PPACA by convincing just a few wavering Democrats to cross party lines But by 2017, it might be too late. Most of PPACA's provisions will have been in place for two years or more, making it difficult for Republicans to garner the support of key health care stakeholders who have already reconciled themselves to life under PPACA and have adjusted their practices accordingly.[111] The subsequent upheaval would be particularly disruptive to the health care industry and to millions of patients. Still, one should "never say never" in politics. A Republican administration and Congress might seek to repeal most of PPACA while preserving a few provisions that are popular with the public. This is the essence of the Patient CARE Act approach.

Even if the Affordable Care Act does not survive, it will have a lasting impact on the thinking and terms of debate over health policy. Both Democrats and Republicans acknowledge the need for government subsidy to make insurance affordable, even though they disagree on the size of that amount. The rules on insurers that bar widespread use of experience rating and that prohibit denying coverage on the basis of health conditions seem to be firmly in place. Both parties and the broader public have embraced these changes (though Republicans would permit certain exceptions). It is difficult to see how the country could go back to what had gone before. Both parties also accept the idea of competition and consumer choice in health insurance coverage, at least for employed Americans. But they disagree on whether these arrangements should extend to government insurance programs for senior citizens, the poor, and disabled. Further changes to medical practice and health care delivery are certain to come, as the pilot programs encouraged and funded by PPACA begin to provide concrete results on what works and what does not.

The more fundamental questions surrounding the nature of health care and role of government in its provision remain unsettled in the United States. If health care is a basic human right that all can lay claim to, then it is not simply a private commodity for those who can afford it, nor is it an act of charity to the least fortunate. If PPACA survives and becomes the foundation of a new consensus, then it suggests that the United States has moved closer to the position of all other industrialized nations, which view health care as a right.

CHAPTER THREE

Germany: Modernizing Social Health Insurance to Meet New Challenges

The Federal Republic of Germany pioneered national health insurance system in the modern world and has served as a model for many countries.[1] Germany's variant of national health insurance (NHI) is termed social health insurance (SHI) because it is part of the broader social insurance system that encompasses government pensions and unemployment and accident insurance. Health insurance coverage is mandatory for all those below a legally set income threshold. But rather than a single government health plan covering the entire population, which is single-payer NHI as exists in Canada, Germans obtain health coverage from a multitude of employment-based non-profit insurance funds. These funds are not government bodies; however, they operate under strict government supervision. Historically, the different health insurance funds stratified the population along occupational, class, and status lines. This changed in the 1990s, when health care reforms allowed for the free choice of insurer. Employers and employees bear the primary responsibility for financing health insurance through income-related contributions, though state actors play an important supplementary role. A small private insurance market is available for those above the legally defined income ceiling. Associations representing providers and insurers have primary responsibility for health care administration, as part of a system of governance known as *corporatism*, but they operate under tight state oversight and supervision.[2]

German political institutions and processes have left their imprint on the health care sector. Coalition governments at the national level, federal structures that bind together national and state actors in networks of cooperation, and corporatist representation of organized interests in policymaking and implementation have produced a "semi-sovereign state" that encourages and institutionalizes processes of negotiation and compromise. The pattern of policy change is one of ongoing adjustment and gradualism.[3]

Like the other countries in this book, Germany confronts major challenges in continuing to balance the goals of universal access, affordability, and high quality health care. As the German population ages and requires expensive care for chronic conditions, there will be fewer workers to pay for the health care of themselves and their elders. In addition, the financing of health insurance from payroll taxes on wages and salaries in an era of slower wage growth adds to the financing concerns. At the same time, new forms of work undercut the security of employment-based insurance. To date, governments have largely worked through the existing institutional arrangements of employment-based social health insurance and have sought to make the system more responsive and efficient through competition and choice, while safeguarding its solidarity and equity. Policymakers have also repaired and even extended the corporatist underpinnings of the health care system. Some of the reforms of the new millennium, have grafted institutional innovations onto these long-standing structures.

This chapter proceeds as follows. The first section "Main Features of German Social Health Insurance" sketches the historical development of SHI and describes its main actors and institutions. The next section describes how the political system—its structure, representation of interests, and political culture—has shaped health care institutions and policies. The third section "Health Care System Performance and Challenges" assesses the strengths and weaknesses of health care system performance and highlights the major challenges it faces. The last section analyzes the more recent policy reforms that governments have introduced to address these challenges, outlining their aims, content, and the underlying politics that explain these reform choices. The chapter's conclusion considers the implications of the reform path for German health care in the future.

Main Features of German Social Health Insurance

Historical Origins

The basic institutional contours of social health insurance based in employment have their origins in the nineteenth century. Chancellor Otto von Bismarck (1871–1890) enacted the social health insurance law as part of his comprehensive system of social security for German workers in the 1880s. Germany thus can boast the first comprehensive welfare state of the modern era, which spanned government-sponsored old-age pensions, accident insurance, unemployment insurance, and health insurance. Just over a century later, German policymakers added long-term care insurance to the country's social insurance system. In constructing the SHI system, Bismarck built upon the preexisting web of mutual funds that arose from the preindustrial guild tradition for many German professions and occupations. The 1883 Act on Health Insurance for Blue-Collar Workers required these workers to obtain coverage through government-approved "sickness funds"[4] organized on class, occupational, or employment lines. These contributions were paid as payroll taxes to the sickness funds. Employees covered two-thirds of the premium, while employers paid one-third. Workers and employers enjoyed a similar ratio of representation on the governing boards of these funds.

Many mistakenly assume that social democratic forces have been the chief architects of the welfare state, as with Britain's National Health Service or Canada's single-payer national health insurance. However, the creation of the German welfare state was not the result of a democratic impulse from the political left but was instead a conservative creation. Indeed, Bismarck's justification for such social protection was based on the grounds of national security: Germany's place as a major world power depended on a healthy and productive workforce and armed forces. Moreover, Bismarck's pioneering action in social insurance occurred against the backdrop of an authoritarian regime unwilling to extend political power to new classes arising from the Industrial Revolution. Imperial Germany had the facade of democratic institutions, but parliament was weak and real power rested with the chancellor and, ultimately, the emperor he served. The regime faced demands from the burgeoning working class and its Socialist Party for genuine rights both in the workplace and in the political arena. But Bismarck responded with a two-pronged approach: he offered workers social protection as a way to buy their loyalty to the regime, even as he denied them political rights and outlawed their Socialist Party. Bismarck also forged a strategic alliance with the Catholic Center Party to secure parliamentary passage of his social insurance programs. The Center Party's motives were a blend of pragmatic politics and theology: a Catholic Center Party pushing a social welfare agenda hoped to head off worker defections to the atheistic Socialist Party. At the same time, Catholic social teaching valued the dignity of each individual. So the Center Party sought to carve out a third way between the miseries of unregulated market capitalism and the statism of communism, both of which it viewed as antithetical to individual well-being.

The design of health insurance financing and administration reflected broader class politics and regime changes in Germany. The local funds, recognized by the government to act as insurers of last resort, became the largest and most influential of the health insurance funds, albeit in ways that Bismarck did not intend. By offering workers two-thirds representation in the administrative boards of the local funds, Bismarck hoped to cement their loyalty to government national health insurance and woo them away from voluntary schemes run by the trade unions. Yet neither Bismarck nor the Catholic Church succeeded in their intentions, as workers remained wedded to their Socialist Party and unions. In fact, administrative jobs in the local funds proved to be important tools of recruitment, professionalization, and patronage for the trade unions and the Socialist Party (later renamed the Social Democrats).[5]

Health care was an arena of conflict among workers, employers, political parties, insurance funds, and physicians from the Imperial era (1871–1918) and continuing under the short-lived democratic Weimar Republic (1919–1933) through the subsequent Nazi regime and into the postwar era. The 1883 health insurance legislation brought previously private mutual societies and union funds under the corporatist umbrella as public-law entities, but did not extend this status to health care providers. Doctors were independent entrepreneurs who fought to preserve fee-for-service reimbursement and patients' free choice of physician. They resisted sickness funds' divide-and-rule strategy of selective contracting and tight fee schedules to control health care expenditures. The trade union-dominated local funds gained further influence when these insurers established their own national-level peak organization. Physicians responded to this threat by forming their own union, the Leipziger Verband in 1900, and engaged in strikes over the ensuing decades. Governments sought to bring a semblance of order and peace to this highly conflictual sector through corporatist arrangements that recognized the legitimacy of organizations representing key health care stakeholders while at the same time setting limits to their power. By the early 1930s, the corporatist institutional framework was in place. Under this, the government gave legal recognition to a limited number of associations to represent doctors and insurers, and set them up to face each other as countervailing power.[6] However, the Nazi regime further centralized the regulatory framework of SHI and destroyed the internal democracy of the sickness funds and provider organizations. The government fired trade union employees from the local funds, purged Jews from physician associations, and replaced these with party members.[7] Shortly after the establishment of the nascent democracy in 1949, the Federal Republic of Germany restored democratic institutions and governance in the health sector that had been in place prior to the Nazi takeover. With the Self-Governance Act of 1951, the members of physician associations and sickness funds could once again elect their officers to their internal governing boards. But to labor's dismay, the law mandated equal contributions *and* representation of employers and employees alike on sickness fund governance bodies. The center-right coalition government at the time held that parity representation would encourage social partnership rather than class conflict among business and labor. It would also circumscribe the trade union movement's control over social policy.[8] In 1955, policymakers designated the associations of sickness funds and ambulatory sector physicians as public-law bodies with authority to administer SHI under government oversight.[9]

Structure of Contemporary Social Health Insurance

At first, German SHI covered only blue-collar workers (and their dependents) since political leaders viewed the productive capacity of this class as vital to Germany's national security. However, governments extended health insurance coverage to other groups of workers in the 1920s, including white-collar employees, so that by 1925, just over half the population was covered. Subsequent extensions to new groups meant that by the 1960s, 83 percent of the population had coverage in the Federal Republic (West Germany); this rose to 88 percent by 1988, the year before German unification. With the 2007 reform law (discussed below), Germany made a commitment to achieve universal coverage by 2009. In 1900, over 23,000 sickness funds existed, but their numbers decreased over time so that by 1960, there were only a little over 2,000 funds. Legislative reforms in the 1990s further accelerated this trend and encouraged mergers among the funds; as of 2010 there were only 165 funds and their number has shrunk further since then.[10]

Today, German SHI continues to retain the institutional arrangements established under Bismarck. Health insurance is largely employment-based with employers required to contribute to the health insurance of their workforce. Since 2007, self-employed individuals and freelancers must carry their own minimum insurance coverage either through SHI or private insurance. As of 2014, approximately 86 percent of the population had health insurance coverage through one of 132 nonprofit government approved SHI funds, 11 percent under private insurers, with the rest, such as the military, police, prisoners, and asylum-seekers, having separate government coverage.[11] The funds originally segmented the population along class, occupation, and status lines. By 2014, there were six types of funds: one single fund for miners and maritime employees (the result of a merger of these two different occupational funds in 2008), one fund for agricultural workers, six guild funds covering the professions, 107 company funds set up by larger firms to insure their own employees and dependents (akin to self-funded employer-based plans in the United States), six substitute funds primarily for white-collar salaried employees, and 11 local funds, which had historically served as insurers of last resort for those unable to obtain coverage from another fund. The local funds are the largest among the national health insurance funds. Until 1996, white-collar employees had free choice of fund but blue-collar workers were assigned to a fund based on their class, region, occupation, or company affiliation. Since then, free choice of insurer has been extended to the rest of the population. Only a few company-based funds continue to restrict membership to their own employees and dependents, as do agricultural funds. Most funds have opened their doors to all.[12]

Contributions to social health insurance are calculated as a percentage of income. This system of financing pools risks among all members of a sickness fund, with each fund levying a contribution rate for its members regardless of gender, age, health status, or family size. This is the essence of social insurance: younger, healthier, and wealthier individuals who are not parents cross-subsidize the more expensive health care costs of those members who are older, sicker, poorer, or have children. Experience-related premiums, which would discriminate against the most vulnerable, are explicitly prohibited in NHI. State unemployment or social assistance offices pay for those outside of the labor force, such as the unemployed, students, and the disabled, while retirees pay their share of health insurance contribution from their pension.[13]

For most of the postwar period, each sickness fund set its own contribution rate to cover the health care costs of its members. In 2009, however, the federal Ministry of Health began setting a single uniform contribution rate for all sickness funds, but distributing risk-adjusted payments among them to account for the health status of each fund's membership. In 2014, the average contribution rate was 14.6 percent of wages, split evenly among employers and workers. The law fixes the employers' share of the contribution at 7.3 percent, but the employees' share can be slightly higher under specific circumstances.[14] These changes are discussed in greater detail in the section "Policy Responses: The 1993, 2004, and 2007 Reform Laws, and Beyond."

A small private insurance sector, which insures 11 percent of the population, exists alongside SHI. All persons whose income falls below the legally set ceiling (4,462.50 euros per month in 2014) must be insured through one of the sickness funds in the social health insurance system, but those whose income exceeds the legally set ceiling for at least three successive calendar years may opt for coverage from one of 42 private insurers. The self-employed must get coverage through a private insurer, unless they had coverage with a sickness fund prior to becoming self-employed. In that case, they may choose SHI coverage instead. Still, as many as 75 percent of those eligible for private insurance choose SHI coverage. Among them are the self employed, persons whose incomes exceed the

SHI threshold for membership, and civil servants. They elect coverage from SHI funds because of the generosity of the benefits and the greater certainty of contribution rates as compared to private insurance.[15] Private insurers charge risk-related premiums for each individual they insure, so that premiums vary by health status. They also offer widely different benefits packages and, until 2004, could deny an applicant coverage based on his or her health status. Like the SHI system, employers contribute to an employee's private insurance premium. Supplemental private insurance policies are also available to cover costs and services not included under SHI or civil servants' schemes.

The pricing and benefit design under private insurance are attractive to those with higher incomes, good health, and no dependents, as they will pay lower premiums than older and sicker individuals and those with dependents. However, once a person opts for private coverage, the law requires that she must stay in that system. This restriction prevents people from gaming the system by selecting cheaper private coverage when they are young, healthy, and single (and thereby removing themselves from the SHI risk pool), and later entering the system when their health care needs become more expensive because of illness or the addition of dependents.

The minimum benefits package under Germany's social health insurance is remarkably generous by international standards. Federal framework legislation as outlined in the Social Code Book (SGB V) covering SHI requires that sickness funds cover all medically necessary benefits. This has been interpreted to include medical care in hospital and ambulatory settings, prescribed drugs, occupational and physical therapies, dental care, as well as homeopathic and alternative medicines and even two-week stays at spa clinics if prescribed by a doctor. The actual catalog of benefits is not spelled out in any law but is instead the product of negotiations between associations representing sickness funds and providers at federal level.[16] Yet there is little variation among benefits packages; 95 percent of the health plans offer identical coverage.

Payroll contributions finance the lion's share of health care expenditures. Yet government plays an important supporting role. State governments finance hospital capital expenditures from taxation, though sickness funds cover hospitals' operating costs for patient care. To relieve the burden on labor costs that payroll-based financing represents, the federal government since 2009 has contributed general and other taxes, such as tobacco taxes, to cover the children's portion of health insurance (see the section "Policy Responses: The 1993, 2004, and 2007 Reform Laws, and Beyond").[17] Private sources constitute 23 percent of total health care expenditures, on a par with the United States. This figure includes insurance premiums as well as out-of-pocket payments for treatments not covered under NHI. Still, cost sharing at the point of service is quite modest compared to the United States. Germans pay minor co-payments for hospital stays and drugs, larger cost sharing for spa treatments and dentures. From 2004 to 2013, patients paid a 10-euro co-payment for the first visit to an office-based physician or to a specialist without referral for each quarter in a calendar year. Vulnerable groups receive financial protection through hardship exemptions; thus, children up to age 18 pay no co-pays, preventive services are exempt from co-payments, and co-payments for individuals with chronic medical conditions or low incomes may not exceed 1 percent or 2 percent of gross annual household income, respectively.[18]

The delivery of health care services reflects a varied structure and relationship involving private and government actors. Ambulatory sector, that is, office-based, physicians are in private practice. Most are primary care doctors, though there are also some specialty physicians in this sector, such as ear, nose, and throat practitioners and gynecologists. Specialist physicians are mostly in hospital-based practice. In Germany, the ratio of primary care to specialty care physicians is roughly equal.[19] The predominant form of practice in West Germany in the ambulatory sector was solo or in small group settings. This was not the case in East Germany, however. Under the communist regime of the German Democratic Republic (GDR) in the East, integrated care through multispecialty practices (polyclinics) tied to hospitals was the norm, and the population received coverage under a tax-financed single-payer health insurance fund. German unification in 1990 brought in its wake the introduction of West German health care institutions of multiple insurers and small-scale medical practices, and many multispecialty clinics disappeared. In the twenty-first century, however, the government reversed course and now encourages multispecialty practices throughout the country that resemble the communist-era polyclinics in the former GDR.[20]

The hospital sector has varied ownership. In 2012, 48 percent of beds were in the public sector, most run by local governments. The nonprofit sector is also substantial, comprising 34 percent of all hospital beds. Many of these facilities are run by religious entities. Private for-profit hospitals made up 18 percent of beds.[21]

Health care providers are remunerated in a variety of ways. Ambulatory care physicians receive a combination of lump-sum payments and fee-for-service reimbursement within a cap. Hospital specialists are in salaried employment, though hospital chief doctors can offer clinic sessions under fee-for-service. Hospitals receive payments under a dual system of financing. State governments finance their capital expenditures through tax revenues while sickness funds cover patient care and hospital operating costs under a diagnosis related group (DRG) system of prospective payment that replaced per-diem payments.[22] The DRG system was phased in gradually and became fully operational only in 2010. At the federal level, the German Hospital Federation and the Federal Association of Social Health Insurance Funds define each DRG for SHI, and private insurers also abide by this system. In each state, the hospital association negotiates the financial value of each DRG with the associations of sickness funds. For prescription drugs, the Federal Association of Social Health Insurance Funds sets a reference price, or maximum amount funds will pay, for drugs with similar ingredients or comparable effect. If a drug costs more than that, patients then pay the difference. Deciding which drugs belong in a particular reference group falls to the Federal Joint Committee, a national-level body that brings together health care stakeholders (see below).[23]

German Social Health Insurance as Conservative Corporatism[24]

A common misconception about national health insurance is that it is simply socialism. Socialized medicine entails a predominant role for the state: the government owns hospitals, doctors are public salaried employees, and health care is financed by general (mainly income) tax revenues. The German social health insurance system, however, is part of an altogether different type of welfare state that originated with conservative political forces and that accords interest groups important roles in policy implementation and administration. As described above, office-based physicians are private providers and hospitals operate under a variety of ownership models. A mix of sources, primarily employers and employee contributions, finance health care. Rather than a single government program, Germans can choose coverage from a multitude of nonprofit sickness funds.

The most distinctive feature that sets Germany apart from socialized medicine is the role of the state and interest groups. In Germany, the state plays a more restricted albeit critical role in statutory national health insurance through *corporatism*.[25] The federal government acts as the guarantor of universal access to affordable, high quality, medically necessary care by enacting general framework legislation at the national level. Such laws and other regulations covering SHI are set out in the Social Law Book V, which dates from 1911. However, the state does not own all health care facilities, employ providers, or issue detailed directives on how they should meet the goals set out in legislation. Rather, the state supervises the major health care interest groups through the Federal Ministry of Health (Bundesministerium für Gesundheit, or BMG) and delegates to them the authority to implement the laws through negotiations among themselves. These associations represent the key actors in the health care system, such as physicians, hospitals, dentists, pharmaceutical manufacturers, and allied health professions. Their organization parallels the federal structure of the German political system. Thus, a single organization represents each interest at the national level and these national associations have a federated membership structure of associations operating in each of the 16 German states. Figure 3.1 illustrates the corporatist relationships in German health care.

In the SHI system, the corporatist associations for physicians and sickness funds operate at both state and federal levels. These are compulsory-membership organizations with substantial self-regulation of individual practitioners' fees and practice patterns. For the doctors, there are 17 Associations of Social Health Insurance (SHI) Physicians (Kassenärtzliche Vereinigung, or KVs), one for each of the 15 states plus two for the densely populated state of North-Rheine Westphalia. The KVs license physicians to practice in national health insurance, conduct formal reviews (medical audit) of individual physician practice patterns, and negotiate fees and other terms of service with associations representing the sickness funds. The Federal Association of Social Health Insurance (SHI) Physicians, or KBV, is the peak association that represents the KVs in politics and in negotiations with its sickness fund counterpart, the Federal Association of Social Health Insurance Funds, at national level. These two national-level bodies work in conjunction with other national level provider associations to determine which services to include in the schedule of covered benefits under the national health insurance system (see the section "Policy Responses: The 1993, 2004, and 2007 Reform Laws, and Beyond").[26] The six types of sickness funds each have their own organization at state level. Before 2008, each type of fund was also represented by its own peak association at national level; since then, a single umbrella association, the Federal Association of Social Health Insurance Funds (Gesetzliche Krankenversicherung Spitzenverband, or GKV-SV), represents them at the federal level.[27] A similar arrangement exists in the hospital sector. The German Hospital Federation (DKG) is the peak association for the 16 state-level hospital associations plus 12 other associations representing university, public, and private for-profit hospitals. Although these hospital organizations are private associations, governments have increasingly granted them legal authority and obligations to administer the hospital sector under SHI.[28]

The institutional embodiment of corporatist representation of interests is the Federal Joint Committee (Gemeinsamer Bundesausschuss, or FJC), which stands at the apex of the SHI system. The FJC has the duty and

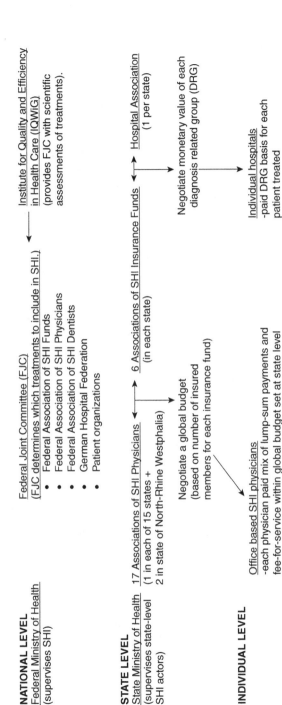

Figure 3.1 Corporatist structure of German social health insurance (SHI).

Source: Adapted from Hoyer, *Social Health Insurance in Germany and the Market Position of the TK* (2009); D. Sauerland, "The legal framework for health care quality assurance in Germany," *Health Economics, Policy and Law* (2009), p. 87; Obermann, Müller, Müller, Schmidt, Glazinski, *Understanding the German Health Care System*, PowerPoint, p. 76; and author's own rendering.

authority to determine which services should be covered under SHI. The committee's members include all of the major health care stakeholders, including the KBV, the peak association of sickness funds, and the national association of hospitals, dentists, pharmaceutical companies, and allied health professionals. The committee also receives input from accredited associations representing patients.[29]

Government supervision of these otherwise autonomous and powerful associations lies at the heart of corporatism, and ensures that private interests conform to the public good. Without government supervision, these associations would simply exploit their position to pursue their own interests. Under corporatism, associations of providers and insurers are neither wholly public nor private entities but are, in fact, both. Their official designation is "corporatist associations with public obligations," or public-law bodies, which imposes a dual mandate as private associations representing their members' interests while also reconciling these to the common good. The state grants these associations significant powers and legal monopoly to represent their members in politics and to provide health services or insurance under the SHI system. The state accords them considerable autonomy, or self-administration (Selbstverwaltung), in running that system and in regulating the behavior of their individual members to ensure that they conform to SHI laws and regulations. But in exchange for this privileged status and self-governance, these associations must implement the health care laws as part of their duty to fulfil the public good, as defined by the state. If they fail to do so, then the health ministry has the authority to intervene in SHI administration by decree. Normally, the mere threat of government intervention has been sufficient to convince insurers and doctors to come to an agreement on how to implement the law.[30]

In sum, corporatism is a regulatory approach that grants the state powerful leverage over the behavior of health care actors without resorting to detailed intervention into the day-to-day administration of the health care system. By relying on a few large associations with compulsory membership, the corporatist structure has worked to channel conflicts in more predictable ways than before. It is easier for state actors to interact with a few peak associations than with multiple, competing groups. Governments have relied on corporatist regulation for nearly a century, and have even extended its scope throughout the health care system. It is the dominant approach to health care regulation in Germany. However, policymakers have increasingly resorted to new instruments, such as competition and direct state intervention in health care administration in specific areas, to correct what they viewed as deficiencies of corporatism.[31]

Political Underpinnings of the German Health System: Institutions of Government, the Role of Civil Society, and the Social Market Economy

Government Institutions

The development of German SHI mirrored a broader history of contestation over the role of the state and society in social provision. But as described above, after World War II, these questions were settled in favor of a polity that dispersed state power, provided strong societal representation through corporatist interest associations, and institutionalized the values of the social market economy in a comprehensive welfare state. Given these varied influences, health policy is seldom if ever the vision of a single party; rather, compromise among various parties and stakeholders is the norm.

The Federal Republic of Germany represented a conscious break from the excessive concentration of state power that had marked the Nazi dictatorship. At the same time, the specter of the German Democratic Republic to the East served as a constant negative reference of state centralization under communism. The political system that West Germans created in 1949 was a parliamentary democracy, with a prime minister (chancellor) drawn from the legislature following parliamentary elections. But this polity incorporates important checks and balances on executive power that stand in sharp contrast to, say, Britain's centralized executive.

One such check is the Federal Republic's requirement of coalition governments. Like other parliamentary democracies, the executive branch is formed following elections to the lower house of parliament, or Federal Diet (Bundestag). But owing to its mixed electoral system, in which a party's overall number of seats in the Bundestag reflects the percentage of the popular vote it receives, Germany has a multiparty system.[32] Because of the existence of several parties in the Bundestag, it is extremely rare for a single party to win an absolute majority of seats and then form the government (i.e., appoint a cabinet) alone. Instead, the largest party must enter into a coalition government with another party. This places real checks on the chancellor's power. Rather than ruling alone with a compliant party in parliament, the chancellor instead must negotiate and compromise with her coalition partners in the executive branch and in the Bundestag to ensure passage of legislation.

German federalism places additional constraints on national executive power. The Federal Republic requires power sharing by national and state governments. The 16 states (or Länder) directly appoint members of the upper house of the parliament, or Federal Council (Bundesrat), and thus have a direct voice in writing legislation at the national level. Bundesrat delegations reflect the partisan composition of their state governments and must vote according to the latter's instructions. Because state elections follow their own calendar and do not coincide with national parliamentary elections, divided government, in which the chancellor and his coalition partners possess a majority of seats in the lower house but face an upper house controlled by the opposition parties, is not only a distinct possibility, but often the reality. Furthermore, the constitution requires that legislation that directly affects the interests of the states receive Bundesrat approval or else it cannot pass. Though not all health care legislation falls under this domain, much of it does, especially in matters relating to hospital policy. On such legislation, negotiation and compromise between the different houses of the parliament, and between it and the executive branch is imperative if the bill is to avoid a Bundesrat veto.

A powerful and independent judicial branch acts as a third important check on executive power. Unlike the Nazi regime, which disregarded the constitution and colonized the judiciary with Nazi Party loyalists, the Federal Republic created a state based on the *Rechtsstaat* (rule of law). This means that the constitution is taken very seriously. Judges, moreover, are to be independent of politics and are appointed for their expertise rather than their party views. Significantly, the Federal Constitutional Court, the highest court of the land, possesses the power of judicial review, which gives it the authority to strike down laws passed by the parliament and executive if it violates the German constitution.

The Role of Civil Society: Interest Groups and Political Parties

In the postwar Federal Republic, peak associations representing the major classes and sectors of civil society are key actors in the formulation and implementation of policy. When crafting legislation or regulations for the health care system, government politicians and civil servants must consult relevant interest associations for their opinion. Known as the remiss procedure, such consultation is required by law at the stage of policy formulation. In other words, this guarantees that health care interest groups have a "seat at the table," so to speak, and may influence the content of policy at the formulation stage. But this does not necessarily translate into a policy veto by these interests: while they must be consulted, the government is not legally required to adopt their recommendations. In rare cases, governments may go against these constituencies if they believe conditions require that a major reform must be enacted. Corporatist associations also influence policies at the stage of implementation at both state and federal levels. As discussed above, the health sector provides an example. The state delegates the responsibility to run the health care system to provider and sickness fund associations on its behalf. Sometimes interest groups will use this power to delay or block implementation of legislation that their members oppose. If that happens, the health ministry may invoke its powers to intervene and issue directives by decree, on the grounds that the health care interests have abandoned their broader public obligation to fulfill the law.[33]

Interest groups also try to influence health policy deliberations by more customary methods, through their links to the political parties and their lobbying activities. The political parties, in line with their class and ideological orientations, are traditionally closer to some healthcare stakeholders than others. The two largest parties in the Federal Republic are the Christian Democratic Union (CDU) and its Bavarian counterpart, the Christian Social Union (CSU), and the Social Democratic Party (SPD). The CDU/CSU, a classic "catchall party" that bridges religious and class divisions, must heed both its business and Catholic trade union wings. The union wing is a staunch defender of social policy. Under CDU-led coalition governments, a politician from the party's trade union wing has generally headed the health ministry, which gives the local funds and workers a greater voice in health care policies. The CDU has dominated the politics of the Federal Republic, serving in government far longer than the SPD. The SPD, garners strong electoral support from manual workers, trade union members and salaried white collar. The SPD is close to the local funds that insure manual workers. The Free Democratic Party (FDP), which advocates economic and political liberalism (i.e., small government, free markets, and political liberty) is a smaller party that draws electoral support primarily from the self-employed and the professions and has close ties to the associations representing pharmaceutical companies and physicians. It has served as the junior partner in coalition governments with both the CDU and the SPD. As the kingmaker in coalition governments, the FDP has been able to extract concessions from its larger coalition partners that advance the interests of its health care provider constituents. The Green Party is also a smaller party. Its advocacy of environmentalism, women's rights, direct democracy, and social justice have appealed most to university-educated urban professionals often in the public sector, such as educators. The party promotes equitable financing of health care. The Greens have served in coalition at national level with the SPD and in state-level coalitions with a range of parties.

Depending on the party composition of the government, different interest groups can exert more or less leverage on health policy. When

Center-Right governments composed of the CDU and FDP have been in power, policymakers have tended to be more attuned to the preferences of the business community and health care providers. Yet the CDU has also had to walk a delicate balancing act to reconcile these interests with its trade union wing. Conversely, when Center-Left governments (the SPD and Greens) have been at the helm, the concerns of patients and unions have had more influence than those of providers. Finally, in cases of "grand coalitions," either formal coalition governments or involving informal cross-party cooperation between the CDU and SPD, health politics have been marked by sweeping deals that seek to balance concerns for economic competitiveness and health care efficiency with equitable sharing of burdens of any painful health care reform. This usually means that the interests of employers and unions have taken precedence over those of providers. Such grand coalitions have delivered the most radical changes in the health sector, as in 1993 and 2007. This may seem a paradox, given the catch-all nature of these two parties. But the outcomes make sense if we remember that these two parties are not beholden to health care providers as the FDP is, and that as catch-all parties they have more in common with each other than one might expect. Moreover, the simple math shows that such grand coalitions have huge share of the seats in the Bundestag. Along with the requirements of party discipline in a parliamentary system, passage of controversial reform legislation is far more likely, so long as a deal has been worked out among the two parties at the formulation stage. As discussed below, the CDU and SPD share a consensus on the core values underpinning the health care system and the broader welfare state and economy in which it is nested.

The Role of Ideas: The Social Market Economy

Since World War II Germany has committed itself to building a *social market economy (SME),* and to a distinct set of core values regarding the appropriate role of the state, interests, and market forces in the economy and in social provision. The SME acknowledges that the market economy is the best way to allocate resources to their productive uses and to generate wealth. But it stops short of leaving the distribution of wealth or the meeting of social needs to market forces. The social market economy in practice justifies a generous welfare state to help those who might lose out in a market system or who perform socially valuable work such as caring for family members. Hence, the postwar German welfare state provides comprehensive state pensions to all workers and their dependents, universal child allowances (cash payments to families with children), paid parental leave, SHI, unemployment and workplace accident insurance, and social assistance. It also requires state steering, or guidance, of market forces to ensure that capitalism does not undermine the social goal of solidarity. But this is more a matter of setting the framework for competition rather than direct command and control or state ownership of the economy.[34]

The social market economy is the postwar political bargain between the Left and the Right that sought to overcome the country's traumatic history. Both the CDU and SPD in the new democracy wanted to avoid repeating the disasters of unrestricted capitalism of the 1920s and 1930s, which they saw as responsible for the mass unemployment of the Great Depression and the brutal Nazi dictatorship that followed. These same politicians also had no stomach for communism's crushing of individual human freedom. The mainstream parties of both the Left and the Right therefore embraced the social market economy as a "third way" between unbridled capitalism and communist authoritarianism, both of which threatened to destroy human dignity and freedom.[35]

The social market economy also drew from the wellspring of social Catholicism as articulated in papal encyclicals and promoted by the Catholic Center Party in the late nineteenth and early twentieth centuries, and later adopted by the postwar CDU. This strand of Catholicism arose in reaction to the destructiveness of free-market capitalism and the misery and inequality that had accompanied the Industrial Revolution. Social Catholicism championed the cause of workers organizing into unions and ameliorative social policies to preserve the dignity of all human beings. While asserting the dignity of the individual, social Catholicism also viewed all persons as members of a broader human community rooted in solidarity. This view of human society also celebrated the idea of subsidiarity, which saw social protection as a hierarchy based first in the family, then the local organization (the union or church), and finally the state as the provider of last resort and as supporting these civil society groups in their tasks.[36]

The health care system expresses the ideas of the social market economy in its administrative and financial arrangements. Consistent with subsidiarity, the state plays an arms-length role in setting out the rules of the health care system and then delegating responsibility to employers, unions, and sickness funds and KVs to finance and administer the health care system. In a similar vein, multiple insurers based in employment, and private health care providers (such as nonprofit religious institutions that own and maintain hospitals and nursing homes) act as an alternative to a single state-run national health service financed by taxes. As noted, health insurance contributions based on income pool risks and rely on the stronger to cross-subsidize the weaker members of society, thus embodying the idea of solidarity.

Both the Right and the Left accept the basic contours of the social market economy; their differences have been more a matter of degree rather than of kind. For the CDU, the social market economy embodies cherished conservative principles of family, order, and paternalism. The SPD came to terms with the social market economy only in 1959, when it abandoned its commitment to nationalization of industry and accepted the welfare state nested within capitalism. Although the SPD has favored greater state intervention in job creation and employment, it accepted the SME for its restraint of capitalism within a net of workers' rights and broad social protections.

In sum, all of these political factors are in play in health sector policies and institutional arrangements, creating a politics marked by compromise and negotiation. The dispersal of power in the German political system encourages a particular pattern of policymaking that often entails drawn-out negotiations and compromise among governing parties, the states, and interest groups. Coalition governments limit the freedom of action of a single party and instead necessitate cross-party deals. The remiss system ensures that interest groups will have a voice and an opportunity to influence the content of policy, though it stops short of guaranteeing them a veto. Federalism gives a voice to the states in determining national policies that affect their interests. Corporatist administration of the social health insurance system accords associations of providers and insurers a very strong position to influence the implementation of health policy. Finally, the core values underpinning the broader social market economy find expression in the institutional arrangements of German social health insurance. The notion of solidarity supports universal access to care based on need and income-based insurance contributions in which the healthier and wealthier cross-subsidize coverage for the sicker and poorer. Subsidiarity legitimizes the delegation of government authority to associations of doctors and insurers to implement policy health sector on its behalf and also legitimizes the principle of self-governance, which grants them considerable freedom of action in health care administration.

Health Care System Performance and Challenges

Germany's SHI has performed well when set against general health care system goals and the performance of other industrialized nations. Health care expenditures in Germany in 2009 were 11.6 percent of GDP and $4,213 per capita. This puts Germany in the upper ranks of OECD countries, but well below the United States, which devoted 17.4 percent of GDP and $7,960 per capita to health care. (The OECD averages are 9.6 percent of GDP and $3,233 per capita.) And even though Germany spends far less than the United States, it covers nearly all of its population through statutory or private insurance. Health outcomes are also good, as measured in terms of life expectancy and infant mortality. But like other industrialized countries, Germans suffer from chronic conditions, such as cardiovascular disease, diabetes, and lung cancer due to smoking. Still, given the Germans' penchant for consumption of beer and chocolate, their health outcomes are respectable.[37] The system has also been relatively responsive to consumers who have long enjoyed free choice of office-based physicians and a statutory minimum benefits package that would be the envy of most Americans. Indeed, critics of the German health care system argue that it gives the population too much choice and is too generous, leading to overuse of medical services.

External Economic and Demographic Pressures

But there are problems. The biggest challenge is assuring the long-term financial viability of the health care system in the face of demographic pressures. In 1995, 4.4 workers supported 1 retiree, but by 2020 this is projected to be 2.1 workers to 1 retiree.[38] An aging population living longer with chronic medical conditions will need expensive care. But Germany's stagnant birth rate means that there may not be enough working age persons to cover the health care needs of their elders.

A second source of trouble is Germany's reliance on payroll taxes to finance health insurance. This form of financing has been one of the hallmarks of the conservative corporatist welfare state but it will be an insufficient funding base for rising health care needs.[39] This problem first revealed itself in the slower economic growth following the 1970s oil shocks. Though high oil prices were the immediate cause of recession, longer term processes were also at work. The gradual shift out of manufacturing toward a postindustrial service sector economy starting in the mid-1980s led to wage growth rising more slowly than GDP and the appearance of structural unemployment. Taken together, fewer workers were paying into the social insurance system from a smaller pool of wage income. Job protection rules that made it difficult and expensive for employers to lay off workers, and generous unemployment insurance and early retirement arrangements financed from payroll taxes, created a vicious feedback loop that drove up nonwage labor costs, threatened German competitiveness in the global economy, and exacerbated. Long-term unemployment and low labor force participation rates were especially notable among women, the unskilled, immigrants, and older persons.[40] In short, Germany was creating too few jobs and too many dependents on social insurance in an unsustainable pattern.

German unification in 1990 aggravated and made painfully apparent the limitations of payroll-based financing of social insurance. Political unification was followed by deindustrialization and a massive economic collapse of the Eastern economy starting in the mid-1990s. By 2000, unemployment had hit a postwar record of 5 million. Jobless rates in the Eastern states, at 20 percent of the workforce, were twice that of the West. Mass unemployment strained the budgets of local governments, which had to cover social insurance and assistance for the jobless. eastern workers also paid higher social insurance contributions than their Western counterparts. Indeed, to cushion the blow of economic dislocation in the east, the government relied heavily on social insurance to finance early retirement pensions, unemployment insurance, and health insurance of the unemployed. As a result, social insurance contributions of all employers and workers jumped from 35.6 percent of gross wages in 1990 to 41 percent by 1996. Over the same period, the average contribution rate for health insurance rose from 12.6 percent to 13.6 percent. Financing German unification through social insurance worsened the destructive feedback loop between labor costs, competitiveness, and unemployment.[41]

Subsequent public policies and wage restraint by unions helped reverse this trend, but did not fully resolve the health care financing question. The Social Democrat–Green coalition government headed by Chancellor Gerhard Schröder pushed through unpopular welfare state and labor market reforms in 2003. These so-called Hartz reforms made unemployment benefits less generous and required the unemployed to be actively seeking work in order to claim benefits. The reforms also introduced new forms of contingent work: "mini-jobs" permit employers to hire workers on a part-time basis and at lower wages than those negotiated by unions, and to terminate contracts without cause in the first two years of an employment contract. The government also picked up the social insurance contributions of employers in these types of jobs. These reforms, along with buoyant demand for German industrial exports among newly industrializing countries, led to a rebound in employment. Yet wages and salaries have lagged behind profits and the reforms created a new segment of labor force more commonly seen in the United States and Britain: the working poor whose wages are so low that they must continue to rely on forms of government social assistance to survive.[42] German exports regained their price competitive and employment recovered with the Hartz reforms, but stagnant wages meant that payroll taxes alone were still insufficient as the sole source of health care financing.

The shift out of manufacturing to a postindustrial economy based on services has also precipitated changes in the occupational structure, making health insurance less secure for some workers. Most Germans have long had a regular employment relationship and have thus had access to statutory NHI through their workplace. But this was not the case for those in the new forms of flexible and contingent employment in the postindustrial economy, such as part-timers, temporary workers, and free-lancers, many of whom were young and lacked stable ties to an employer and the health insurance that came with it. Some of them could obtain coverage through the private insurance market or SHI. But many to bear the full cost of the premium; if they could not afford it, they simply went without coverage. Though their numbers were small, at 0.2 percent of the population or 200,000 persons in 2007, their share was growing and was a concern to policymakers.[43]

Structural Weaknesses of the Health Care System[44]

At the same time, the structures of the health care delivery system had long been a source of inefficiency. The strict separation of ambulatory and hospital sectors fostered duplication and poor coordination of care. Likewise, the dominance of solo or small group practice among ambulatory physicians, long championed by the KVs, militated against coordinated care. Patients enjoyed free choice of doctor, but such consumer responsiveness allowed for self-referrals to specialists that may not have been warranted. Hospital financing did not help. The health insurance funds paid for inpatient care on a per-diem rate, which encouraged excessively long lengths of stay, while the state governments financed capital projects separately. Such bifurcation of hospital financing militated against coordinated planning of care in that sector. In addition, at the behest of the KVs who sought to protect physicians' monopoly on ambulatory care, hospitals were legally prohibited from offering less expensive alternatives to inpatient stays like outpatient day surgery. Prescription drug prices were higher in Germany than in other countries, though not as high as in the United States. The generosity of SHI meant that many treatments were covered even though they lacked scientific evidence of their clinical effectiveness.

Nor did the corporatist framework always ensure a balance between health insurers and providers as intended. The idea behind corporatism was to organize the unruly ambulatory care physicians and insurers into large associations that would counteract and balance one another at state and national levels.[45] In practice, the KVs often had the upper hand in the relationship. One manifestation of this imbalance was the fact that health insurance funds lacked specific information on patient care that they ultimately paid for. The information asymmetry lay in the peculiar arrangement for reimbursing ambulatory physicians. The schedule of benefits covered under SHI as well as a point values for each procedure, is determined by the national associations of the SHI doctors and funds. At the state level, each KV negotiates a budget to pay physicians for ambulatory care with the peak associations of health insurance. But doctors bill their state-level KV, not the sickness funds, for care they provide to patients. This means that the funds do not know which services they are paying for. The KVs also exploited their stronger bargaining position relative to the insurance funds. Until 1977, doctor's associations concluded separate contracts with each type of fund, which led to outbidding among the funds and higher fees for doctors. A further problem lay in the open-ended nature of fee-for-service reimbursement of KV doctors. If doctors did more procedures, the insurance funds and the KVs would simply negotiate a more generous budget for the following year. Required by law to cover their costs, the insurance funds would simply raise insurance contribution levels on employers and employees to accommodate this generosity. Taken together, these arrangements for physician reimbursement spurred cost inflation in the ambulatory sector in the 1960s and 1970s.

In response, governments introduced a series of measures to constrain health care costs and redress the imbalances in the corporatist framework. The Health Care Cost Containment Act of 1977, enacted by the coalition government of the SPD and FDP, established a national roundtable, the Concerted Action in Health Care, to make recommendations on health care spending based on broader economic indicators. The body's membership included peak associations of providers, insurers, employers, trade unions, and government officials at all levels. State-level associations of insurers and providers were supposed to follow the roundtable's recommendations when negotiating reimbursement agreements. In 1985, the CDU-FDP government led by Chancellor Helmut Kohl (1982–1998) added a Council of Experts composed of doctors, social policy experts, and health economists to advise the broader Concerted Action. Policymakers presumed that the provider associations and insurers would voluntarily abide by such recommendations and control their members' incomes to prevent more intrusive government intervention in their domain of health care administration. This was, after all, how corporatism was supposed to work. But the roundtable's recommendations were not binding on health care stakeholders, and the law even permitted KVs and insurers to reject the Concerted Action's advice and conclude their own agreements. The weakness of the Concerted Action to enforce its decisions rendered it an ineffective instrument to enforce cost discipline on health care actors.

Governments had more success in addressing the inflationary effects of fee-for-service reimbursement of ambulatory care. The 1977 law introduced an *all-payer system* of collective bargaining, which brought coordination to the sickness funds and strengthened their bargaining position relative to the KVs. Since then, the KVs no longer conclude separate contracts with individual sickness fund associations. Instead, the peak associations representing each type of fund negotiate a single budget for physician reimbursement with the KV in each state. Another important change to physician reimbursement came in 1987 with the introduction of prospective budgeting and its linkage to broader economic indicators. This required the KVs and insurance fund associations to calculate ambulatory care budgets based on the number of members in each insurance fund, the amount of health spending in the previous year, and the development of wages and salaries in the wider economy. Prospective budgeting meant that the monetary value for each physician service would no longer be fixed but would now float in order to keep the KV budget solvent for the entire year. Thus, if the budget ran low in the last quarter, physicians would receive correspondingly less for the same type of service that they had provided earlier in the year. Prospective budgeting succeeded in slowing the rate of growth in ambulatory care expenses in the 1980s, but the scheme had its disadvantages. Doctors complained that capped fee-for-service led to uncertain incomes in the latter part of the year. They also argued that the reliance on economic indicators did not take into account the degree of illness in the patients they treated. Hence, policymakers introduced a new formula in 2007 that accounts for patient morbidity in physician practices (see see the section "Policy Responses: The 1993, 2004, and 2007 Reform Laws, and Beyond.").

The corporatist framework in ambulatory care meant that individual physicians could not charge what they wished for their services but had to be reimbursed by their KV out of the budget that the association negotiated with insurers. Some doctors still attempted to circumvent the state-level budgets by increasing the volume or complexity of services. In response, the KVs developed a peer review system that dates from the 1930s. A peer review board or committee monitored physician practices and reviewed those practitioners whose treatment decisions were above the norm. Physicians did not face any sanctions if they could justify their behavior to the review board. But if they could not, the board could take action ranging from education or a warning to reduced reimbursement the following quarter. Still, the peer review system was not as effective in controlling individual physician behavior as one might have expected. This was because peer review committees were composed entirely of physicians who were reluctant to pass judgment or punish their own colleagues. This review system also left insurers in the dark on doctors' treatment decisions (since the KVs did not share the results of such reviews with them) and with no voice in the process. The 1977 reform law addressed this imbalance by mandating that health insurers comprise half of the membership of the review committees, but the advantage still lay with physicians because the chair of the review board was always to be a physician, who would cast the decisive vote in the case of a deadlock. A more serious issue was the lack of good data on which to base reviews. The review boards relied on the average treatment and prescribing patterns of each subspecialty, rather than on clinical guidelines based on scientific evidence of treatment effectiveness, as the measure to determine whether an individual doctor was providing medically necessary or quality care.[46]

The legislative actions of the 1970s and 1980s also failed to deal with the escalating expenditures on hospital care and prescription drugs. Both areas continued to outstrip the growth of ambulatory care spending; indeed, pharmaceutical spending in the latter half of the 1980s rose at twice the rate of ambulatory care.[47] High hospital spending lay partly with the per-diem payment of hospitals that encouraged long inpatient stays. Other causes were the more intensive and expensive health needs of an aging population and breakthroughs in medical technology and drug therapies. But a major reason for the cost explosion in these two sectors lay in the incomplete reach of corporatism. Unlike the KVs, hospital and pharmaceutical associations were voluntary membership bodies with few powers over their members, and insurers concluded reimbursement agreements with each hospital rather than with a state-level hospital association. Such realities denied the federal government the ability to enforce a coordinated cost containment strategy spanning the entire health care system.

The organization of the SHI system was not only inefficient, it was also an affront to equity. Due to historical legacies in the evolution of SHI, white-collar salaried employees enjoyed free choice of health fund, but blue-collar workers did not; the latter were assigned to an occupational, company, or local fund and could not change insurers. For manual workers and their trade union representatives, this situation was clearly a violation of the idea of equity. At the same time, the captive membership of health insurance funds fostered serious disparities in contribution rates. As noted, contribution rates are calculated as a percentage of income and had to cover the health care expenses of all members of a health insurance fund. This was a boon for substitute funds, whose members tended to have higher incomes and better health. Their contribution rates thus took a smaller share of their income than their blue-collar compatriots in the other types of funds. The local funds, in particular, were insurers of last resort whose membership was disproportionately composed of manual workers, those with lower incomes, and those with poorer health. With the onset of deindustrialization, the local funds had to levy higher contributions on a shrinking base of employed workers to cover the health care needs of their jobless members. Though the average contribution rate among all types of sickness fund was 12.5 percent in 1990, the particular rate ranged from 11 percent for some substitute funds to more than 15 percent for some local funds.[48] This structure was not only grossly unfair, but it also locked in inefficiency. With a captive membership, none of the health insurance funds had any incentive to offer lower premiums, develop better customer service, or offer innovative forms of care to their subscribers.

Policy Responses: The 1993, 2004, and 2007 Reform Laws, and Beyond

Both sets of problems—those inherent to the particular arrangements in SHI as well as external demographic, economic, and labor market trends—converged to push policymakers on a path toward major reform of health care beginning in the 1990s. But there has not been a single law ushering in a radical health care overhaul; in fact, the German pattern of health care reform has spanned nearly three decades and several laws, with adjustment through legislation enacted every few years. Through these successive reform laws, policymakers have sought to ensure that the health care system is affordable for the long haul but without sacrificing quality and solidarity. They have pursued these goals through a multipronged strategy that promotes competition and choice in the pursuit of efficiency and equity; enhances the corporatist regulatory framework to extend its ability for more coordinated decision making; and requires treatment and coverage decisions be subject to rigorous scientific evidence of clinical and cost effectiveness. In some instances, this has required short-term and even more enduring state intervention in health care administration.

The reform path has been marked by periods of ongoing adjustment interrupted by rare instances of radical change and high drama. Some of the more controversial reform ideas took a decade or more of debate before becoming law. In some cases, policymakers modified radical reform proposals into compromise solutions in order to garner the requisite political support. Policy outcomes reflected the forces of coalition politics, federalism, and corporatism, which required negotiated solutions among parties, state governments, and representatives of health care interests. Yet some reform laws also took direct aim at the rigidities and weaknesses of corporatist administration in the health sector. In those instances, particularly in 1993 and 2007, party politics trumped interest group politics, with the governing parties bypassing recalcitrant interest groups (and even their own coalition partner) in drafting reform legislation.

Within this pattern of ongoing reform, three laws stand out from the rest for their scope of innovation in the health sector and their focus on the core aims of the reform strategy outlined above. They are the 1993 Health Care Restructuring Act of 1993, the Social Health Insurance Modernization Act of 2004, and the Social Health Insurance Competition Strengthening Act of 2007. In addition, the laws illustrate the range of politics at work in German health care: the politics of inclusion and compromise for less controversial measures (in 2004), the victory of political parties over interest groups (1993), and the intricacies of coalition politics, federalism, and the interests of key health care stakeholders (2007).

The 1993 Health Care Restructuring Act[49]

The 1993 Health Care Restructuring Act enacted by the CDU–FDP government of Chancellor Helmut Kohl was primarily an attempt to rein in skyrocketing health care costs and payroll contributions in the face of mass unemployment. But it was also a response to the weaknesses and rigidities of the corporatist arrangements in the social health insurance system itself. In addressing the cost explosion, the law authorized the health ministry to impose emergency budgets on providers by decree to cover ambulatory physicians, hospitals, dentists, pharmaceuticals, and allied health professions. The caps were tied to the revenues of the health funds. Yet policymakers resorted to such heavy-handed action only after corporatist self-governance of the health sector had failed. Four years earlier, the Health Care Reform Act had mandated sickness funds and hospital associations to develop a new reimbursement system based on lump-sum payments (DRGs) to replace per-diem payments for inpatient care. The DRGs would be a fixed payment that reflected the average cost of care for a specific diagnosis or episode of care. The 1989 law had also directed insurance funds and KVs to negotiate clinical guidelines for prescribing drugs and treatments and for use by the boards that reviewed the treatment decisions of individual doctors. But the provider associations and insurers had proven unable or unwilling to come to agreement on these provisions through their collective bargaining. Hence, the 1993 law authorized the federal health ministry to introduce sectoral budgets and begin to develop DRGs by decree, but only for three years. After that period, the government hoped that insurance funds and providers would find the resolve to negotiate responsible budgets and develop clinical guidelines through their own negotiations.

Beyond simply prodding the corporatist associations to do their job, the Kohl government intended to modernize the century-old SHI system by introducing two new policy instruments: competition and evidence-based medicine. Policymakers preferred corporatism's arm's-length supervision of SHI to micromanagement by state decrees. But they also hoped that elements of market competition would shape the behavior of insurers and providers in a more efficient and responsive direction. And, by requiring providers and insurers to develop treatment guidelines based on scientific evidence, the government hoped to curb wasteful SHI spending on treatments that yielded little or no therapeutic benefit.

Managed competition ushered in free choice of insurer for all Germans. Policymakers hoped that freedom of choice would encourage sickness funds to woo members primarily by offering efficient, high-quality health care, consumer responsiveness, and to a lesser extent, lower contribution rates. Free choice of fund on an annual basis began in 1997.[50] Prior to requiring funds to open their doors, however, policymakers introduced a risk-adjustment scheme in 1994. The scheme profiled the health risks of all fund members based on age, sex, disability, and employment status, and required funds with healthier and wealthier members to make financial transfers to those with sicker and poorer members. The reasons for this risk-adjustment scheme were twofold. First, risk-adjusted payments would counteract attempts by sickness funds to compete by accepting only healthier, more profitable enrollees. Second, the scheme would shore up the position of the local funds and level the competitive playing field among different types of funds. Without the prior equalization of risks, the local funds, whose rates had historically been higher than other types of funds, would have faced a mass exodus of members to funds with lower rates. Managed competition came with several other constraints. One was that health insurers open their doors to new members to accept all applicants, regardless of their class, occupation, or health status. Another was the requirement that all social health insurance funds had to offer a comprehensive minimum benefits package so that they would not be tempted to attract only good risks with minimal catastrophic plans. For the same reason, experience-rated premiums remained illegal under national health insurance, and contributions continued to be based on income. In sum, the government set strict rules on the parameters of competition so that it would not destroy the solidarity of SHI.

Finally, the 1993 law contained minor co-payments for prescription drugs, hospital stays, and some therapies that had been introduced four years earlier. The government maintained that co-payments would discourage patients from seeking unnecessary health care. Still, the co-payments were minor, amounting to roughly $5–$10 per prescription drug and $10 per day for the first 14 days of hospitalization. Children, the unemployed, and students were exempted from such co-payments, while adults with chronic conditions or fixed incomes would not pay co-payments beyond 1 to 2 percent of their income respectively.[51]

The enactment of the Health Care Restructuring Act represented a sharp departure from the normal politics of inclusion. Chancellor Kohl and his health minister, Horst Seehofer, took the unusual step of bypass-ing the Free Democrats in the coalition government to cut a deal with the opposition Social Democrats on the basic outline of reform in closed-door negotiations. The CDU then presented the deal to the FDP as a *fait accompli*. Provider groups got their chance to weigh in during subsequent formal consultation, but their opinions mattered little since the CDU and SPD had already concluded a deal.

Political realities shaped the chancellor's strategy. First, the SPD held a majority in the upper house of the legislature, and Kohl needed the Bundesrat's assent for the reform to become law. Second, the Free Democrats were close allies of the medical profession and pharmaceutical industry, both of whom had proven very protective of their incomes thus sabotaged much of the 1989 law. The KVs, moreover, had proven them-selves obstinate in implementing clinical guidelines and other cooperative tasks that the 1989 law had mandated. Kohl and his health minister had to bypass these actors if they were to enact meaningful reform. In essence, the CDU worked with the SPD in an informal grand coalition to get the law passed. In doing so, both parties made compromises. For instance, the SPD and their local fund and trade union allies lauded the health ministry-imposed budgets on health care providers as a way to stabilize insurance contribution rates, but were not enthusiastic about co-payments. What made it palatable for the SPD and their allies was the exemptions from co-payments for those most vulnerable, which satisfied their sense of equity as did the granting of free choice of fund to manual workers.[52]

The 1993 Health Care Restructuring Act represented a first step to use competitive mechanisms and considerations of both clinical and cost effectiveness to slow health care spending. But it did little to address the uncoordinated features of health care provision. Moreover, Germany's continued reliance on payroll taxes had not solved the problem of long-term financing of national health insurance, even with the turnaround in employment in the new millennium. More Germans were now find-ing work, partly due to the global economic boom, partly due to the job search and work requirements of the government's labor market reform policies. But the mini-jobs permitted under the Hartz reforms made access to health insurance more precarious for some workers than in the past. Such jobs were part-time, temporary, or involved freelance work that did not always come with the health or other social insurance guarantees of stable full-time employment.

Successive governments addressed these problems with a number of laws, the most significant of which were enacted in 2004 and 2007. The policy aims of such legislation were to guarantee the long-term finan-cial viability and accessibility of national health insurance and to encour-age more coordinated care that would be both of high quality and cost effective. While working within the existing corporatist framework, policymakers also made some significant structural changes to it by extending competition and choice. They also ventured beyond the social health insurance system the territory of for-profit private insurance in 2007.

The 2004 Social Health Insurance Modernization Act

Corporatist Coordination at Federal Level[53]

The Social Democrat–Green coalition government led by Chancellor Gerhard Schröder (1998–2005) initially focused its energy on the delivery rather than the financing of health care. The 2004 law upgraded and reinforced the corporatist scaffolding at federal level to foster more coordinated decision-making. Hence, the law replaced the Concerted Action in Health Care and the separate federal-level committees for different areas of the health care system with the Federal Joint Committee (FJC). Like its predecessor, the Concerted Action, the FJC brings together the major health care stakeholders. But the FJC's membership is broader, extending beyond insurers, providers, and government to include accredited associations representing patients, especially those with chronic illnesses. Policymakers streamlined the decision structures of the FJC in 2008. Since then, the responsibility for making all coverage decisions for SHI related to ambulatory, hospital, and dental care rests with a single body within the FJC, the Plenary Group. The Plenary Group's membership brings together representatives designated by the federal-level associations: five representatives of the health insurance funds, two representatives of the KV doctors, two hospital representatives, one dentist, and five non-voting representatives of federally accredited patient organizations. Three full-time neutral members also sit on the Plenary Group. Since 2012, only relevant provider representatives can vote on decisions affecting their particular sector.[54]

The FJC carries out quality assurance for the entire SHI system and, more significantly, makes decisions on which treatments should be covered under social health insurance. Its directives must ensure that treatments are "adequate, appropriate, and efficient."[55] And unlike its Concerted Action predecessor, the FJC's coverage decisions and directives are legally binding on all actors in social health insurance. To fulfill these important tasks, the FJC is assisted by the newly created Institute for Quality and Efficiency in Health Care (IQWiG). This institute reviews the state of scientific knowledge on diagnoses and treatments of selected diseases, evaluates new drugs, reviews clinical guidelines, and provides reports to the FJC and information to the public on health care quality. The institute must consult outside experts when carrying out its tasks. Significantly, IQWiG's remit does not extend to evaluations of the cost effectiveness of treatments. Nor can it make binding recommendations on which treatments should be included in SHI coverage; that responsibility rests with the FJC. Still, it supplies the FJC with information on the clinical effectiveness of treatments and guidelines that the latter incorporates when making coverage decisions.

The composition of the its decision processes seek to address different types of legitimacy. First, the FJC meets some measures of democratic legitimacy and accountability by including all stakeholders in its deliberations and meetings. Moreover, its proceedings and that of the IQWiG are transparent; the media widely reports on the FJC's meetings, which are open to the public, so that citizens have access to information about its work. To be sure, it falls short of full democratic participation since the patient representatives on the FJC lack voting power on coverage decisions. But open meetings, patient representatives, and media scrutiny perform oversight functions over a decision process that might otherwise be hidden behind closed doors.

Second, the FJC's reliance on scientific evidence to determine coverage seeks to avoid uninformed or arbitrary decisions. To be sure, the FJC's coverage decisions involve deliberations and negotiations among its members, who may sometimes bring their own values or material interests, or those of their constituents, to bear. But the FJC is legally required to consider the latest scientific evidence as furnished by IQWiG when fashioning its directives. This requirement is significant because as societies strive to keep health care spending within manageable bounds, coverage decisions grounded in clinical evidence rather than simply a single-minded pursuit of cost containment, will likely garner public confidence in the process and outcome.

Equity considerations constitute a third type of legitimacy. Since FJC coverage decisions apply to the entire SHI system and apply to everyone alike, the public is more likely to view the decisions as fair. Additionally, delegating coverage decisions to health care stakeholders who must weigh the scientific evidence available rather than giving the job to elected politicians, may depoliticize what may be difficult and controversial matters. The FJC's structure and decision rules not only deflect blame away from the government but also prevent politicians from intruding on fundamental decisions about health that affect the quality and longevity of individual human lives.

Finally, the FJC's development of clinical guidelines, which are distinct from overall SHI coverage decisions, are not simply a blunt instrument to force doctors and patients into submission. Such clinical guidelines are developed and disseminated nationally, but they are ultimately put into practice at the microlevel, in a doctor's office or a hospital, providing clinicians with information they can draw upon to help them make appropriate treatment decisions. Guidelines also assist physician practice review boards, giving them more accurate scientific information on clinical efficacy that is superior to data that simply provides peer averages. Guidelines need not be rigidly applied, but instead can and should allow for exceptions in practice, as long as the clinician can justify these on the basis of their patient's medical condition. Ulla Schmidt, the SPD health minister who led the drafting of the 2004 law, summed up Germany's corporatist structure of decision-making through the Federal Joint Committee, which balances expertise, inclusion, and oversight:

> This is the approach we prefer in Germany: consensus building under a form of self-regulation, but [also] under general government oversight. The federal government provides a general legislative framework for our universal health insurance system. But precisely how to implement it is left to the experts and representatives of the various stakeholders in health care. No political committee can decide whether a new medical procedure should become part of universal coverage or not. We feel that this should be left to the experts who, in our case, are hospitals, physicians, dentists, and sickness funds. The Joint Federal Committee also has patient representatives as well, so that patients can be heard, too.[56]

Coordinated Care at the Local Level[57]

The 2004 law gave incentives to insurers and providers to pursue coordinated care at the local level and furthered the introduction of quality measures. This effort comprised four new practice models, participation in which is voluntary for physicians and patients. Some of these innovations predate the 2004 law. Legislation in 2000 and 2002 permitted health funds to offer some types of integrated care, including disease management programs and gatekeeper models, as well as the possibility for selective contracting with specific groups of physicians, rather than the KVs, to provide them. Initially, insurance funds and physicians were slow to take up these new freedoms. Since the introduction of the 2004 law, however, such innovations have taken off.

The first new model of coordinated care is *integrated care contracts* (ICCs) between insurance funds and providers. Under these arrangements, patients must seek treatment from within a specified network of providers. To date, most of the ICCs address only particular types of care such as cardiovascular and orthopedic services.[58] ICCs may also extend to allied health professions like physical and occupational therapists as well as physicians. To encourage doctors and funds to develop such contracts, the government set aside 1 percent of the total ambulatory and hospital care budgets for ICCs. This start-up financing from the government totaled 800 million euros and was available to providers and insurers up through 2008. The financial incentives have yielded results: starting with only 600 integrated care contracts in 2005, they numbered more than 5,000 in 2008, having treated nearly four million patients.

The *gatekeeper (or family doctor) model* is the second form of integrated care. Under this model, patients select a family practitioner to coordinate their care. They must be referred by that physician to appropriate specialists. However, patients may directly visit gynecologists, pediatricians, and eye doctors for certain services. To become a gatekeeper practice, physicians must abide by a number of quality of care provisions that include the use of evidence-based clinical guidelines, having a quality assurance program in place, and participating in quality circles. In keeping with the patient-centered focus and the broad nature of primary care, gatekeepers must also receive relevant training in communication with patients and in the diagnosis and treatment of mental illness as well as geriatric and palliative care. Gatekeeper plans have been popular with patients because of the discounts that come with them. By 2007, 5.8 million patients had enrolled in such plans. They have been particularly attractive to elderly patients and those with chronic conditions.[59]

Polyclinics constitute the third model of coordinated care. They are multispecialty practices that offer outpatient services from primary care and specialty physicians under one roof, and may also include allied health professions such as pharmacists, physical therapists, and occupational therapists. Either hospitals or doctors may establish these practices. Polyclinics have been popular with younger and female doctors who prefer regular hours and salaried employment to self-employment in solo practice, and with patients who value the convenience of one-stop medical care. Most polyclinics remain small practices consisting of only four doctors on average. But their numbers have grown substantially since their introduction, rising from 70 clinics and 251 physicians in 2004 to 2,006 clinics and 13,000 doctors (representing 10 percent of all ambulatory doctors) in 2013. The vast majority of these physicians are salaried employees.[60]

Coordinated care has made big advances under the fourth model of *disease management programs* (DMPs). DMPs cover diabetes, coronary heart disease, breast cancer, asthma, and emphysema, which are the major chronic diseases afflicting the populations of industrialized nations. To receive federal accreditation, the programs must follow evidence-based treatment guidelines; have quality assurance systems in place; document and evaluate treatments, outcomes, and costs; provide proper training for providers and patients; and follow specified patient enrollment procedures. By 2013, over 6 million patients were enrolled in 10,501 regional disease management programs.[61]

These new forms of care constitute a challenge to long-standing practices in German national health insurance, particularly the position of the KVs in corporatist administration and in setting physician reimbursement. Health insurers can now bypass the KVs and contract directly with groups of physicians to provide coordinated care. The new forms of care offer possibilities for payment innovations, such as shared savings, performance-related payments for achieving quality measures, and additional reimbursement for documentation of such measures and coordination of care. Thus far, such payments remain rare,[62] perhaps due to their complexity and the caution of physicians concerned with the uncertainties of assuming financial risk for patient care. Outside of these specialized contracts, the KVs remain the negotiating partner with the health insurance funds at state level in determining the reimbursement of ambulatory physicians. Should selective contracting become more common, however, it would circumscribe the power of the KVs in determining the terms and conditions of medical practice and remuneration. Likewise, polyclinics have challenged the KVs' cherished model of solo practice. Having been the mode of medical organization in the communist East Germany, they were abolished following German unification. But with the 2004 law, they have made a comeback. The law essentially resurrected these multispecialty clinics, and they are spreading throughout the country.

More Patient Cost-sharing

The law sought to contain costs through controversial patient cost-sharing measures. First, to discourage unnecessary treatments and doctor-hopping by patients, patients would have to pay a 10-euro fee for the initial visit to ambulatory doctors and dentists in each quarter. The co-payment would also apply to every visit to a specialist if patients had not first obtained a referral from their primary care doctor. Out of equity considerations, pre- and postnatal care and children's care remained exempt from cost sharing, and co-payments were capped to 2 percent of annual household income, and 1 percent for those with chronic conditions. Second, the law sought further savings by striking some items from the essential benefits package, such as eyeglasses and over-the-counter drugs.[63]

The law also introduced a 0.9 percent surcharge on employee contributions as a way to restrain labor costs. This surcharge, along with the new co-payments, made employees responsible for a greater share of health care financing. This was not the final say on this question, however. Subsequent legislation repealed the copay for doctor visits in 2013, and revisited the question of additional contribution rates for employees.[64]

Reform Politics

The politics of the 2004 reform were relatively placid compared to those associated with the 1993 and 2007 reform laws. The composition of the federal government had changed in 1998, when a Social Democrat–Green coalition government assumed power following the federal elections. Yet the practice of achieving health care reform through consensus between the two largest parties in German politics remained in place. With Chancellor Schröder leading the moderate wing of the SPD, the coalition parties agreed on delivery system reform with the CDU, which held a majority of seats in the Bundesrat. Health insurers' desire for greater freedom of contracting for new forms of care was also in synch with those of the coalition partners. The usual defender of the doctors, the Free Democrats, exerted no influence since they were a not in government. The SPD and Greens were sympathetic to the needs of patients and the pursuit of solidarity, but they also faced concerns over health care cost containment and the competitiveness of German firms.[65] Hence, the coalition government's introduction of the employee contribution surcharge mollified employers and their allies in the CDU-led Bundesrat, but did not curry favor with the left wing of the SPD or its allies in organized labor.

The 2007 Social Health Insurance Competition Strengthening Act[66]

If the 2004 reform law confined itself mainly to the delivery of health care, the 2007 Social Health Insurance Competition Strengthening Act made health insurance financing its primary concern. The underlying reform politics was also markedly different. Whereas in 2004, the SPD–Green government largely agreed with the opposition CDU on the need for and contours of delivery system reform, in 2007 the parties were deeply polarized on how best to guarantee the immediate and longer term financial viability of social health insurance. The gulf not only separated the CDU from the SPD but also divided the SPD internally. Forces on the Left and Right initially offered widely different proposals that reflected dramatically different visions on the proper role of public versus private, and individual versus collective responsibility in obtaining and paying for health insurance. In the end, the two sides forged a complex compromise that borrowed elements from both. The deal reflected broader political realities following the 2005 federal elections that yielded a formal grand coalition government of the CDU and SPD headed by CDU chancellor Angela Merkel. The coalition agreement on health care reform also revealed that the two main parties still adhered to the basic principles of the social market economy. That being said, passing the law came about only after protracted negotiations between the two coalition partners and in an environment of vocal opposition from health care stakeholder associations.

The overriding aim of the 2007 legislation was to put national health insurance on a more secure financial footing for the future. Related to that was ensuring that all residents had continued access to affordable and comprehensive health care coverage. To realize these goals of affordability and access, policymakers devised a complex plan that introduced new structures and financing arrangements for national health insurance and also imposed new requirements on the for-profit private insurance sector. The reform also promoted greater competition among insurers and extended models of coordinated health care introduced in 2000 and 2004 to ensure that the quest for affordability would not sacrifice the quality of care. The law went into effect in 2007 but many of its provisions were phased in over a four-year period.

Shoring up the Financial Base of
National Health Insurance

After decades of discussion and debate, the 2007 law finally addressed the problems of adequately financing health care in the face of an aging population and a shrinking revenue base. Policymakers also recognized the need to deal with the broader economic effects of payroll-based financing of the welfare state, which burdened firms with potentially uncompetitive labor costs and was one cause of structural unemployment. The Hartz reforms addressed the latter two problems by labor market deregulation, which introduced more flexible and low-wage forms of employment and which pushed the unemployed to seek and accept work more readily. The 2007 health care reform tackled the insufficiency of payroll-based financing of health care, by broadening the financing base of SHI beyond wages and salaries.[67] First, the law removed children's health care from payroll taxes. From now on, the federal government would pick up the tab for this care through general tax revenues. Second, the legislation broadened the base of taxable income subject to national health insurance contributions. Hereafter, health insurance contributions would be financed not only from taxes on wages and salaries but also on nonwage income like rents and dividends.

To address employers' concerns over rising labor costs, the 2007 law also fixed the employer's share of health insurance contributions and shifted responsibility for absorbing financing increases to employees. The government also tightened the ability of persons to opt out of national health insurance for private coverage. Prior to the 2007 law, a person whose income exceeded the legally set threshold for one year could opt for private insurance, and many did so. Since private for-profit insurers levied experience-rated premiums, their rates were lower for younger, healthier individuals with higher incomes than if they remained in the SHI system. Under the 2007 law, an individual now had to meet or exceed the income threshold for three consecutive years before switching to a private insurance, and could return to SHI only if their income fell below the threshold. Policymakers hoped that these changes would keep a greater number of healthier and wealthier people in social health insurance and thereby improve risk pooling and stabilize contribution rates for all members of that system.[68]

Intensifying Competition Among Sickness Funds

As its name indicated, the 2007 law intensified managed competition in the social health insurance system. The aim was to use competitive mechanisms rather than the blunt and intrusive tools of government-set budgets and directives to get more efficient health care from insurers and providers. Choice of fund would also give patients an escape from a fund that raised its rates. But this strategy also depended on the government setting out clear rules for competition to safeguard the solidarity of SHI.

The first element of this pro-competition strategy was to grant health insurers some scope to offer new benefits packages to attract new members and reward them for healthy lifestyles. Insured persons continue to enjoy free choice of fund and all funds must continue to offer the basic comprehensive benefits package as before, but the funds can compete on extra benefits or new payment arrangements at the margins. This is especially important now that contribution rates are uniform for all funds (see below). Proponents of the schemes believe that they will encourage individuals to take more responsibility for their health and reduce unnecessary trips to the doctor. Toward that end, health funds can offer patients deductible plans rather than care that is free at the point of service, indemnity-type contracts whereby members pay for their health services and then submit bills for reimbursement; contribution rebate schemes to members whose annual health care costs remain below a preset target; and additional benefits at extra charge such as gym memberships to promote wellness. By shifting some financial risk for health care to patients, some of these options are a safer bet for younger and healthier members than for older and sicker ones.

But some of the new health plans appeal to the chronically ill and not just those who are healthy. Such innovative plans include gym memberships, chronic disease management programs, integrated care contracts, and gatekeeper models. Health insurers could offer many of these programs as far back as 2000 and the 2004 law provided funding to encourage them to do so. But the 2007 law required funds to make such alternatives available to members, although participation by patients and doctors remained voluntary. Insurance funds and providers were also eligible for government funding for such programs, such as start-up money through 2008 for disease management programs, and additional risk-adjusted payments to health insurance funds and providers who participate in them. The 2007 law also expands the basic benefits package for SHI to include preventive services like immunizations free of charge. Rehabilitative services for the elderly and disabled as well as palliative care are now also covered.

The reforms have their critics. Some worry that the new benefit packages will serve as subtle tools of cream skimming by insurers. Yet policymakers expect that new improvements in the risk-adjustment mechanism (discussed below) will sufficiently counteract such temptations. Others worry that developing all of these new insurance products, above and beyond the standard benefits package, could drive up administrative costs if funds have to create large underwriting departments to devise such plans.[69]

Greater competition and choices among insurance products also required new rules to safeguard solidarity. Otherwise, insurers would compete by wooing only healthier patients. Moreover, new forms of care like disease management programs required buy-in by insurers and providers. They would only offer such treatment options for chronically ill patients if they were rewarded rather than punished for doing so. The 2007 law therefore introduced novel financing arrangements and also vastly improved the risk-adjustment system that had been in place with the 1993 reform law.

The earlier risk-adjustment scheme had significantly narrowed contribution rates among funds so that they varied by only 1 percent. But the system did not capture all risks perfectly, so that contribution rates still varied according to the health status of the funds' membership. In a break from past practice, the law created a central Health Fund (Gesundheitsfond) at the federal level, which became operational in 2009. Prior to this, each insurer set its own contribution rate as a percentage of income of the fund's members that was sufficient to meet their health care expenditures. The 2007 law stripped this authority from the funds. Instead, government now calculates a uniform contribution rate for all funds. For the first two years, the federal Ministry of Health set the rate; since 2011, it has been set by law. Employers pay half of the share of a uniform income-based contribution rate set by the health ministry for all funds and employees pay the other half. At the same time, the law fixes the employers' contribution but allows the employees' side to float, as discussed below.

The flow of contributions into and out of the Health Fund works as follows: Under previous practice employers sent payroll tax deductions directly to the health insurance funds their employees chose (or were assigned to). Now they send these payments directly to the Health Fund. The Health Fund, in turn, distributes to each insurer a lump-sum capitation payment based on the number of members, plus an additional risk-adjusted payment that accounts for their health status (see Figure 3.2).

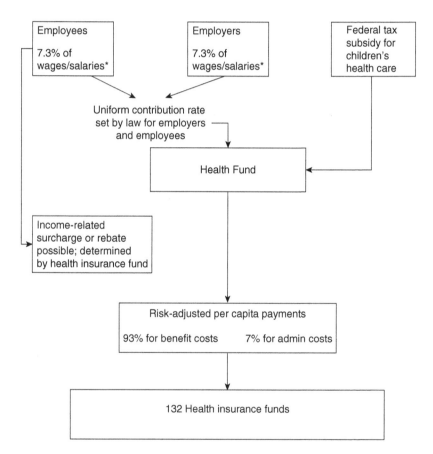

Figure 3.2   Financing flows in German social health insurance since 2009.

Sources: Adapted from Hoyer, *Social Health Insurance in Germany and the Market Position of the TK*, 2009, p. 16; and Lisac, "Health Care Reform in Germany: Not the Big Bang" (2006); and Busse, Reinhard and Miriam Blümel. 2014. *Germany: Health System Review*, vol. 16, issue 2, *Health Systems in Transition*. European Observatory on Health Systems and Policies.

The risk-adjustment equalization scheme, first introduced in 1994, was an imperfect instrument to reduce contribution rate differences based on health status. It only took into account the age, sex, number of dependents and pensioners, income differences, and number of members receiving unemployment benefits or social assistance. And some of the insurance funds proved more adept than others in attracting healthier patients through the use of various marketing strategies. Since 2009, however, the scheme has been fine-tuned to account for the average health care costs of 80 expensive chronic and acute conditions, so it better counteracts cream-skimming.

Payroll contributions flowing into the Health Fund cover roughly 95 percent of the health care costs incurred by the health insurance funds. But with the health ministry setting a uniform contribution rate for all funds, what would happen if one of them faced a deficit or a surplus? The 2007 law had an answer. If an insurer faced a deficit, it could impose a surcharge on members of eight euros per month, up to limit of 1 percent of income. Members who faced this surcharge would also have the freedom to leave that fund for another. Conversely, if a fund had a surplus, it could reward its members with a rebate.[70] This mechanism allows for some degree of price competition among the funds and also gives them a strong incentive not to raise their prices if they wish to retain their membership. It also makes employees responsible for any shortfalls or surpluses of insurers, since the contribution share paid by employers is fixed.

In 2014, the uniform contribution rate was 14.6 percent, so employers and employees each paid 7.3 percent. The addition of new tax revenues to cover children's health care has stabilzed contribution rates. But so has the possibility of patients switching to a new fund if their current insurer levies a surcharge. As a result, the average payroll contribution rate for NHI fell from 15.5 percent in 2009 to the uniform rate of 14.6 percent in 2014.[71]

While critics worried that the Health Fund would amount to a huge expansion of government bureaucracy, this has not been the case. The responsibility to set the contribution rate and develop the risk-adjustment scheme rests with the Federal Health Insurance Office working in conjunction with the federal health minister and the Federal Association of SHI Funds. Altogether, there were only 21 persons in the federal insurance office in 2009.[72]

Adjustments to Remuneration of Ambulatory Physicians

Government efforts to better compensate for health risks was not confined to insurers but also extended to ambulatory sector doctors with the introduction of a morbidity-adjusted remuneration system in 2009. This important change to physician reimbursement had been announced in the 2004 law, but implementation difficulties led to its reintroduction in the 2007 law. Prior to its introduction, the KVs and health funds negotiated a budget for all ambulatory sector physicians at state level. This regional budget was a capitation amount for each patient or insurance fund member in that state, essentially capping overall physician reimbursement. From this regional budget, the KV paid each physician fee-for-service or a lump-sum payment per patient. But physicians were unhappy with this system for a number of reasons: the capitation formula did not capture the health status of their patients, and their reimbursements would decline toward the end of the year to stay within budget. This essentially penalized them financially for treating a higher number of patients with severe illnesses, especially at the end of the year.

The new reimbursement system addresses some of these concerns. It provides doctors with financial incentives to treat sicker patients and provide preventive services. The overall budget for KV physicians remains capped at state level. But it is now calculated on the basis of morbidity factors as well as the number of members in the health insurance funds in each state. From this overall budget, each doctor receives a prospectively set target for the volume of services. The volume target is adjusted for physician specialty as well as the morbidity of the patients in his or her own practice. The price for each item of service is fixed in euros and follows a national fee schedule set by the federal associations of SHI physicians and insurers. But the volume target sets an upper limit to how much each doctor can earn and thus keeps overall physician compensation within a cap. Should a physician provide services that exceed the targeted volume above a certain threshold, he or she will receive reduced payments for those services. The new reimbursement system also increasingly substitutes lump-sum (or bundled) payments (calculated on the age and sex of the patient, and for specialists, the diagnosis) rather than fee-for-service. To balance this trend toward lump-sum payment, the health insurance funds also remunerate doctors for unexpected medical costs, such as those associated with an epidemic, and do not count such payments against their volume targets. In addition, the health funds pay fixed fee-for-service prices for preventive services like immunizations and screenings, as well as ambulatory surgery, all of which remain outside the physician's volume target. Physicians also receive additional separate payments if they participate in disease management programs, essentially rewarding them to care for chronically ill patients.[73]

Responding to Insecure Access to Health Insurance

As previously noted, Germany has experienced long-term structural unemployment since the 1980s. While the Hartz reforms have allowed more temporary, part-time work and self-employment, such policies and a changing economy have introduced new health insecurity. German SHI had long assumed stable employment, but the new forms of work had created a small but rising pool of uninsured. The highest estimate of the uninsured in 2005 reckoned that 300,000 people (out of a population of more than 69 million) lacked health insurance. The uninsured are primarily the wealthy, the self-employed, or those who had been voluntarily insured but had failed to pay their premiums.[74] The 2007 law responded by creating both new rights and obligations in health insurance coverage. There is now an individual mandate alongside the longstanding employer mandate. Those uninsured who were last covered by the social health insurance system have to return to it. The law also bars SHI funds from dropping a person for nonpayment of her contribution. Since 2009, those not eligible for SHI coverage must take out private insurance. But the law provides tax-financed subsidies to the self-employed and those on low incomes to make insurance affordable in both the private and SHI systems.

The government has also introduced new regulations on for-profit commercial insurance companies so that those who are privately insured but who have expensive medical conditions can get adequate and affordable coverage. Since 2009, private insurers must offer all clients a basic benefits package (Basistarif) equivalent to the minimum benefits coverage under social health insurance. The premium cannot be higher than the maximum contribution rate for SHI, nor can private insurers levy surcharges based on an individual's medical condition. New subscribers to private insurance can opt for the basic benefits package without medical underwriting; existing members who are aged 55 or older or former members who can no longer afford experience-rated premiums can also switch to the basic benefits option. Private insurers must also participate in a risk-adjustment scheme if they cover high-risk individuals who are ineligible for SHI insurance (such as pensioners or self-employed persons) or who cannot afford the basic premium. The risk-adjustment scheme is separate from the one for SHI funds.[75]

Continued Coordination of Care and of Corporatist Decision-Making

Building on the 2004 law's encouragement of integrated care, the 2007 reform extended new forms of coordinated care outside the traditional medical field. Integrated care contracts can now include long-term care services and encompass the allied health professions. Contracts for coordinated care permit the health funds to bypass the KVs and engage in selective contracting with individual physicians. These new forms of care obviously encroach on the KVs' jurisdiction.

At the same time, the 2007 law requires greater coordination between insurers and providers throughout the SHI system. In 2008, the government abolished seven separate federal associations for each type of fund and replaced them with a single umbrella association at national level, the Federal Association of Social Health Insurance Funds. In 2009, the government mandated greater cooperation among corporatist associations of insurers and providers by designating the Plenary Committee within the Federal Joint Committee as the single decision-making body for coverage decisions for SHI.

Reform Politics: Early Polarization and the Reassertion of Negotiated Solutions

The politics underpinning the 2007 law were turbulent because the reform of health care financing brought up politically fraught questions on the role of government, the private sector, and the degree to which health care is an individual responsibility or one of the broader society. These questioned the fundamental structures of the 120-year old SHI system. The debate was also years in the making.[76]

Formal consideration of health care financing issues followed the September 2002 reelection of the SPD–Green coalition government. In November 2002, SPD health minister Ulla Schmidt convened the Commission for Financial Sustainability of Social Security Systems (the so-called Rürup Commission). The commission included representatives of the governing coalition as well as scientific experts, economists, employers, unions, sickness funds, private insurers, and state and local governments. Bert Rürup, an economics professor and SPD member, headed the commission. The members were deeply divided on the future of SHI, how best to finance it, and whether it should include the entire population. Unusual for German policymaking, the commission failed to reach a consensus. And its final report in August 2003 presented two divergent proposals, both of which were radical in their own way.[77]

A *citizens' insurance* (*Bürgerversicherung*) was the idea of Karl Lauterbach, a health economist, physician, and SPD member of the Bundestag who served on the Rürup Commission. National health insurance through the nonprofit sickness funds would now cover the entire population, including those who had previously been privately insured-civil servants, the self-employed, and those with incomes above the SHI threshold. In short, citizens' insurance would effectively eliminate private for-profit health insurance. The rationale for such radical action was that private insurance tended to attract younger, healthier, and given the income threshold, wealthier segments of society. The current SHI system, by contrast, had more members with expensive medical conditions. Making those in private insurance now part of SHI would strengthen the risk pooling in that system. Eliminating private insurance and folding it into SHI would also end what some saw as "two-class" health care system. Citizens' insurance would continue to calculate contributions based on ability to pay and not health status. Hence, insurance contribution rates would continue to be calculated as a percentage of income. But it would also broaden the income base for social health insurance financing to include not only wages and salaries but also nonwage income like dividends, rent, and interest. Further, the maximum taxable income for social health insurance would be raised by nearly one-third to match the level for national pensions. Taken together, all of these changes would shore up the financial base of the SHI system. In sum, citizens' insurance was intended to ensure the financial sustainability of national health insurance and its solidarity in the future. The idea for citizens' insurance was probably borrowed from the Netherlands, which had broadened its funding base for its social health insurance system and also included private insurers.[78]

Rürup himself favored a very different alternative, that of *flat-rate premiums* (*Gesundheitsprämie*). Under this proposal, health insurance would be compulsory for all individuals, who would pay the same flat-rate premium regardless of their health status or income. General tax revenues would subsidize premiums to make them affordable for those with low incomes. Employers would no longer contribute to health insurance, thereby reducing their nonwage labor costs. This proposal for tax-financed individual insurance resembled the existing Swiss system of national health insurance.[79]

The debate over health care financing continued after the 2005 parliamentary election. The poll yielded an inconclusive result with the CDU and SPD in a virtual tie. After much wrangling, the two rivals agreed to form a "grand coalition" government headed by the CDU's Angela Merkel. The new government formalized the long-standing unofficial cooperation between the two catchall parties on matters of social policy. The coalition enjoyed a comfortable majority in the Bundestag to enact reform. But any agreement had to satisfy both coalition partners, as well as the Bundesrat, which represented the state governments, whose interests sometimes diverged from those of the federal government, even when the same party enjoyed majorities in both chambers.

After protracted private negotiations among the coalition partners that included Chancellor Merkel, the government reached an agreement that became the basis of the 2007 SHI Competition Strengthening Act. It was a complicated compromise that combined elements of both alternatives outlined above but stopped short of wholesale adoption of either one. The CDU, bowing to employers' labor cost concerns, secured the provision to fix employers' share of health insurance contributions. At the same time, the party rejected the flat-rate premium model on the grounds that it would place a greater burden on lower income persons. Also, taking employers out of health care financing could have placed a heavy burden on taxpayers to subsidize premiums for those on low incomes. This dual position reflected the party's cross-class appeal and an internal structure that gave a voice not only to business but also to trade unions, particularly on social policy matters. The CDU also rejected the citizens' insurance model for fear that it was a slippery slope toward a single-payer government insurance system like that of Canada or Britain. The party preserved the separate existence of private insurance for technical rasons as well, citing the difficulty of breaking contracts between clients and their insurers. After all, like employers, private insurers were an important constituency of the CDU.

The SPD had to make some concessions, but secured others. The party's left wing opposed freezing employers' share of insurance contributions because it feared that employees would end up bearing a greater share of health care costs. The left wing also wanted to absorb private insurance into citizens' insurance. On both measures, the SPD conceded defeat. However, the SPD succeeded in retaining income-based contributions and broadening the income base for SHI, both of which it viewed as essential to preserve the solvency and solidarity of SHI.

Health care stakeholders did not receive all they wanted either. Social health insurance funds and labor unions opposed the Central Fund on the grounds that it added an extra layer of bureaucracy. The unions disliked the idea of having employees pay an additional surcharge to funds if the uniform contribution rate was insufficient to cover health care expenses, and favored the integration of private insurance into SHI. But the government did not heed their concerns. Still, some of their preferences found their way into the law, such as the broader taxable income base for SHI and the removal of the cost of children's health care from insurance contributions. Health insurance funds welcomed the ability to negotiate new forms of care and engage in selective contracting with individual physicians. The KVs regarded selective contracting and polyclinics as a challenge to their monopoly position in negotiating physician income and forms of care but they welcomed the morbidity-based reimbursement formula adopted for ambulatory care. They also retained their privileged position in representing ambulatory sector doctors in many areas of health care administration: the KVs continue to negotiate the bulk of physician reimbursement at state level, while their federal association remains the representative of physician interests in key decisions on the FJC.

Once the legislation was enacted, the courts weighed in. Private insurers unsuccessfully brought a suit before the Federal Constitutional Court challenging the new regulations. The high court upheld the requirement for a minimum benefits package as consistent with the constitution. The court ruled that the constitution's designation of the Federal Republic as a social state gave the federal government the obligation and authority to regulate private interests to safeguard the social welfare of the people.[80] The law thus brought private insurers' practices closer to those of social health insurance, but stopped short of creating a full-fledged single national health insurance system. Nonetheless, even if the two sectors remained legally separate, in practice the line between them had become blurred.

In the end, the 2007 law also conformed to the usual pattern of German policymaking. It was the product of protracted negotiations over ideas that had originated in discussions and proposals a decade earlier. By settling on a compromise, policymakers stopped short of fully embracing one radical solution in its entirety. The government did not replace the existing system of employment-based insurance with compulsory tax-financed individual insurance. Nor did it eliminate private insurance. It retained much of the existing system but added new elements. The compromise offered something to every stakeholder, but none of them got everything they wanted.

Further Wrangling Reasserts the 2007 Settlement[81]

Subsequent governments have revisited the question of health care financing but little has changed since the 2007 law in this regard. Due to electoral politics, health policy has seesawed somewhat but has thus far ended in a stalemate.

The 2009 election saw a new coalition government that reverted to past practice. The CDU was again the largest party in the Bundestag and chose to return to its old coalition partner, the FDP. The Free Democrats now headed the federal health ministry and resurrected the idea of compulsory individual insurance with flat-rate premiums. The scheme sat well with the FDP's ideology of individual responsibility. By removing health care from employment, it also appealed to the CDU's business wing. The coalition enacted a health reform law in 2011, but the proposal for individual insurance was conspicuously absent. The reason for this was opposition from within the governing coalition, particularly within the CDU camp. The Christian Social Union (CSU) is the expression of the CDU in Bavaria and has been in every coalition government as part of the Christian Democratic grouping. More conservative than the CDU on social issues, the CSU also expresses the Catholic values that underpin the social market economy. Because individual insurance based on a flat-rate premium would hit those with lower incomes hardest, the CSU rejected the proposal as an affront to solidarity and social justice.

Still, the 2011 law contained some inequities as a trade-off to preserve labor cost competitiveness. The law removed health ministry discretion in setting the uniform contribution rate for national health insurance funds and also raised it at 15.5 percent of wages and salaries. But employers would only pay 7.3 percent while employees would shoulder 8.2 percent. As before, any deficits that the health funds incurred could be passed on to their members as a supplementary premium. This represented a further departure from equal financing of health care from payroll contributions. Employees would not only pay 0.9 percent more than employers at the outset, but might also be saddled with an additional community-rated premium levied by the funds.

The parliamentary elections of 2013 restored Merkel's grand coalition between the CDU and SPD. With the Social Democrats again in government, health policy took a more solidaristic turn—up to a point. The new government sought to protect patients from undue health insurance burdens while also addressing the concerns of employers to hold the line on indirect labor costs. The grand coalition tried to balance these two aims with a new law in 2014. Starting in 2015, the law abolished the 0.9 percent additional contribution rate and supplemental premiums on employees. The general contribution rate, lowered to 14.6 percent of income, continues to be set by law and employers and employees once again split that share equally. However, if social health insurance funds run a deficit, they may now levy an income-dependent supplemental surcharge on members to be determined by each individual health fund. This essentially locks in employers' share of health insurance financing but holds employees financially responsible for any additional health care costs above that general contribution rate. Although not as imbalanced as the CDU–FDP's 2011 reform, it continues the break from the practice and principle of equal financing. Employees will continue to pay (minor) co-payments, and in the future will be responsible for a surcharge on their health insurance contributions, unless they exercise their right of choice of fund and find an insurer with a lower rate. In essence, the law restores the 2007 settlement and seeks to balance equity in health care with the broader economic competitiveness of German industry.

Conclusion

The health care system in Germany has been the object of ongoing adjustment by policymakers in consultation with health care stakeholders to meet new challenges. These stakeholders include a wide range of interests beyond simply insurers and providers. Employment-based financing also brings employers and labor unions into the policy mix. Policymakers have also had to address the interests of state governments. Yet amid all the policy change, the basic contours of the SHI system, as well as the core principles that underpin the social market economy, remain intact. A review of the major reforms provides evidence for this conclusion. The mandate on individuals to carry insurance affects relatively few people; most Germans continue to obtain health insurance through employment. New requirements on private insurers to offer basic coverage bring that sector into alignment with the principle of solidarity in SHI, namely, universal access to health care based on medical need rather than ability to pay. The introduction of choice of insurance fund and new forms of care are major innovations that seek to enhance efficiency and patient choice and equity. But some changes may work against responsiveness to patients: gatekeeper models, after all, restrict patients' choice of doctor. The use of contribution rate surcharges (not to mention copayments) signals a break from the principle of parity financing. Even so, the limits on the play of competitive forces, and improvements in risk-adjustment for funds and physician compensation, safeguard solidarity and encourage funds and providers to accept sicker patients. German SHI still includes hardship exemptions from cost sharing to protect the vulnerable. The quest to promote more coordinated care, particularly for those with chronic medical conditions, and to bring evidence-based medicine into treatment and coverage decisions also offers the possibility of delivering higher quality care at a lower cost than under the previous model of fragmented, reactive treatment of disease at an advanced stage.

Germany's approach to health care reform has been to modernize its nineteenth-century framework based on employment-based insurance and corporatist governance to meet the challenges of the twenty-first century, particularly those posed by an aging population and the limitations of payroll-based financing. A mixed or "hybrid" model has emerged, incorporating new policy tools into preexisting corporatist governance.[82] SHI continues to rely on payroll taxes for most of its financing, but the "income" subject to taxation has expanded. The government is also supplementing payroll contributions with general tax revenues to cover the cost of children's health care. Both measures have worked to stabilize payroll contributions and indirect labor costs: the 2014 uniform rate is 14.6 percent of wages, down from 15.5 in 2012.[83]

Policymakers have also grafted limited market competition and more enduring state intervention in health care administration onto the corporatist scaffold. The basic framework of corporatist administration, whereby the state sets the basic rules and parameters of social health insurance but relies on associations of healthcare providers and insurers to work out the details of their implementation through negotiated agreements and coordinated decision making, persists. In its role as the guarantor of universal access to affordable quality care and as the supervising authority over health sector associations, the state has had to make more frequent forays into SHI administration than in previous decades. The health ministry's temporary imposition of budgets in SHI subsectors is one such example, but it is consistent with the state's oversight role under corporatism. However, recent reforms have made the state's presence in health care administration more permanent. The setting of a uniform contribution rate for all SHI funds by law and the health ministry's operation of the central fund to distribute risk-adjusted payments to insurers are clear examples of enduring state intervention. At the same time, the state still relies on corporatist associations to administer most of the SHI system, and has even increased their remit and authority with the Federal Joint Committee, which encompasses all parts of the SHI system and whose directives are binding on all of its actors. This balance between state, corporatism, and competition could change in the future, should new forms of integrated care and selective contracting become more widespread and challenge the monopolistic position of the regional Associations of SHI Physicians.[84]

German health care remains among the most generous and expensive in the world. Yet government efforts to promote more coordinated care and to wed clinical and cost effectiveness suggest that policymakers take the question of affordability very seriously. The reforms represent promising steps on the path of best practice and financial sustainability. Although Germany has begun to move away from equal financing of health care, its health care system still retains much of its solidarity. Whatever the future holds for health policy, policymakers will face the ongoing challenge to reconcile equity with affordability and quality, and to ensure that the burden of adjustment is borne fairly. How this will play out in the future is, of course, a matter of politics.

CHAPTER FOUR

South Africa: Confronting the Legacies of Apartheid

The Republic of South Africa illustrates the triumphs and challenges of democratic transformation in the postcolonial era. For three centuries, white European settlers and their descendants, who comprised a minority of the population, had imposed a political, economic, and social system based on racial hierarchy, which they enforced by the repressive denial of basic human rights of the indigenous black majority. In 1948, the system of legal segregation and disempowerment of blacks and other nonwhites, called apartheid (the Afrikaans word for "aparthood"), became official policy under the rule of the National Party (NP). Despite global opprobrium, apartheid lingered until 1994, when South Africa held the first free all-racial elections in the country's history. This first important step in the path of political democratization was all the more remarkable because it was the outcome of difficult negotiations rather than the bloodshed of all-out civil war.[1]

Economically, South Africa counts many advantages. It possesses bountiful natural resources and a capitalist economy based in mining, agricultural exports, and financial services established under white rule. While still part of the developing world, South Africa ranks among the middle-income countries (the so-called BRICS, which comprise Brazil, Russia, India, China, and South Africa) and is the second-largest economy on the African continent (Nigeria ranks first). Under white minority rule, the fruits of economic gains had been denied to the black majority. Poverty and inequality endure to the present day, despite the end of white minority rule.

Since the 1994 election, the African National Congress (ANC) has led governments that have embarked upon ambitious programs and policies to address the broad and deep manifestations of white minority rule. They have sought to dismantle race discrimination in all areas of life, address rampant poverty and inequality, and modernize the economy. Notable progress has been made. The South African constitution adopted in 1996 explicitly acknowledges a broad range of civil liberties and even social rights, including a right to health care. ANC governments repealed the apartheid-era laws that enforced separation of the races and instituted affirmative action programs to boost economic opportunities for blacks. In the area of health, the ANC has extended basic services (sanitation, electricity, and housing) and built thousands of new primary care health clinics in the poorest areas of the country. The government also significantly expanded the welfare state to cover all of the population with a public pension as well as targeting cash payments and income assistance to those most in need, such as the disabled and pensioners.

Notwithstanding these substantial accomplishments in only two decades of democracy, the apartheid legacy of separate and unequal continues to express itself, particularly in population health outcomes and in the structure of the health care system of South Africa. The statistics are sobering. Despite being the second-largest economy in the African continent, South Africa's child mortality rate since 1994 has actually worsened and its maternal mortality rate has shown next to no improvement. HIV/AIDS and tuberculosis (TB) are twin scourges that have sharply reduced life expectancy. The country's rate of new HIV infection, at 12.2 percent or 6.4 million people, ranks first in the world. Its infection rate for TB, at 860 per 100,000 people in 2013, is among the highest in the world.[2] The figures mask significant racial and income disparities in the experience of disease, with black South Africans bearing the brunt of these illnesses.

Gaping disparities in health outcomes today reflect the lingering impact of "boundary institutions," or rigid identities based on race, that were constructed during apartheid.[3] In South Africa, as elsewhere in the world, levels of health are largely socially determined. But poverty, inequality, and their effects on ill health are much broader and deeper in South Africa than in the richer industrialized democracies. Indeed, South Africa has one of the highest levels of income inequality in the world.[4] Such disparities in resources pose substantial challenges to health policy. As a middle income country, South African policymakers confront the health care problems found in developing countries as well as those of wealthier industrialized nations. On the one hand, infectious diseases—not only HIV/AIDS but also those more common to developing nations such as TB, malaria, and diarrheal diseases in children—are rampant. On the other hand, South Africa faces a rise in chronic noncommunicable diseases such as heart disease, diabetes, and stroke, which are often associated with the industrialized world.[5] Some of the rise in noncommunicable diseases lies with increasing longevity in South Africa.

But it is also due to broader social conditions associated with poverty and inequality that lead to poor diet, lack of exercise, and lack of access to necessary health services. Indeed, the urban and rural poor bear the heaviest burden of noncommunicable diseases. Yet, as a lower middle-income nation, the South African government lacks the fiscal resources that wealthier Western countries possess to respond to such ills. At the same time, bowing to the rules of a free-trade global economy, such as balanced budgets and the reduction of trade barriers, ANC governments have pursued economic liberalization as well as social justice, with some-times contradictory results. Critics of this Janus-faced approach maintain that the government's strategy has not sufficiently addressed the ill health that continues to plague the majority of the country's citizens. They go further and argue that economic liberalization has actually worsened unemployment and poverty, thereby aggravating the health problems in the country. Moderates among them call for a better balance between growth and redistribution rather than economic policies that only satisfy domestic and foreign businesses, and international creditors and develop-ment agencies. Radicals demand more aggressive redistribution measures and nationalization of key industries.

Not all of South Africa's health problems can be laid at the doorstep of external economic forces. Some of South Africa's health care challenges are traceable to government policy choices during and after apartheid. The glaring example was the ANC government's initial response to HIV/AIDS. In the first few years of the new millennium, the government's policy was to deny the scope and threat of the disease, and refuse to adopt evidence-based treatments. This policy let the virus to spread in an uncontrolled fashion, contributing to hundreds of thousands of deaths. Yet even this seemingly inexplicable policy response can be traced back to the nation's experience of apartheid. Apartheid sowed seeds of mutual distrust among policymakers both black and white, which contaminated their health pol-icy decisions. This deep mistrust warped the framing of HIV/AIDS policy, from defining who was at risk for HIV/AIDS, what should be done to address the disease, and whose advice should be heeded in this regard.

One of the major sources of the country's health woes is the health care system itself. As a result of the apartheid era, South Africa possesses two distinct systems, separate and unequal. The first system is a private one of commercial insurance and state-of-the-art health care facilities that cater to a minority of the population (primarily whites and the small emer-gent black middle class). This system is well funded through private insur-ance contributions and employs the majority of the country's doctors and nurses. The second system is publicly funded and provided and serves the black majority. As it was during apartheid, it remains under-resourced. A significant policy challenge is to rebalance the public and private health care systems so that all South Africans can enjoy equitable access to quality health care. Toward that end, the ANC has committed itself to establishing a national health insurance system. It has also articulated a policy agenda that addresses serious deficiencies in health care delivery, especially its institutional fragmentation, lack of managerial expertise, and dearth of health care providers in the public system. In this quest, the country's policymakers are in line with the United Nations and the World Health Organization (WHO) strategies for universal coverage.[6]

This chapter proceeds as follows. The first section "The Dual Health Care System" describes the present dualistic health care system in South Africa and its historical development. It makes clear that colonialism and capitalism under white minority rule have powerfully shaped the health disparities and disease patterns that afflict the country today. The second section "Political Factors Underpinning Health Policy" describes the major political forces underpinning health policy in South Africa. This includes the structures of the current political system, the leading political parties and civil society organizations (domestic and international), the competing ideologies of white supremacy apartheid on the one hand and black liberation movement majoritarianism of the ANC on the other, and the policy legacies of the apartheid era that have created the health care challenges facing governments since 1994. The third section "Policy Responses to Health Care Challenges Since 1994" examines the record of ANC governments in addressing health challenges since the end of apartheid, showing how politics have shaped policies. The last section assesses South Africa's health policy record to date and offers a prognosis for the future.

The argument in brief is this: The legacies of the past affect the institutions that finance and deliver health care in South Africa to this day. ANC governments have sought to ensure that all South Africans have access to quality care. They have made some important gains in improving population health, but they still have a very long way to go. Even though they operate under significant constraints and face daunting odds, if policymakers practice politics as the art of the possible they can yet realize their ambitious goal of health equity.

The Dual Health Care System: Current
Features and Historical Origins

South Africa's Two Health Care Systems

South Africa has two health care systems that one finds in many other developing nations. A private system caters to a small elite segment of the population (whites, civil servants, and the emergent black middle class).

The rest of the population relies on an underfunded and overstretched government system, foreign aid workers, traditional healers, or some combination of all three for their health care needs.[7] Yet South Africa's health care systems differ in some important respects from the poorer nations of the Global South. As a middle-income developing nation, South Africa devotes significantly more resources to health care than do the poorest countries. South Africa devotes 8.5 percent of its GDP to health, or $942 per capita.[8] Following the advent of black majority rule in 1994, the country has also made significant strides in making basic primary care free to all of its population.

The structure of the public or government health system since 1994 conforms to the model of a national health service (NHS). In this model, the government plays the main role in financing and providing health care and in administering the public system. The NHS is financed from general tax revenues out of the national budget. Patients receive health care in public facilities; doctors, nurses, and other health care workers are public employees. The administration of the NHS mirrors the country's federal political system, with the national level Department of Health (DOH) at the apex responsible for strategic decisions and allocating funds to lower levels. Below the DOH, nine provincial departments are responsible for health care for the population in their provinces. At the local level, district health authorities are responsible for primary care.

The National Health Act of 2004 centralized administration and deprived local governments of important responsibilities by transferring primary care and local health services to the provinces. Despite this structural change, questions over responsibilities and money remain. These center on the allocation of money between provincial and local levels as well as the extent to which the national DOH will allow provincial governments some freedom to devise their own policies.[9]

The public sector health care system that the ANC inherited upon taking power in 1994 suffered from a century of a deliberate government policy of deprivation. Severe imbalances between primary and specialty care compartmentalized the system. Health care provision emphasized services in urban hospitals, especially those providing tertiary care or affiliated with a medical school, at the expense of primary care. In 1993, 76 percent of public expenditures went to hospital services while primary care received only 11 percent. Such priorities largely benefited the white minority in the cities. In response, the ANC government under Nelson Mandela expanded primary care by upgrading 248 existing clinics and constructing 485 new facilities in less than five years. The government also made health care free for children under age six, pregnant women, and mothers who were breastfeeding, and required new physicians and pharmacists to do community service in underserved areas beginning in 2001.[10] Yet significant disparities in public health spending between the richer urban provinces and the poorer rural ones still persist.

Two decades after apartheid's end, the numbers tell the story of enduring inequality between the two health care systems. In 2013, private insurance accounted for 42.7 percent of all health care spending but only covered slightly more than 16 percent of the population. By contrast, the public health care system accounted for 48.4 percent of health care expenditures while caring for roughly 84 percent of South Africans. A majority of physicians (79 percent in 2007) and nurses practice in the private sector, thus depleting the public system of much-needed personnel.[11] A number of factors are driving the personnel shortage: migration into the private sector due to voluntary severance packages in the public sector in the mid-1990s, better pay in the private sector, migration overseas, the closure of nursing schools in the late 1990s (leading to fewer graduates), retirements, and relatively flat spending on public health since the mid-1990s.[11] In short, the public health care system must work from a revenue base that is woefully insufficient to meet the constitutional right to health care for all citizens.

Not only does the public system face insufficient resources, it also deals with vastly greater problems than the private system. The responsibility for caring for those with infectious diseases like HIV/AIDS and TB falls largely to the public sector. In addition, the public health care system suffers from insufficient managerial expertise, unclear lines of responsibility, and problems of coordination among the national, provincial, and local governments responsible for health care.

The private health care system is not without its problems. First, private spending on health care has risen rapidly even as public funding has remained flat. Between 1996 and 2006, per capita private spending rose from 3,000 rand to roughly 5,500 rand; during the same period, public funding stood at just below 1,000 rand.[13] The spending explosion in private health care has a number of causes. One is fee-for-service reimbursement, which encourages higher volumes and more complex procedures. Another factor is overspecialization and an emphasis on hospital-based curative care. The result is an oversupply of specialist physicians, who are associated with a more intensive and expensive practice style than primary care. The second problems is that private insurers require beneficiaries to pay substantial out-of-pocket costs. Finally, the large number of private health plans for such a small portion of the population has undermined risk pooling, leaving members of some plans who are sicker and poorer paying a much higher premium than those with healthier risks and higher incomes.[14]

Origins of the Dual Health Care System[15]

South Africa's dual structure of health care financing and provision origi-nated with European conquest and subsequent capitalist development. The health care system, and the pattern and distribution of disease, closely followed and served the needs of the mining industry, which became the most prominent sector in South Africa's industrial economy.[16] European colonists repressed the indigenous black population from the beginning of their imperial project in the late seventeenth century. Then, in 1948, Afrikaners (descendants of the Dutch) established apartheid under National Party governments. Apartheid separated the population into rigid racial categories of European (white), colored (mixed race), Asian (South Asia), and Bantu (black). The categories served as the basis for subsequent dis-crimination against all nonwhites in social relations, education, employ-ment, and residency. Apartheid also profoundly shaped health policy.

The discovery of precious minerals in the mid-nineteenth century spurred South Africa's industrialization based on mining, with severe con-sequences for the indigenous population. Like the plantations before them, the profits of the mining magnates rested on a vast labor force consisting of largely black migrant workers whose pay was below subsistence levels and remained so well into the next century.[17] Tax and land ownership laws essentially pushed black men off the land and into overcrowded mining boomtowns; severe punishment of those who deserted ensured that they stayed. A capitalist economy based on mining that relied on black migrant labor undermined black family structure. Women were left to raise the children alone on the homelands or move to the cities to find work as domestic servants.[18]

South Africa's dual health care system developed in tandem with the nation's political and economic systems. Employment-based private insur-ance began in the mining sector. In 1889, mining companies began to offer coverage but only to their white employees. Employment-based insurance remained the exclusive preserve of whites until the 1970s, when health plans opened their doors to nonwhites. The first hospitals in South Africa were run by religious missionaries or were company facilities to serve only their employees. The 1980s saw the growth of private for-profit hospitals to serve those with private insurance. Hospitals located largely in white urban areas had advanced technology; indeed, the world's first heart transplant took place in Cape Town, South Africa in 1967.

A separate public health care system served the black, Asian, and mixed-race populations. White governments deliberately and systematically underfunded that system, which also suffered from fragmented admin-istration and provision of services and poor quality of care. Curative and preventive services were not integrated and different levels of government had responsibility for different types of services. At the national level, there were four health ministries, one for each racial category. Each of the 14 homelands, in turn, had its own health department. While health care spending in the richer urbanized provinces was as much as $100 per capita in 1986–1987, it stood at only $11 per capita in the poorest rural homelands.[19] Following the advent of free and fair elections in 1994 that introduced black majority rule, the ANC government consolidated the separate and uncoordinated health care systems in each homeland under a National Health Service model of administration and provision.

Historical Roots of Current Disease Patterns and Health Disparities

Health and disease are not simply the result of genetics or lifestyle; they are also socially determined. In South Africa, the particular patterns of capitalist development and systematic racism have been major contributors to health disparities between blacks and whites that persist today. An economy heavily based in mining and reliant on black migrant labor has created a causeway for the spread of infectious diseases within the black population. Black men from rural areas in South Africa, and from neighboring countries, work as migrant laborers in the mines. They are warehoused in squalid, overcrowded hostels where infectious diseases like tuberculosis can spread rapidly. Because they are also away from their families for long periods of time, it is not uncommon for them to engage in extramarital sexual relations, having both a "town wife" and a "rural wife,"[20] which allows HIV/AIDS to spread to rural areas beyond the impoverished urban neighborhoods. Gender inequality also accounts for the spread of the disease to heterosexual women. Sexual violence against women, men refusing to use condoms, and the practice of older men having younger women as their sexual partners has allowed HIV to infect women of child-bearing age.[21] Indeed, women have borne the brunt of the disease burden, with HIV prevalence among women aged 20 to 24 at 17.4 percent, compared to only 5.1 percent of males in that age group in 2012. The prevalence rate for teens and young women aged 15 to 19 was 5.6 percent, compared to 0.7 percent of male counterparts.[22] Pregnant or lactating women who have HIV, in turn, have transmitted the virus to their children[23]

The legacies of apartheid are responsible for other health problems in the black population, particularly those associated with poverty. With younger able-bodied men working in the far-off mines, women, children, the elderly, ill, and disabled remain behind in the rural areas, where poverty is the norm and sanitation and basic health facilities are lacking. Indeed, women headed more than 40 percent of black households in 2003, and single-parent households tend to be poorer than those with two wage earners. The children in these homes experience higher rates of stress, neglect, and abuse, which in turn, affect physical and emotional health.[24] The country also suffers from chronically high unemployment that began in the early 1970s and has hit the black population the hardest. South Africa's official unemployment rate stood at 23.8 percent in 1993, the last year of white minority rule, and at 25 percent in 2012. The unofficial jobless rate, which also includes those who have given up looking for work, is estimated at 33 percent.[25] Apartheid's systematic denial of education and jobs to the black majority has been the primary reason behind the unemployment statistics.

Such broader social and economic inequalities translate into severe health disparities among whites and blacks. For example, while infant mortality rates for all South Africans have improved since the advent of black majority rule, racial differences persist. In 1993, the infant mortality rate for whites was 13 per 1,000 live births; for blacks it was 130 to 1,000. The 2002 figures showed a halving of the rates for both races, but large differences remained: the infant mortality rate for whites stood at 7 per 1,000 and for blacks at 67 per 1,000. Life expectancy figures have been even more alarming. In 2002, life expectancy for black women was only half that of white women.[26]Average life expectancy for all South Africans plummeted from 62 years in 1994 to 52 years between 2004 and 2007, recovering somewhat to 57 years by 2013.[27] The averages mask stark racial differences: life expectancy for whites was 72 years but only 47 years for blacks in 2008–2009.[28] The HIV prevalence rate in South Africa in 2013 was 6.3 million or 19.1 percent of the population, down from a peak of 30.2 percent in 2005. Yet even after accounting for this improvement, South Africa has the highest HIV prevalence rate in the world.[29] Moreover, these average statistics hide the fact that such diseases have hit blacks and women hardest. In 2012, 15 percent of blacks but only 0.3 percent of whites was infected with HIV.[30]

In sum, the higher mortality and morbidity rates among the black majority testify to the effects of the long hand of history in South Africa that began with colonial rule and that continues to be felt today. The reliance on migrant labor, first in agriculture and later in mining, government policies of forced resettlement of blacks onto rural homelands and urban slums (townships), the pass laws that controlled free movement of blacks, and the systematic underfunding of education and health facilities have all been powerful social determinants of health. Since the advent of black majority rule in 1994, ANC governments have made the painful discovery that history cannot be quickly or easily reversed. Even so, apartheid is not the only explanation for these health disparities. As we will see below, the economic and health policy choices of ANC governments have also contributed to the spread of HIV/AIDS in the black population.

Nor are HIV and tuberculosis the only health problems facing South Africa. South African society also suffers from shockingly high rates of violence. This not only reflects high murder rates and violent crime, but also extremely high rates of domestic violence, with women the main victims. South Africa's injury death rate is double the global average and the murder rate of women by intimate partners is six times the global rate. These problems are rooted in widespread poverty and inequality, but also, especially in the case of domestic abuse, in patriarchal attitudes.[31] At the same time, as a middle income country, South Africa must also contend with the growth of noncommunicable diseases like heart disease, diabetes, stroke, cancer, and mental illness that are common in wealthier nations. Such diseases reflect an aging population, but also lifestyle changes, such as a diet high in fats, associated with urbanization.[32] While these are significant health challenges, this chapter's primary focus is on the health problems arising from infectious diseases and the health care system's inadequate response. Both problems are rooted in long-standing racial inequities.

Political Factors Underpinning Health Policy

Health care system structures and health policy decisions in South Africa are, as elsewhere, the product of politics. This section briefly describes the main political factors and actors that have shaped health policies in South Africa since 1994.

Parliament and Federalism

The political system of postapartheid South Africa is modeled on democratic principles. As a parliamentary democracy, the lower house, the National Assembly, is directly elected every four years on the basis of proportional representation, which yields a multiparty system. The upper house, the National Council of Provinces, is elected by the nine provincial legislatures and gives them a voice in South Africa's federal system. However, the Council's primary remit is to safeguard cultural minorities and real legislative power rests with the Assembly. The president (who is actually the prime minister notwithstanding the confusing terminology) heads the executive branch. Like prime ministers in all parliamentary systems, South Africa's president is not directly elected but instead comes from and depends on the support of the majority party in parliament.

The country's federal structure allows for significant decentralization of power to the nine provinces. The structure of the public health care system adheres to the federal political structure. The provincial governments have important responsibilities in implementing health policies set by the national Department of Health.

In an effort to break with its apartheid past, the Republic of South Africa since 1994 has been committed to the rule of law and civil liberties. The constitution adopted in 1996 recognizes the country's diversity by naming eleven official languages and contains a bill of rights. Notably, health care is a right specified in the constitution. The judiciary is generally independent and acts as a vigilant defender of the civil rights of citizens. Likewise, the media is independent and takes seriously its role to scrutinize the government and its policies.[33]

Civil Society and Political Parties

South Africa also boasts a vibrant civil society. The legacy of the antiapartheid movement, there are many NGOs and human rights groups, as well as a powerful trade union movement, the Congress of South African Trade Unions (COSATU). In health policy, the various health professions as well as private insurers have their own groups to represent their interests. Business associations and labor unions are active in health policy. Employers who provide health insurance to their workers are a force to be reckoned with in health care policy debates, particularly on questions of health care financing. NGOs like the Treatment Action Campaign (TAC) have been particularly vocal and visible in their effort to influence government AIDS policy.

But health policy is not the exclusive domain of domestic actors and interests. This is especially so in the Global South, where countries must often rely on assistance and investment from abroad. International development agencies and NGOs are often key partners with national governments in the development and implementation of heath policy. For example, the WHO and UNICEF have provided technical assistance to the ANC government in its development of policies to achieve a universal health care system. More broadly, the rules and actors of the global economy can curtail national autonomy over economic policies, which have consequences for health policy. As we shall see, ANC governments have adopted structural adjustment policies as a way to encourage foreign investment. But such economic discipline has limited the amount available for health care and social spending. Multinational corporations and the networks of NGOs spanning different nations have also been major players in South African health policy, particularly on the question of making essential medicines for AIDS treatment more affordable. Sometimes, the relationship between international actors and national policymakers is more conflictual, as with President Thabo Mbeki's disagreement with the mainstream international scientific community on the proper policy response to AIDS.

Partisan politics have also been a major force in shaping health policy. From 1948 until 1994, policies were the exclusive domain of the dominant National Party representing Afrikaner interests. With the advent of universal suffrage in 1994, the dominant party has been the African National Congress, winning every parliamentary election (and nearly all provincial elections) since then. Although a proportional representation electoral system allows smaller parties to win some seats in parliament, the party system centers on the ANC and the Democratic Alliance (DA). Because most black citizens have voted for the ANC in every national election since 1994, the party has garnered comfortable parliamentary majorities, allowing it to rule under single-party government. The Democratic Alliance, which garners about 20 percent of the vote in parliamentary elections, is the main opposition party. Although it has tried to woo black voters, it remains primarily a party of whites (British descendants as well as Afrikaners from the now defunct National Party) and other minorities. The ANC's electoral power is also buttressed by its alliance with the South African Communist Party and the trade unions. Further, the ANC has built up a formidable electoral machine at national, provincial, and local levels to campaign and get out the vote.

The electoral dominance of the ANC has been a major factor explaining the content of health policy since 1994. With such overwhelming parliamentary majorities (just shy of the two-thirds needed to alter the constitution), the legislature has been an ineffective institutional check on executive branch power. One-party dominance has sometimes encouraged the ANC leadership to be dismissive of dissenting voices within and outside the party. In office for over two decades, the ANC has increasingly exploited its powers of appointment to create a formidable network of patronage, awarding civil service jobs and public procurement contracts to party members based on loyalty. Widespread corruption has fostered incompetent governance in the public sector, which has harmed health care system performance.[34]

Competing Ideologies: White Supremacy vs
National Liberation

South African health policy has been the object of competing ideologies, that of white supremacy under apartheid, and the national liberation movement (NLM) ideology of the ANC since 1994. The ideology of white supremacy began with the advent of European colonialism and intensified under apartheid. Its residue continues to shape South African health politics and policy today. As noted above, government policies under the imperial and apartheid eras imported the racial divide into health care, creating two distinct and unequal health care systems. Much of the debate today over how to establish health equity revolves around what the size of the financial transfers from the white minority should be to meet the massive health care needs of the mostly black majority.

Aside from formal institutions, the legacies of apartheid are manifest in other ways. Postapartheid era government policies and practices, such as affirmative action programs and the national census, continue to use these racial categories to identify subgroups of the population. The racial divide has also inhabited the attitudes and identities of many policymakers and the broader public. The story of AIDS policy is illustrative. The rigid racial categories initially made it difficult for the public and policymakers to view AIDS as a national threat and instead encouraged an "us versus them" attitude in assessing who was most at risk.[35] The legacy of mistrust between whites and blacks informed, at least in part, President Mbeki's hostile response to the international scientific community over the correct response to the epidemic.

The second ideology, that of a national liberation movement, directly challenges apartheid value system and practices. The ANC's experience as a national liberation movement has shaped its worldview, creating a distinct definition of democracy and claims to legitimacy that have affected its governance of the country since 1994. The party, which was banned and its leaders imprisoned or forced into exile between 1964 and 1990, saw as its primary aim the end of white minority rule and the installation of black majority rule. In the postapartheid era this has led some ANC leaders to define democracy in majoritarian terms and ignore minority views.[36] It has also allowed leaders to dismiss minority views within the ANC itself. Mbeki's disastrous AIDS policy is one example.

To be sure, not all ANC members subscribe to this particular worldview. Antiapartheid movement leaders such as President Nelson Mandela envisioned the new postapartheid South Africa as a rainbow nation, united in its diversity.[37] Moreover, the ANC's official ideology is that of non-racialism and party membership is open to all races, even if in practice most ANC members are black. The party itself is also a broad tent, with competing factions and opinions.[38] And ANC leaders have exhibited pragmatism in office, as abandoning the party's commitment to socialism illustrates. Still, the NLM ideology remains a force within the party and explains at least some of the government's policies. And the ANC's electoral successes and effective one-party rule for over two decades have only further entrenched such attitudes.[39]

As a national liberation movement, the ANC also pledged to thoroughly "transform the state" once in power. The party not only promised to nationalize industry, but also to extend ANC control to all areas of the state bureaucracy, including the army, police, state-owned companies, and public broadcasting. Two years after taking power, the ANC retreated from its nationalization pledge and the media remains free. But the ANC has extended its power over the state by appointing party loyalists to the bureaucracy and state-owned enterprises.[40]

The NLM ideology partly explains the Mbeki government's policy of denial toward HIV/AIDS, which sidelined critical voices within and outside of the ANC. And some of the incompetent administration of the public health care system lies with the government's practice of putting party loyalty ahead of expertise in civil service. But the ANC is not solely to blame. Some of the health care system's administrative woes rest with an inferior public education system that fails to provide graduates with the managerial skills they need. Some of it rests with the superior pay and working conditions in the private health care system that the public sector health care system cannot match. Both of these latter problems are the legacies of apartheid rather than to the ANC's NLM ideology, which justifies a winner-take-all mentality.

Now that we understand the major political factors that impinge on health policy, we turn our attention to government responses to the major health policy challenges it has faced since the advent of democratic politics. The first is confronting and vanquishing infectious diseases, particularly AIDS and TB. The second challenge consists in the establishment of a comprehensive health care system that meets the needs of all South Africans, particularly mothers and children in impoverished rural areas and urban slums. This second task actually consists of two components. It requires the construction of a national delivery system rooted in primary care that also links up to specialty care when needed. And it requires equitable and sufficient financing of health care. After a disastrous start, ANC governments have begun to turn the tide on HIV/AIDS, but it would be premature to claim victory. The second task also remains unfinished, and it is much more contentious. Whereas a broad consensus now exists among South Africans on how to tackle AIDS, the country remains divided on how to finance health care in an equitable manner. But the conquest of infectious diseases ultimately hinges on the construction of a viable, health care system over the long haul, one that will provide equitable access to quality care at an affordable price to everyone, not just the well-off. Before delving into these two major challenges, we briefly summarize the ANC government's successes in health policy.

Policy Responses to Health Care
Challenges Since 1994

ANC governments have scored some notable health policy successes since coming to power. Of note is the country's acknowledgement that health care is a universal human right. The 1996 constitution explicitly enshrines access to health care as a right of all and places responsibility on governments to realize this right within its available resources.[41] In reality, heatlh care for all has not been fully achieved. But, ANC governments have committed themselves to creating a universal health care system that provides quality care in an equitable manner.

In the meantime, the government introduced a number of specific measures to address the health needs of vulnerable populations. Some have been explicit health policies, such as the elimination in 1996 of patient cost-sharing for health care for children up to age six and for pregnant women, the guarantee of free primary care for all, and the construction of over 1,300 primary care clinics.[42] Others fall under the broad umbrella of social policies that certainly affect health. Thus, households with access to sanitation rose from 50 percent in 1994 to 73 percent in 2007. Access to clean drinking water increased from 62 percent of households in 1994 to 87 percent in 2007. Electrification of households increased from 35 percent in the late 1980s to 72 percent in 2006/2007. The government also provides free water and electricity to the poorest households. The ANC has also expanded the welfare state to ameliorate the poverty of the most vulnerable. Cash grants for children, disability grants, and old-age pensions together reached 12.4 million South Africans in 2007/2008, up from only 2.4 million in 1996/1997.[43]

Still, more than twenty years after the end of the apartheid regime, the health statistics continue to tell a grim story. The mortality rate for children under five years of age has actually increased since 1990, and rates of maternal mortality have stagnated. This is in spite of the fact that women and children have access to free health care. Much of this mortality is caused by HIV/AIDS.[44] This in turn reflects severe weaknesses in the financing and delivery of care in the public health care system that serves most South Africans, as well as maldistribution of health care resources between public and private systems. The latter garners a disproportionate share of money to treat a fraction of the population that the public system serves.

In the 2011 policy paper, *National Health Insurance in South Africa*, the government acknowledged four major health burdens on the country: the HIV/AIDS and TB epidemics; high rates of maternal, infant, and child mortality; the burden of noncommunicable diseases associated with an aging population and lifestyle changes associated with urbanization, a sedentary lifestyle, and changes in diet; and high rates of injury and violence, particularly toward women and children. The government pledged to finish building a national health care system with its foundation in primary care and community services, as well as introduce a national health insurance scheme to ensure adequate financing of the needs of all South Africans.[45]

In the sections below, I analyze three of the main health policy challenges, all of which are intertwined and affect each other. The first concerns addressing the heavy burden of HIV/AIDS and TB. The second is constructing a robust health care delivery system. The third is the effort to introduce national health insurance to address the inequitable distribution of resources between the public and private health care systems.

Containing Infectious Diseases: The Scourge of HIV/AIDS & Tuberculosis

AIDS in South Africa was first reported among homosexuals in 1982. But from 1990 onwards, cases of AIDS exploded in the general population, due to heterosexual transmission. AIDS has hit the poor the, which, in South Africa, means that the mostly black population has borne the brunt of the disease. Those afflicted have not only been adult men and women, but also babies born to infected mothers. As discussed above, the migrant labor system has been a primary pathway for transmission of the disease, with male migrant laborers spreading the disease to multiple sexual partners.

South Africa also has one of the world's worst rates of tuberculosis (TB). In 2006, the country recorded 341,165 cases in a population of just over 48 million persons; only the more populous nations of China, India, and Indonesia registered higher numbers. Over half of new TB cases in South Africa have been found in patients already infected with HIV.[46] The reasons for this have to do with not only individual transmission of germs and viruses but also broader social conditions. AIDS undermines and eventually destroys the immune systems of those afflicted; hence, many AIDS victims also contract TB. The problem is aggravated by the living conditions of those with the highest rates of these diseases. Many live in overcrowded township slums or mining hostels, which are ideal for the rapid transmission of infectious disease. Migrant workers with AIDS return to their rural homelands and infect their wives, who then transmit the disease to their babies through their breast milk.

Policy Missteps and a Failure of Political Leadership

Government policies during and after apartheid also share a large part of the blame for the dual scourge of AIDS and tuberculosis. National Party governments in the apartheid era initially dismissed AIDS as a "homosexual disease," and public health campaigns failed to inform the broader population of the risks. The government also racialized its AIDS policy by creating separate AIDS programs for whites and blacks. In other words, apartheid's rigid racial categories carried over into health policy.[47]

But ANC governments since the end of the apartheid also had their share of policy failures. President Nelson Mandela (1994–1999) paid scant attention to AIDS or TB. His successor, Thabo Mbeki (1999–2008), and his health minister, Manto Tshabalala-Msimang, initially pursued a policy of misinformation on the causes and effective treatment of AIDS. The Mbeki government refused to give free antiretroviral therapy drugs (ARTs) to pregnant women with HIV, even though such treatment was highly effective at preventing the transmission of the disease to their offspring, until it lost a case before the Constitutional Court in 2001. AIDS activists brought the suit on the grounds that the government had failed to uphold the right to health care specified by the constitution. Further policy changes came in 2003, when the Mbeki government announced that free ARTs would be available for all persons who needed it. A year later, the government declared TB a national emergency and turned the WHO's treatment recommendations into a crisis plan. Yet even after the president shifted course in 2003 and declared that AIDS patients would have access to free ARTs, Tshabalala-Msimang continued to promote alternative remedies to treat and cure AIDS, such as garlic, lemons, beetroot, and vitamin supplements. Finally, in 2007, the government signaled its seriousness by adopting strategic plans to combat AIDS and TB with measures based on mainstream scientific evidence.[48]

But by then, government foot-dragging had done much damage. The government's initial delay contributed to the spread of AIDS and TB, exacting an enormous human toll: between 2000 and 2003, 330,000 people died of AIDS. The government was not solely to blame for the epidemics. The WHO's recommended treatment for TB was also at fault. It may have been cheaper than more effective alternatives, but the WHO's regimen did not help those who had developed drug-resistant strains of the disease.[49] Even so, with AIDS hitting the black community especially hard, Mbeki's stance had the perverse effect of harming his own constituents, leading to untold suffering and thousands of needless deaths.

There are several reasons behind the seemingly inexplicable policy of denial by the Mbeki government. One was that the international scientific community was not united on the cause of AIDS. Peter Duesberg, an internationally renowned molecular biologist who was among the first to discover the link between retroviruses and cancer, was one such skeptic. He argued that the lag between HIV and full-blown AIDS was too long to be explained by a virus, and maintained that recreational drugs were the real cause.[50] In 2000, Mbeki convened an advisory panel on AIDS that privileged the views of dissident scientists who denied that HIV causes AIDS. Duesberg was the head of that panel, and his views carried great weight with the president.

The Mbeki government's initial stance toward AIDS was also rooted in the deep mistrust that apartheid had engendered between blacks and whites. Just as apartheid's false ideology of racial superiority had allowed for the systematic underfunding of health care for those who were not white and had defined AIDS as a black disease, the Mbeki government's response to AIDS was shaped by its struggle against this brutally dehumanizing system and imperialism in general. Some of Mbeki's top health officials remained suspicious of the mainstream scientific community because it was largely urban, white, and Western. They viewed AIDS best practices with suspicion, akin to a new imperialism. For example, Mbeki's head of the commission on African traditional medicine, Herbert Vilakazi, was a sociologist who argued, with some truth, that Western was rooted in an ideology of white superiority that was dismissive of the knowledge of Africans and other nonwhite civilizations. His rejection of Western science and pharmacology led him to argue that ARTs were so toxic that they caused more harm than good and that traditional African remedies were equally effective in treating AIDS. Vilakazi also maintained that ARTs primarily benefited the global pharmaceutical companies that manufactured and profited from them. Mbeki and his health minister Tshabalala-Msimang pointed to apartheid's impoverishment of blacks, and publicly asserted that the poor sanitation and malnutrition that accompanied poverty, were the real cause of AIDS.[51] The president also publicly criticized what he viewed as insinuations among many whites that AIDS was simply the result of promiscuous black Africans and their depraved and inferior culture, a view that apartheid-era governments had popularized.[52] Deep-seated racial divisions had also tainted broader public views of AIDS. May whites viewed AIDS as a black or gay disease. In the black community, conspiracy theories abounded. Such accounts held that the police and National Party governments during apartheid had deliberately spread AIDS among the black populace. Blacks themselves called the disease "Afrikaner Invention to Deprive us of Sex."[53]

To be sure, there was ample historical evidence of Western science in the service of European conquest of the peoples of the Global South.[54] And there were problems with AZT, the first drug to treat AIDS. Given in excessively high doses, AZT could have toxic side effects; it could only keep the disease at bay for a short time; and the appearance of drug-resistant strains undermined the effectiveness of AZT treatment. So the suspicions of Western medicine by Mbeki and his government were not completely unfounded. But in taking their battle against white imperialism and applying it to AIDS, they ignored well-established scientific evidence on the cause and treatment of the disease. In 1996, a new class of ARTs, known as Highly Active Antiretroviral Therapy (HAART), was found to have minimal side effects and could suppress the AIDS virus and keep the immune system functioning for years.[55] This essentially transformed AIDS from a certain death sentence into a treatable chronic disease that need not sacrifice one's quality of life. However, the government did not embrace this treatment approach until 2003, and only after significant pressure from AIDS activists. Another factor hindering an effective government response was the international pharmaceutical companies' exorbitant prices for ARTs, which had placed these life-saving drugs out of reach for many developing countries. Even so, some developing countries like Brazil had found ways to get around this barrier as early as 1996, albeit only after a protracted fight with the drug industry.[56]

Changing Course: The Role of Civil Society and International Institutions

The Mbeki government's refusal to come to grips with AIDS met with vocal opposition from a range of AIDS activists, NGOs, and the mainstream scientific community, both within and outside of South Africa. The government was an opponent of rather than a partner to these groups, at least initially. At the 2000 International AIDS Conference (ironically held in Durban, South Africa), over 5,000 researchers issued the Durban Declaration, which stated unequivocally that HIV caused AIDS. The South African health minister rejected the declaration, calling it elitist.[57] But civil society, already mobilized, continued to ratchet up the pressure in the face of government intransigence. The AIDS movement coalesced around the Treatment Action Campaign (TAC). Founded in 1998 by Zackie Achmat and Marky Heywood, two members of the ANC and activists in the struggle against apartheid, TAC is a broad-based organization that includes as its members religious organizations, labor unions, health care professionals, the young, the poor, and women. While it seeks to bridge racial divisions, its members are mostly black, which is not surprising given that blacks have the highest rate of HIV prevalence in South Africa. Like the antiapartheid movement before it, TAC employed a range of tactics to combat political inaction on AIDS. The organization aimed "'to challenge by means of litigation, lobbying, advocacy, and all forms of legitimate mobilization, any barrier or obstacle, including unfair discrimination, that limits access to treatment for HIV/AIDS in the private or public sector.'"[58] TAC engaged in massive demonstrations and civil disobedience to put pressure on South African politicians to make ARTs available to all, free of charge, through the public health care system. TAC also provided health education about the transmission and prevention of AIDS and offered small ART treatment programs to its members. It also forged alliances with AIDS activists in other countries.[59] AIDS activists in South Africa used the courts to challenge government policies, such as the 2001 case in which the Constitutional Court ordered the Mbeki government to provide free ART treatment to all pregnant mothers.

By the beginning of the twenty-first century, the fight against AIDS had become a global social movement, and TAC found allies at the international level. An array of organizations engaged in coordinated lobbying and advocacy aimed at changing the practices of Western governments, international organizations, and drug companies. Among the most prominent umbrella associations were DATA (Debt, AIDS, Trade, and Africa) and the Global AIDS Alliance. The AIDS lobby was remarkably diverse, ranging from health and social care providers, patients living with AIDS, grassroots organizations, global NGOs like Doctors Without Borders and its Campaign for Essential Medicines, philanthropists like Bill and Melinda Gates, even rock stars (U2's Bono) and evangelical Christians. They sought increased funding for HIV/AIDS prevention and treatment, and improved access to affordable ARTs in the poorest nations with the highest disease burden. Their targets were not only governments and their various summits, but also the pharmaceutical industry that owned the patents on ARTs.

South Africa's AIDS policy, then, was not exclusively a national concern but was subject to international law and global actors. On the legal front, the most significant developments have concerned changes to the Trade Related Aspects of Intellectual Property Rights (TRIPS) agreement. Members of the World Trade Organization (WTO) had concluded the agreement in 1995. TRIPS protects copyrights and patents for a minimum of twenty years and imposes substantial penalties on nations that violate its terms. However, TRIPS contains escape clauses allowing countries to bypass patent protection on essential medicines in the event of a public health emergency. Specifically, if a nation declared a public health emergency, it could now either manufacture cheaper generic equivalents (compulsory licensing) or import them from manufacturers in other countries (parallel importation). In 1997 the ANC government passed the Medicines and Related Substances Amendment Act empowering the health minister to issue compulsory licensing of cheaper generic equivalents or to import them from producers in India and Brazil. Access to affordable drugs was vital to South Africa's ability to provide free ARTs to those who needed them.

The South African government experienced intense cross-pressures. On the one side from pharmaceutical companies and from the governments of Western nations where many of them were headquartered. In fact, the US government put the squeeze on the South African government by imposing trade sanctions as a way to get the law repealed. But on the other side was the array of AIDS advocacy groups not only pushing for the Mbeki government to do more to make treatment available to those with the disease but also pressuring the US government. Their persistence led President Bill Clinton to reverse course, lift the sanctions and publicly express support for free ARTs in Africa. Thirty-seven South African pharmaceutical companies also challenged the constitutionality of the 1997 law. But the case served as a public platform for AIDS activists to confront the pharmaceutical industry, with great effect. AIDS activists organized public demonstrations outside the courtroom and shamed the drug companies by displaying placards of dying victims. Hoping to restore their reputations, the drug companies dropped the suit in 2001 and covered the government's legal costs.[60]

Successive declarations by the WTO have clarified and strengthened the rights of developing nations to bypass patents in health emergencies. The 2001 Doha Declaration on TRIPS and Public Health was an important step forward. It admonished the WTO to take seriously the public health problems posed by epidemics such as HIV/AIDS, TB, and malaria; declared that protection had to be balanced against affordability of critical medicines; and asserted that each country had the right to define a national emergency and to issue compulsory licensing. In 2003, the WTO further strengthened the hand of developing nations in securing access to affordable essential medicines. Known as the WTO Decision on Paragraph 6 (of the previous Doha Declaration), the decision permitted countries to manufacture patented medicines under compulsory license not simply for their own population, but also for export to countries that did not have such capacity. This decision greatly improved access to such medicines in the poorest nations and represented a victory of developing nations against the international pharmaceutical companies and the Western governments that supported them. Prominent AIDS organizations allied with developing nation governments were also critical to this victory.

Even with this decision, developing countries may still face obstacles in their quest to obtain affordable life-saving drugs. This is because bilateral agreements between two countries bypass the WTO and its TRIPS provisions.[61] Still, the price of ARTs has fallen dramatically, primarily due to the widespread availability of generics but also because pharmaceutical companies have agreed to negotiate price discounts with developing countries. The cost of HAART in developing nations was $10,000 to $15,000 per patient per year in the late 1990s; by 2007, the figure had plummeted to a mere $87.[62]

The sustained efforts by activists, developing nation governments, and the scientific community also paid off in the form of new funding sources for treatments of AIDS. The developed nations launched the Global Fund to Fight AIDS, Tuberculosis, and Malaria in 2001. In the United States, Republican President George Bush and Congress established the President's Emergency Plan for AIDS Relief (PEPFAR), and authorized $15 billion over five years. At the international level, UNAIDS is a body that coordinates the actions of UN agencies and national governments on AIDS policies. The WHO has come to recognize that best practice for HIV/AIDS is not prevention alone, but prevention plus treatment. This dual approach has proven to be both clinically and cost effective. ART treatment of those infected with HIV reduces the level of the virus; the weakened virus is less easily transmitted to other adults and to children. It also reduces the likelihood of developing TB and other predatory diseases associated with a compromised immune system.[63]

The changing environment altered the Mbeki government's calculations and its AIDS policy. Under growing pressure from a network of AIDS activists at home and abroad, constitutional court rulings ordering the government to make ART treatment available to those who needed it, and WTO rulings that recognized the government's legal authority to produce or import affordable drug treatments, Mbeki reversed AIDS policy. In 2003, his government announced that all pregnant women who tested positive for HIV would have access to free ARTs. In 2007, with the input of the scientific community and AIDS activists, it adopted separate evidence-based national plans to combat AIDS and TB. The strategic plan for AIDS encompassed prevention, treatment, respect for human rights, and encouragement of research and aimed to cut HIV rates by half and start ART in 80 percent of those who needed it. The TB program gave priority to treating comorbid HIV and TB and multiple drug resistant tuberculosis (MDRTB), containing and preventing new infections, and encouraging more research. The country has received much-needed funding from PEPFAR and the Global Fund to implement both strategic plans. South Africa's contribution is substantial, with domestic public sources comprising over 75 percent of the funding of its HIV programs.[64] President Jacob Zuma (2009–present) has continued the new AIDS policy approach. Although Zuma was initially cavalier in his public statements on AIDS, he has since been tested for the disease and has urged other citizens to do the same. In 2010, he also announced government initiatives to expand a campaign for HIV testing and counseling.[65]

The policy shift has begun to make a difference, albeit slowly. According to UNAIDS, South Africa's HIV prevalence rate in 2013 was 6.3 million persons, or 19.1 percent for adults between the ages of 15 and 49. Over half of those living with HIV, or 3.5 million, were women. In that year, 200,000 persons died of AIDS-related causes. Tuberculosis rates closely mirrored HIV rates. From a low of 289 per 100,000 people in 1994, new TB cases rose to 585 per 100,000 in 2000 and peaked at 977 per 100,000 in 2008. AIDS and TB still overwhelmingly afflict those who are black, female, and poor.[66]

These figures, while staggering, are better than at first glance. The rising HIV prevalence rate can be explained by the fact that more people are receiving treatment and living longer than in the past. In just three years, the number of AIDS-related deaths had been halved, from 410,000 in 2010 to 200,000 in 2013. Although South Africa has not attained its 2007 goal to achieve 80 percent HAART coverage in five years, more than 60 percent of those with AIDS were receiving ARTs in 2011. New cases of HIV infection had fallen from an annual peak of 720,000 in 1999 to 340,000 in 2013. The incidence of new TB cases had declined to 860 per 100,000 in 2013. South Africa has also made major strides in addressing HIV in mothers and children, achieving more than 75 percent coverage in services to prevent the transmission from mother to child in 2011. New infections in children dropped sharply from 76,000 cases in 2005 to 16,000 in 2013. In 2012, the government embarked upon an integrated five-year plan to address HIV, TB, and other sexually transmitted diseases.[67] This coordinated strategy should be more effective than separate plans for the different diseases that often occur together. In sum, South Africa has made significant progress since 2007. But caring for those with HIV/AIDS and TB will impose high costs on the health care system for many years to come and will reduce resources available for other health needs.

Addressing Health Care Delivery System Shortcomings

Structural deficiencies in the public sector health care system pose a second major challenge for policymakers. And this problem is inextricably intertwined with the first challenge just discussed. Absent an efficient, effective, and comprehensive health care delivery system that meets the needs of all South Africans, particularly the impoverished black majority that bears the burden of infectious disease, it will be difficult to bring AIDS and TB under control.

Since coming to power, ANC governments have articulated sound policies aimed at constructing a coordinated, comprehensive health care system that brings affordable quality care to all. In its 1994 document, *A National Health Plan for South Africa*, the ANC government followed Britain's National Health Service (NHS) as a model for its public sector health care system. As in Britain, health care is tax-financed, directly provided by government, and administered by managers in a hierarchical structure. The ANC also adopted the standards set out by the WHO emphasizing primary care. The structure of the public system is tiered. At the apex is the Department of Health at national level. It is responsible to set health policy nationally. At the provincial level there are nine departments of health. At the local level, community health services are responsible for health promotion and prevention, while nurse-run clinics provide primary care. Hospital services also adhere to this hierarchical structure. District hospitals provide general inpatient care at the local level, with regional hospital and then tertiary hospitals providing more specialized hospital care.

But in practice, the health care system does not run as smoothly as the blueprint would imply. Some of the difficulty lies with introducing a hierarchical health system into a country with a federal political structure. Not surprisingly, confusion has followed. Lines of authority and definition of responsibilities between different levels of administrative entities (national, regional, and district) and between these entities and elected provincial and local governments remain murky. Provincial and local governments on the one hand, and health authorities on the other, are competitors as much as collaborators in determining and implementing health policy. The National Health Act of 2004 sought to define responsibilities more clearly. But in placing responsibility for primary care and district health services with the provincial authorities, it perhaps unwittingly undermined the authority and diminished the role of district authorities. The system also suffers from insufficient input from local citizens on health policy decisions.[68]

The federal health ministry has outlined sound policies, but in many cases these do not translate into effective implementation on the ground. Much of the failure lies with severe shortages of health care providers and facilities, as well as underdeveloped data and communications systems, and a lack of follow-through on protocols. Attracted to better pay in the private sector, there are too few doctors and nurses working in the public system. The same is true for management, which also suffers from insufficient training. As a consequence, district management teams, which are supposed to be the linchpin of the health care system, remain undeveloped. These delivery system failures have resulted in many preventable deaths, particularly among mothers and children. An example of this is the insufficient reach of postnatal care, which reaches only 10 percent of mothers and babies. This dismal figure, in turn, stems from a lack of coordinated care between clinics and mothers after birth. Let us trace the process. While most women give birth in either a clinic or hospital, they are often discharged six hours following a routine delivery, due to a shortage of beds in the facility. The expectation is that they will receive the necessary follow-up care in three days, but this often does not happen because clinics lack both the staff to do home visits and a communication system with the hospital to inform them when the mother has been discharged. Yet the three days following birth is a vital window: it is when maternal and infant mortality is most likely to occur. And it is also the time when new mothers need information on proper feeding choices to ensure good nutrition and to prevent transmission of HIV to their babies.[69]

In short, many maternal and infant deaths could be reduced if a better care system was in place. One possible solution to the lack of sufficient workforce is to have community health workers do the home visits and serve as a liaison between mothers and the clinics. Community health workers are local residents, and may even be family members or friends of patients, who are trained in basic primary and preventive care and who link medical treatment in facilities to care in the home and community. Because they are local residents, they understand the conditions in which patients live. As locals, they are known to the patients they serve, making them better able to forge a relationship of trust with their patients than a foreign aid worker might. By doing home visits, they can identify people who are ill and arrange to get them to a clinic. They may also address health needs that arise from social conditions, bringing nutritional supplements to patients to combat malnutrition arising from poverty. Community health workers are an inexpensive yet effective way to address the broader social as well as individual medical determinants of health.[70]

The policy challenge, then, is to follow through on the commitment to build a health care system throughout the country that gives primary and preventive care priority and, integrates medical and community care, and addresses the social determinants of health. This requires, first, not only more doctors, nurses, and mid-level health care providers, but also their better geographical distribution to underserved areas. Toward that end, the government has introduced loan forgiveness and training programs.[71] Second, the health system needs to shift resources away from tertiary hospital care in the larger urban areas to hospitals, clinics, and community interventions in poorer rural areas. Third, the government must improve administrative capacity at all levels, including communications and patient records systems as well as the training of managers. Fourth, better cooperation and coordination of the public health care system with nongovernmental organizations, both local and international, is needed. For example, community health workers can deliver much-needed primary and preventive care at a lower cost than clinic-based care by doctors or nurses. Yet many community health workers are employed by NGOs and their work is not well coordinated with public providers.[72]

Finally, policymakers must integrate the work of the health care system with other sectors if they are to improve overall health. This requires not only better integration of the health care and social services systems at local and provincial level, but a readiness on the part of the government to address the broader social determinants of health and illness that arise from poverty, unemployment, domestic violence, and a labor migration system that fuels the spread of HIV. These kinds of policy interventions must extend beyond the health care system to education, employment, and social welfare policies at all levels.[73] The government has made substantial strides in reducing poverty through its social grants cash programs to the elderly and disabled. But it must do more to improve education and job readiness. Indeed, the lack of improvement in education and unemployment has led many to question whether the government's economic strategy is part of the problem or the solution.[74] Some also question whether the government has done enough to alter the maldistribution of wealth and opportunity that dates from the apartheid era.[75] This is a larger political debate over the roles and responsibilities of domestic and international economic actors and has engendered opposition from within and outside the ANC itself. It is addressed in detail later in the chapter.

Achieving Equitable Health Care Financing

Many of the health policy challenges discussed thus far reflect pervasive inequities in resources between the public and private health care systems, which in turn reflects broader inequalities in wealth and opportunity in South African society. Redressing the disparities between the private and public health care systems has been a primary policy aim for the ANC. In its 1994 *A National Health Plan for South Africa*, the ANC called for the establishment of a broad-based commission of national inquiry to study the feasibility of national health insurance (NHI) and to "undertake detailed planning for implementation of an NHI if there is sufficient consensus on this option."[76] The commission had to consider several different models of national insurance, from a single-payer scheme administered by either the government or private actors, to building on the existing system of private health insurance schemes and improving risk pooling among them.

This is not the first time that national health insurance has been on the political agenda in South Africa.[77] Governments before and during the apartheid era had considered such proposals. In 1928 and again in 1935, government commissions recommended NHI for urban workers in formal sector employment, but policymakers did not act on them. The National Health Service Commission of 1942–1944 (popularly known as the Gluckman Commission after the physician who chaired it) called for universal health care financed by taxes and based in primary care health centers. The government established 44 such centers, but these were abolished by the National Party after it came to power in 1948.

The end of apartheid and the election victory of the ANC in 1994 brought the question of national health insurance back onto the political agenda. In that year, the ANC-led government resurrected the Gluckman Commission's primary care health center model and made it the cornerstone of the public health care system as outlined in *A National Health Plan for South Africa*. Serious discussion on health care financing reform also began anew. In 1994 and 1995, two government commissions recommended compulsory private insurance, initially for those in formal sector work, but eventually expanding it to other segments of the population. Under these proposals insurance would be provided through work and financed primarily from payroll contributions, and private insurers would become the main vehicles for expanding coverage. Providers could operate in either the public or private sector. In 2002, a commission of inquiry added a proposal to establish a tax-financed national health fund to channel resources to cash-starved public facilities through the annual government budget process. At this point then, South Africa might have adopted a model looking much like the Patient Protection and Affordable Care Act in the United States. There, for-profit private insurance provides the bulk of coverage but operates under a regulatory framework requiring community-rated premiums and risk-adjusted payments among insurers. The government provides separate tax-financed coverage for the poor. The mixed system of public and private providers also remains in place.

However, many in the ANC were not enthusiastic about this model. At its party conference in Polokwane in 2007, the ANC called instead for the adoption of a single-payer national health insurance scheme. This became the basis of the 2011 policy discussion paper, *National Health Insurance in South Africa*.

National Health Insurance in South Africa: The 2011 Plan[78]

Ostensibly a discussion paper, the government has made it clear that it is moving forward with *National Health Insurance in South Africa*. Toward that end, it established pilot projects beginning in 2013. But important questions, particularly on financing health care, are not yet settled. As we shall see below, the document is a work in progress.

For the ANC, single-payer NHI is the solution to many of the flaws of the current dual health care system. Yet the 2011 document not only addresses the issue of health care financing but also proposes measures to improve the delivery of services. The discussion paper and its allies say that NHI will bring universal coverage and ensure an adequate funding stream to achieve this goal. NHI will also rectify the severe imbalances between the public and private health care systems and bring much-needed resources to the public system that serves the vast majority of South Africans through financial transfers from the privileged minority who enjoy private insurance and private medicine. NHI will also address the major flaws in private insurance, particularly the fragmentation crated by multiple insurers, which undermines risk pooling and results in substantial out-of-pocket costs borne by members. NHI will also wean the private system from its overreliance on specialization, hospital care, and fee-for-service reimbursement, all of which have made private health care far more expensive than public sector care.

The 2011 *National Health Insurance in South Africa* document lays out the fundamental principles underpinning the future NHI system: a *universal right* to health care that the government will guarantee; *social solidarity*, which justifies cross-subsidy from rich to poor and healthy to the sick; *effective* care, which necessitates evidence-based treatments; *appropriateness* of care, especially tailored to local needs; *equity*, which requires the elimination of financial and other barriers to care for the most vulnerable; *affordability* of services, which recognizes that health care is a public good, not simply a commodity, and therefore must be affordably priced so as to be widely available; and *efficiency* in administration. Achieving these principles requires a national health insurance system that provides universal *access* to quality care; pools risks among insurers through the creation of a single fund; relies on a single payer possessing the requisite market power to procure affordable services for the entire population; and strengthens the public sector health care system by providing it with adequate resources.[79]

At less than 60 pages, the document is not a detailed plan for health system transformation. It does, however, set out the core ideas of the government's vision. On the delivery side, it reiterates the need for a primary care focused health care system and lists specific measures to strengthen primary care. An important innovation here is the creation of district clinical specialist support teams, comprised of an obstetrician/gynecologist, pediatrician, family practitioner, anesthesiologist, midwife, and nurse, which will work in localities with the highest disease burdens. The teams will focus on reducing maternal and child mortality rates. They will also serve to better coordinate primary care with hospital-based specialty care. Another innovation is the creation of primary health care agents, i.e., community health workers, at ward level to work with families and communities at risk of illness. In addition, on-site health services will be established in the poorest schools. To ensure locally appropriate services, district health authorities will be given the responsibility to plan and purchase health services for a given population and will be independent of the providers. District health authorities will be able to purchase services from public and private providers. The existing structure of tiered hospitals will remain, with more complex services provided at successively higher levels.[80]

To restrain medical inflation and unnecessary provision of services, provider reimbursement will move away from fee-for-service. Primary care providers will receive capitation along with performance-related payments. Hospitals will initially receive global budgets but will transition to diagnosis-related groups (DRGs) i.e., lump-sum payments per diagnosis.

To ensure universal access to quality care, national health insurance provide a minimum benefits package of medically necessary services. NHI will be compulsory for all South African citizens and legal permanent residents. To ensure adequate financing, the government plans major changes that will affect the private sector. The government has stated that private sector insurance will exist alongside NHI, but will repeal the tax subsidies that those with private insurance have enjoyed up to now. Faced with the loss of tax subsidies for private insurance, most of those privately insured will likely opt for cheaper NHI coverage instead. Those who choose to continue with private coverage will have to pay some form of tax to help finance NHI.

At the apex of the public system, the document proposes a single-payer National Health Insurance Fund. This will be a public entity with subnational branches that will negotiate contracts with health care providers. If implemented as planned, it will have significant assets to control costs. As a single-payer government insurance plan, the fund will possess monopsony power to negotiate lower prices from health care providers. As a nonprofit plan, it will have lower administrative costs than private insurers and will not have to worry about paying out dividends to shareholders.[81]

Still, the government could not ignore the reality of the existing private sector of insurers and providers. This has required the ANC to consider other forms of universal coverage, even though the government prefers the single-payer model and stated so publicly in 2011. To reassure the private sector, the plan permits the exploration of universal coverage through a social insurance system (SHI) with multiple insurers.[82] If multiple insurers are allowed, the central fund presumably will administer a system of risk-adjusted payments among them, as in Germany.[83] Since most practitioners are in private employment, the plan will allow them to continue to treat patients with privte insurance as well as those with SHI or NHI coverage as long as an independent body, the Office of Health Standards Compliance (OHSC), accredits them.[84]

Constructing the National Health Insurance
System: Developments thus Far

The 2011 document sets out a timetable to introduce the new health care system over a 14-year period, from 2011 to 2025. During that time, different elements of the system will be piloted through demonstration projects. A white paper, which will set out the final proposals and serve as the basis of legislation, is supposed to follow a period of consultation with all health care stakeholders. Given the ANC's large parliamentary majority, the legislation is likely to pass.

However, the policymaking process has been anything but smooth and the timetable has not always been followed. In April 2011, the Department of Health established 11 pilot districts in the poorest communities and in all of South Africa's provinces. Between 2011 and 2013, the health minster met with more than 15,300 stakeholders in the pilot districts. The department also hosted an international conference to explore models of universal coverage existing in other nations.[85] However, the white paper, which was supposed to be published in 2013, has yet to be released. Some of the delays in meeting the timetable stem from technical issues, but many of them are political.

The reaction to the 2011 plan has been decidedly mixed. While the ANC's allies, such as the TAC and the trade unions, supported the general direction of reforms, other actors were critical. Stakeholders across the political spectrum expressed support for the basic principles contained in the document regarding the need for universal access to quality and affordable care. But criticism has centered on the consultation process and the specific content of the paper. The Helen Suzman Foundation, a prominent human rights organization, expressed concern over the lack of transparency and inclusion in the development of the plan. Instead of following the usual procedure of appointing a broad-based commission of inquiry to develop policy recommendations, the ANC had formulated its proposals behind closed doors in the four years after its 2007 Polokwane declaration. After the document was released, the government initially allowed only a two-month period for public comment, which many considered far too brief for a policy change of this magnitude. Although the Foundation was satisfied with the government's extension of the consultation period to four months, it insisted that the plan should be viewed as a starting point for further discussion rather than an agreed-upon endpoint requiring only minor changes. The foundation also criticized the compressed legislative timetable and argued that a much longer consultation period involving the broader public and key stakeholders would be prudent.[86]

The content of the 2011 paper, as well as the process of its development, raised the hackles of many stakeholders. The Helen Suzman Foundation charged that the ANC's plans were too centralized and violated the constitutional authority and powers of provincial governments. It questioned whether single-payer NHI would address the problems of quality care and argued for reform of the public sector health care delivery system instead. Specifically, policymakers had to address the public system's inefficiencies, lack of accountability, and poor management. The foundation held that private health insurance and private providers should be preserved but called for better coordination between the two as the foundation for universal coverage.[87]

Academic experts in public sector management, such as Alex van den Heever, found the plans flawed. In his critique, van den Heever took issue with the data for its mistakes, vagueness, and inattention to the technical challenges involved. He viewed the document as scapegoating the private health care system for all of South Africa's health care problems. He rejected single-payer NHI, and warned that the government's plans to remove tax subsidies for private coverage would trigger a mass exodus out of private insurance and overwhelm the public system. van den Heever recommended preserving both the private and public systems but called for reforms in each sector. For the private sector, better regulation and risk pooling were in order. For the public sector, the solution was more public spending and eliminating patronage and resultant inefficiency. Toward that end, he urged a truly independent OHSC, maintenance of provincial responsibility for health care provision, and the strengthening of the capacity of district level providers. Like the Helen Suzman Foundation, van den Heever viewed the paper's proposals for centralized administration of NHI as an unconstitutional encroachment on provincial government powers.[88]

Private providers also took a dim view of single-payer NHI. The South African Private Practitioner Forum, which represented specialists, argued that the private sector health care served as a safety valve for unmet need that an overstretched public sector could not provide, and that the higher pay prevented doctors from leaving the country. The group called for public sector reform, such as multispecialty polyclinics, better pay to attract primary care doctors to rural areas, and improved management. It also contended that the country's deep poverty would not provide sufficient tax base to finance NHI. The forum instead proposed compulsory social insurance for those in formal employment and continuation of the separate tax-financed public system for the poor.[89] The South African Medical Association worried about physician reimbursement and wanted to preserve fee-for-service in some form.[90] Discovery Health, a for-profit company specializing in health care administration, called for public–private partnerships and a system of multiple insurers rather than a single-payer model, and offered its services in this regard.[91]

Other private sector health providers said much of the same and recognized opportunities for partnering with the public sector.[92]

In the government's defense, it should be pointed out that the plan did outline proposals for reform of the public sector delivery system that envisioned more autonomy down to district level. And the Department of Health has forged ahead to implement improvements in the health care delivery system. According to the Department of Health, by 2013 one-quarter of 40,000 community health workers had received training in the community-oriented primary care approach. The national and provincial governments were upgrading and constructing new health facilities, training more doctors and nurses, and recruiting specialist physicians from Cuba and the United Kingdom. The WHO was assisting the government in devising training programs and standards for managers. However, significant work still remained in the development of information technology and electronic medical records.[93] And there were still too few doctors working in the public sector. By 2014, 56.4 percent of the positions on district clinical specialist support teams had been filled, with over 80 percent of pediatric nurse and midwife staff hired. But the teams had hired only half of the needed specialist physicians.[94]

The basic questions centering on the financing NHI and the future of private medicine remain unsettled. They raise issues of sufficiency and equity. The Treasury Department has considered payroll tax contributions by employers and employees, increased sales tax (value-added tax), an income tax surcharge, or some combination of all of these. This question has been at the heart of the health care reform debate. As the WHO and Oxfam have recognized, payroll-tax financing is not a sufficient basis for universal health insurance in developing nations. Payroll taxes can cover (most of) the health care costs of those in formal employment, but they would have to be very high to cover the health care costs of the entire population, including those in informal work as well as the unemployed. Those who work in the informal sector are paid "under the table" and do not contribute to payroll taxes. In South Africa, the informal sector comprised 2,205,000 persons, or 16.2 percent of the labor force in 2012. Broad unemployment, which includes the jobless who are actively seeking work, and the long-term unemployed who have given up looking for work ("discouraged workers"), stood at 33.2 percent in 2012.[95] Limiting NHI to those in formal sector employment paying payroll taxes will therefore exclude a sizeable portion of the population. Private sector insurance, which covers only 16 percent of the population, may be too small to spread risks adequately. In any case, confining risk adjustment to the private sector, which some critics of single-payer NHI have proposed, does not pool risks across the population as a whole, the vast majority of whom are uninsured.[96]

General tax revenues will likely have to be the major source of funding for NHI. These could take the form of either income taxes, or indirect taxes levied on the purchase of goods and services, such as sales or value-added taxes, or gas taxes. The government has stated that the bulk of financing will come from general taxes, and that these will be progressively levied on income. But since the rich and middle class comprise a small proportion of the population, income taxes alone may not suffice. Sales (or value-added) taxes may also be needed. Sales taxes are somewhat regressive, since all who purchase goods and services must pay the tax, regardless of their income. And through such indirect taxes all contribute to NHI, even those on low incomes and in the informal sector. This regressivity is offset by the fact that sales taxes would capture more revenue from higher priced goods that the wealthy are likelier to buy. The government expects a likely combination of general tax revenues, employer and employee payroll contributions to finance NHI in South Africa.[97]

Certainly, the charges of mismanagement and corruption in the public sector are warranted and serious. But even if the government adopts sensible measures to combat corruption that many experts and stakeholders have offered, it is unclear whether that will be enough to rectify decades of inequality that plague health care and the broader society today. Put another way, does South Africa, as a developing country, lack the tax base to expand coverage? Or is the problem insufficient distribution of resources between the publicly and privately insured? South Africa spends 8.9 percent of its GDP and $1,221 per capita on health care. These are not trifling amounts. Still, measured as a share of the national budget, South Africa may be spending too little. Health comprises 11.5 percent of the national budget, well below the 15 percent target that the country and other African governments agreed to in 2001 and that the WHO recommends.[98]

If the country's health care problems are caused by a combination of poverty, corruption, and a severe imbalance between the private and public sectors, then effective solutions must be multifaceted. Redistribution from private to public health care could be financial transfers as well as coordination and sharing of facilities and personnel. And until the country achieves better growth, South Africa will probably continue to need outside aid from international organizations and donors in the medium term. The government must continue to hire and retain sufficient health care workers, and improve management and coordination within the public sector health care system. Again, the private sector and international actors can lend funds, personnel, and technical assistance. But the ANC must also stop its practices of patronage and corruption in the public sector.

The issue of government corruption, and their effects on health policy, are discussed in the next section.

Broader Political Challenges: ANC Governance

The challenges facing the public sector health care system, and the relatively slow gains of health policy, in part lie with broader economic and social problems that together work in a vicious circle. Policies designed to spur economic growth and investment have met their aims. But economic growth has not been high enough to provide the necessary tax revenues to fund social spending that would reduce health disparities. Moreover, economic policies have unwittingly increased unemployment and inequality, which are then responsible for a host of illnesses. Whether the blame lies with the government's economic strategy, its incompetence and corruption in office, the magnitude of inequality bequeathed by apartheid, or some combination of these factors, is the topic of fierce debate. While a definitive answer to this question is beyond the scope of this book, we can briefly consider these arguments and their implications for health policy.

The Contradictions of Growth, Employment, and Redistribution (GEAR)

Some of the health care challenges in South Africa stem from the contradictions of economic and social policies that ANC governments have pursued. As a national liberation movement, the ANC, along with its Communist Party and trade union partners, was committed to ending white oppression in both the political and economic realms. Universal suffrage and the repeal of apartheid-era laws were the means to achieve political equality. An ambitious economic program of socialism, including nationalization of key industries and comprehensive land reform, was to be the means to reverse the inequities of colonial capitalism. Upon coming to power, however, pragmatists within the ANC prevailed upon the party to reverse course on the economic front. The party adopted a new strategy, termed Growth, Employment, and Redistribution (GEAR), whereby it renounced socialism and accepted capitalism and private property, but with conditions. The ANC would deploy legal and gradual means to achieve economic and social equality within the capitalist framework. The chief policy instruments were affirmative action programs (termed black economic empowerment) for blacks in both the public and private sectors, legal land transfers to black farmers with compensation to white farmers, and government spending on human capital investments in the areas of education, health, and social services. GEAR also committed the government to adopt structural adjustment policies to encourage foreign investment and economic growth and thereby reverse the international ostracism and sanctions that the country had experienced during the apartheid era.[99] The government gave priority to reducing inflation and eliminating its budget deficit and debt.

GEAR has registered some impressive results. The government transformed the apartheid-era budget deficit into a surplus by 2007, the first since the 1950s, and nearly halved the country's debt from 45 percent of GDP to 25.5 percent in 2008.[100] It has used tax revenues to finance expansions in health, education, and social services, to provide free water and electricity to the poorest, and has made health care for children free at the point of service. Taking account of taxes, cash transfers, and direct services, government policies have reduced the share of those in extreme poverty (living on less than $1.25 a day) from 34.4 percent to 16.6 percent of the population, and those in moderate poverty (living on less than $2.50 a day) from 46.2 percent to 39 percent of the population in 2011. Expenditures on social programs in 2011 amounted to 17.6 percent of GDP, which represented a little more than half of the government budget. Those receiving social grants have risen from 8 million in 2003–2004 to more than 15.8 million persons in 2013–2014. Cash grants to children and the elderly have been extremely effective in reducing poverty.[101] The public and private sectors have also introduced a range of affirmative action programs that have led to the emergence of a nascent black middle class.

But disappointments persist. South Africa's economic growth rate was below that of peer middle-income nations like China and India even before the onset of the recession in 2008, which has made matters worse. Since 2011, the country's economic output actually declined and is only expected to rebound to 2.5 percent in 2015. The slower economic growth has further pushed up broad unemployment, which surpassed over 30 percent of the workforce in 2009 and has remained stuck at that level. The recession wiped out the gains in government accounts: the deficit now stands at 4 percent of GDP and debt at 40 percent of GDP. Yet the Zuma government has stuck to GEAR's commitments to inflation and budgetary control by raising taxes and cutting spending. The austerity policies and recent budget deficits and debt have constrained the capacity of fiscal policy to reduce inequality and poverty.[102]

Poverty and inequality in South Africa remain among the highest in the world. Even with the help of social programs, 39 percent of the population lives in poverty, as measured as less than $2.50 a day. Also troubling, income inequality has worsened since 1994. Some of this is due to the success of government affirmative action policies and the creation of a black middle class, which has raised incomes at the top but has been too limited to pull up those at the bottom. The GINI coefficient, a key measurement of income inequality, ranges from absolute equality (a score of 0) to absolute inequality (a score of 1). South Africa's GINI coefficient drops from 0.77 to 0.59 if government cash programs and in-kind services are included. Still, it stands at one of the highest in the world. Even after the effects of social spending and taxes are included, the incomes of the richest 10 percent of the population are 66 times higher than the poorest 10 percent. The richest 20 percent consume 61.2 percent of the nation's wealth while the poorest 20 percent consume only 4.3 percent.[103] In a country of roughly 53 million people a black middle class of 6 million persons counting dependents, remains small.[104] Educational inequities persist and continue to hold back economic opportunities for most black South Africans. Of those employed at the end of 2014, 45.4 percent of whites but only 16.4 percent of blacks had earned a college degree, and more than half of blacks and coloreds had not finished high school. Over 60 percent of white men but only 14.7 percent of their black counterparts had employment in skilled occupations; black men were concentrated in semi-skilled occupations and black women in unskilled work.[105] As Allister Sparks has so eloquently put it, South Africa under apartheid resembled a double-decker bus. The upper level, representing the advanced formal sector of the economy, was for whites only and had many empty seats. The lower level was reserved for blacks and nonwhites and was standing room only. GEAR has allowed a black middle class to join the upper level, but plenty of open seats remain. Meanwhile, the lower level is still black and overcrowded. Many of the passengers in the lower deck are entrepreneurial and hardworking but earn very low incomes because they are employed in the informal sector.[106]

Who or what should bear the blame for the country's continuing problems? There is no agreement on this point. Some critics argue that GEAR has worsened the plight of blacks. Opening the South African economy to global competition has led to mass unemployment particularly in industry and mining, and has swelled the ranks of the informal low-paid sector. Others blame the sheer enormity of inequality that apartheid bequeathed to the country, which has resulted in inferior education and public health systems. Middle-class whites and blacks flee the public education system for private schools charging high tuition. The high mortality rates of women and children not only reflect the ravages of the AIDS and TB epidemics, but also an education system that has failed to provide the skilled doctors, nurses, and managers that the public health care system so badly needs. Likewise, the lower pay scales in the public sector have encouraged the more talented people to seek employment in the private health care sector, where incomes are much higher.[107]

GEAR's detractors come from a number of quarters. Some are within the ANC, among its rank and file members, labor unions, and voters. But some of the loudest voices come from outside the party. A prominent example is Julius Malema, who was expelled from the ANC and went on to form his own party, the Economic Freedom Fighters. These critics blame the ANC's abandonment of socialism and adoption of structural adjustment as a big reason for South Africa's economic and social ills, and see nationalization and forced land seizures as the solution. Other voices—in the media, NGOs, the health policy community, and academia—also worry that GEAR has been too attentive to the interests of the business community and therefore done too little to improve the lives of most South Africans. But they stop short of calling for socialism and instead urge the government to temper the pursuit of balanced budgets and the interests of business with more redistribution and investment in human capital, especially to address the skills gap.[108]

Disagreement over the causes and solutions to the country's problems remain. But there is general consensus that the modest growth rates have prevented the government from spending enough on health care and other social services that are needed to tackle the social determinants of poor health and high mortality in the black population. The government thus faces a Catch-22 situation. A high skills, high wage economy offers the best chance out of poverty and inequality, but this requires massive public and private investments in health and education. Economic growth rates are currently too low to bring in the sufficient tax receipts required for such investments. And deficit spending could undermine the business confidence necessary for investment and growth. All the while, an increasing number of citizens are becoming impatient at the slow pace of change in their living circumstances.

Corruption and Complacency Bred by One-Party Rule

A more serious charge against the ANC has been that the party has allowed incompetence and corruption to flourish, which in turn have undermined effective administration of the public sector, including the health care system. The ANC's practice of "cadre deployment," or the appointment of party members into positions in the public sector based on their party loyalty and revolutionary credentials rather than their qualifications, bears much of the responsibility for the managerial incompetence in the public sector, including the state health care system.[109] Certainly National Party governments under apartheid appointed party loyalists to the public sector, too. But there is no denying that patronage and corruption have run rampant under ANC rule, particularly under President Zuma. Government contracts routinely go to those willing to pay bribes or to party loyalists. Far too many ANC government officials put their own enrichment ahead of the well-being of the nation they are supposed to serve. Such practices have crippled the effectiveness of the public sector at all levels of government, leading to failures in health care and other social services delivery.[110]

So why has the ANC become so corrupt? A major reason is that the party has won every national and most provincial and local elections handily since 1994. The opposition parties in parliament are fragmented and, in any case, lack sufficient electoral support to mount a serious challenge to the ANC's rule. Without an effective opposition to check its power or hold it to account, it is perhaps not surprising that the ANC has resorted to patronage and has tolerated or engaged in widespread corruption. Other explanations highlight the ANC's NLM identity and ideology, which encourage some members to view public sector employment as a just reward for the nearly century-long struggle against apartheid, or as simply part of the party's project to wrest state power from the white minority. But there may be more material reasons as well. In a country where so many blacks lack skills and face poor employment prospects, the public sector has become the only plausible avenue for economic advancement.[111]

In any case, corruption and patronage in the ANC will only undermine the government's efforts to implement policies to improve the health of all South Africans. But many South Africans, both within and outside of the ANC, are disturbed by the corruption and incompetence of public officials. The ANC has been a "broad church" noted for the strength of its internal democracy and its open debates on party policy. A new generation of leaders may become the standard-bearers of a new politics for clean and competent government. Should such leadership fail to emerge, then reform may come from without. One scenario would be a formal split within the ANC or a rupture with one of its partners, such as the trade union confederation. Such electoral fragmentation could provide opportunities for new smaller parties to join forces with existing parties like the Democratic Alliance around a program of clean government. Together, they may be able to form a new coalition government and move the country in a different direction.

Conclusion

Health policy in South Africa since 1994 has reflected the country's larger struggle to overcome the legacies of apartheid and to build a just and equitable society for all of its citizens. The ANC has made notable gains in redressing the health inequalities that apartheid and imperialism before it had produced. Life expectancy is increasing again, as more South Africans have access to life-saving medications to combat AIDS. After a decade of disastrous denial, South Africa's ART program is now the largest in the world and viewed as a model for other countries. The government is continuing to build the foundation of a primary care centered delivery system and has committed itself to achieving a more equitable means of financing of health care.

Certainly, the task of improving health care and health outcomes is formidable. Constructing a robust primary care-based health care infrastructure and addressing the social determinants of health require policymakers to overcome substantial technical problems in policy implementation. The resource constraints in a developing nation with severe levels of poverty make the job harder. Policy mistakes by ANC governments, particularly in the response to AIDS under President Mbeki, have also contributed to needless suffering and death. Government corruption and incompetence also contribute to the public health care system's inefficiencies and delivery failures.

Whether the ANC continues in office or a new coalition comes to power, current and future governments will have to confront and overcome the legacies of apartheid. In health policy, this requires the development of a modern, competent health care delivery system. But it also requires finding mechanisms to finance health care in ways that spread risks equitably and ensure that all South Africans have access to quality care. Of necessity, this will require some redistribution from the rich and healthy to the poor and sick. As a reminder, the public sector serves 84 percent of the population to the private sector's 16 percent, yet both use roughly the same amount of resources. There must be a better and more balanced distribution of resources between public and private sectors if South Africa is to achieve its dream of quality health care for all. Likewise, health policy must be part of a broader coordinated strategy with other policy domains if the country is to attack the broader social determinants of health arising from poverty and inequality.

The task is formidable and the ANC's record thus far is mixed. The current inequities in South Africa's health care system and its broader society are relics of the country's apartheid past. And whatever solutions South Africa adopts to address these problems will certainly reflect the constellation of political forces and past policy legacies. But that does not mean that a country and its people are condemned to remain prisoners of history. Human beings can confront their individual and collective history and write a new chapter if they have the political will. South Africans only need to look at their recent past and the achievements of the anti-apartheid movement as evidence of such possibilities. Similarly, creating a health care system that provides everyone access to affordable, quality care will require hard bargaining and strategic compromises among all stakeholders, including government actors, interest groups, and citizens, along with support from the international community.

CHAPTER FIVE

Conclusions and Prospects

A nation's health care system is in many ways like a city's neighborhoods.[1] One neighborhood may have exclusive high-end stores, gourmet restaurants, and stately homes. The immediately adjacent neighborhood has run-down dwellings, shuttered storefronts, and chains offering fast-food fare. In still another neighborhood, renovated row houses and compact bungalows house a mix of older residents and new families. The main street is teeming with life: shops sell practical items such as housewares; cafes, pubs, and restaurants cater to the taste buds; residents can walk to the nearby movie theatre. The public library and park are open to all. The different neighborhoods, moreover, are more or less connected to each other. The upscale area is deliberately inaccessible except by car. The poor neighborhood cut off from the surrounding suburbs because only one bus line serves its residents and that route stops at the city line. The third neighborhood, by contrast, is well connected to other neighborhoods and the surrounding suburbs and outer counties through a network of local buses and regional commuter rail lines that complement cars. The physical structures, amenities, and character of any neighborhood reflect the relationships between the neighbors, businesses, local governments, and the choices they have made.

So, too, does a nation's health care system. Like a neighborhood, its physical structures and policies reflect the interactions among its stakeholders—providers, insurers, the government, and the public. The design of the health care system also embodies public attitudes about whether health is a private or public good.

This chapter brings together what we have learned from our three cases. We begin by summarizing how politics have shaped health policy in the United States, Germany, and South Africa. We then extract broader lessons from these three countries for health policy more generally. Finally, we consider the main health care challenges facing policymakers in the future.

The Interplay of Politics and Policy

The main goals of any health care system are equitable access to quality care at an affordable price. Achieving a balance among these distinct yet interrelated aims is not easy in quiet times and is more difficult in the face of major change. The world of health policy is not static. Countries confront new challenges in health care and must devise solutions in ways that continue to strive to fulfill these fundamental goals.

In a sector this complex, health policy certainly involves technical issues to be solved. But health care reform is far more than devising a technical solution to a problem. Rather, it is a political struggle about the respective roles and power of government and interest groups in the health sector. The three I's of politics—institutions, interests, and ideas—plus history, fundamentally shape policy. Together they have influenced the policy choices, outcomes, and health care reform of our three countries.

The Three Reform Paths

The United States had been fast approaching the limits of a dual health care system. Employment-based private insurance allowed firms to voluntarily opt out of providing insurance coverage to their employees and insurers to shun the sicker and poorer who were the least profitable. A parallel system of public insurance programs for specific groups outside the labor market followed in the 1960s. But starting in the 1980s, the gradual advance of more flexible forms of employment, along with ever-spiraling health care and health insurance costs, began to erode employment-based coverage. What at first were small cracks soon widened into gaping crevasses. Public insurance programs did not expand enough to capture those who were falling into the abyss. By 2009, nearly a fifth of the population lacked health insurance. By any measure the United States continued to outspend every other country by a wide margin, yet the quality of care provided was uneven. Health outcome measures ranked the United States lower than many of its peers among the industrialized nations. On some measures such as infant mortality, the United States fared worse than some developing nations.

The policy response has been breathtaking in its ambition and scope in seeking to tackle all of these problems. But it does so by building on the existing dualistic structure of the American health care system. The Patient Protection and Affordable Care Act (PPACA) of 2010 makes insurance more affordable for small firms and individuals through premium subsidies and regulated competition among health plans on online marketplaces in each state. It bars insurers from discriminating against sicker members of society. It pools risks through an individual mandate and risk-adjusted payments among health plans in the online marketplaces. The law also extends Medicaid up the income ladder to the working poor and to low-income adults without children. However, the states may opt out, and 20 of them have done so. PPACA also addresses deficiencies in health care delivery in order to slow the growth in health spending and improve the quality of care. For instance, the government is funding payment reforms that replace fee-for-service with a single payment (or bundled payment) for a given diagnosis or episode of care, and that reward providers for achieving good health outcomes. The law also seeks to reorient the system away from its excessive emphasis on specialty care and provides federal funds to train more primary care providers. Lastly, the government is taking a number of steps to promote the adoption of evidence-based treatments.

This complex piece of legislation sprouted from the political environment in which it was planted, one that disperses power and requires bargaining among numerous actors at different levels. PPACA rested on delicate compromises among powerful health care interest groups representing major health care providers and the private insurance industry. The political system's separation of powers exacted compromise between different branches of government. Even with a majority in both houses of Congress, President Obama could not count on Democrats' loyalty. He and Democratic leaders in both chambers had to cut deals to keep waverers from bolting and crossing over to the Republican side. Republicans, by contrast, closed ranks to block enactment of the Democrats' reform, and not a single one crossed party lines to vote for PPACA. But as a minority party, they lacked the votes to succeed. Since then, they have continuously sought to defund, repeal, and replace it. The Supreme Court has also weighed in on key questions of constitutionality of the law. The high court's decisions have altered the law's course in ways that its framers did not intend or imagine by making the Medicaid expansion optional. Federalism has also left its mark by giving state governments important powers to regulate private insurers, create online marketplaces, and set the essential benefits package.

PPACA was also the object of a fierce battle over ideas and values. The law's proponents invoked ideas of fairness by arguing that hard-working Americans should not be subject to bankruptcy and disability because they could not find affordable insurance. They justified the individual mandate in terms of individual responsibility. Opponents portrayed the law as big government out to destroy individual liberty. Specific aspects of the law are quite popular with the public, such as allowing young adults to remain on their parents' coverage for a few more years and reining in industry practices that prevented the sick from obtaining coverage. Yet the public continues to express reservations regarding the individual mandate and its elements of compulsion. And opinion polls continue to find that the public is evenly divided on its support or disapproval of the law as a whole.[2]

Germany largely solved the problem of access to insurance and health care through its social health insurance (SHI) system of compulsory employment-based coverage through nonprofit insurers. On health outcomes, Germans continue to rank among the top tier countries, even as they spend half as much as the United States does on health care. However, Germany faced new challenges arising from its rapidly aging population and the limitations of payroll-based financing of health care. Governments have had to address three specific questions: First, how to meet the growing burden of chronic illnesses of a graying population? Second, how to assuage employers' concerns that rising health insurance and labor costs were eroding their competitive position in the global economy? And third, with fewer workers and more retirees now and in the coming decades, would payroll taxes be sufficient to finance the population's health care needs in the future, or would new sources of financing need to be tapped?

German governments of different partisan complexions have enacted legislation since the early 1990s that constitute a mixed approach to health care reform. They have maintained the existing corporatist framework between providers and insurance funds but have upgraded it to meet new needs. One way has been to coordinate decision-making across the different subsectors of the health care system through the Federal Joint Committee (FJC) at the national level. This body has the authority to make binding coverage decisions for SHI. Coverage decisions do not emanate from the government, but from the committee's membership, which comprises the basic stakeholders of the system—the associations of providers, insurers, and patient representatives. Associations of health care providers and insurers continue to administer the health care system at state level.

The German reforms have also grafted new elements onto the corporatist trunk. Governments have introduced managed competition on the insurers' side to promote choice and efficiency. They have also safeguarded solidarity through a risk-compensation scheme among insurers. And to ensure a sound financial footing for SHI in the future, the government has extended the scope of income subject to payroll contributions.

Constructing the market in SHI has required greater and more enduring state intervention in the administration of that. Notably, sickness funds can no longer independently set their contribution rates. Instead, the uniform contribution rate for all funds is set out in law, and the Federal Health Insurance Office (in conjunction with the health ministry and federal association of SHI Funds) administers a Health Fund at national level that distributes risk-adjusted payments to SHI insurers. To relieve pressure on nonwage labor costs, the federal government has shifted the health care costs of children from payroll taxes to general revenues. This constitutes a new and an enduring state presence in SHI financing.[3]

This process of constant adjustment in health care policy, and the complex compromises thereby required, reflect the institutional and political dispersal of decision-making in Germany. The political system fragments power and requires the balancing of different actors and interests to forge agreements that can be enacted and implemented. Coalition governments bring different parties together in the executive, while federalism gives the states a direct voice in determining national laws and major jurisdiction in health care system regulation. Under corporatism, the government must consult major health care interest groups on legislation and policy changes and also delegates substantial authority to them (albeit under government oversight) to implement these. The dominant values of the social market economy stress solidarity and equitable burden sharing, and are wary of unfettered free-market forces operating in the realm of social well-being. At the same time, subsidiarity (i.e., delegating decisions to the lowest level possible and privileging the main groupings in society) values and legitimizes the role of organizations to represent civil society in politics, the economy, and social life, and proscribes excessive government interference. Such values are broadly shared by the public, the mainstream political parties, and the major stakeholders in health policy (not just providers and insurers but also labor unions and even many employers). Those who advocate a radical break from long-standing SHI arrangements thus far have been marginal and have been overruled by countervailing parties, interest groups, and public opinion.

South Africa faces enormous health challenges that are qualitatively different from those in the United States or Germany. Despite its ranking among the larger emerging market economies, South Africa still must contend with poverty and disease on a scale and depth that simply has no parallel in the Western industrialized countries, with far fewer resources to do so. Infectious diseases are illnesses of the poor; in South Africa, they fall heaviest on the black majority, who live on average 20 fewer years than Americans and Germans. White South Africans, by contrast, enjoy the blessings of affluence and longevity. Their health problems take the form of noncommunicable chronic diseases that are common in the developed world.

These health disparities are reinforced by the existence of two very different health care systems in South Africa. While the more affluent white minority enjoys access to quality medical care from a private health care system, the mostly impoverished black majority relies almost exclusively on an inferior, under-resourced public sector health care system. This is a problem of misallocation between the private and public sector health care systems. The private sector accounts for nearly half of health care expenditures but treats at most, a third of the population. The public sector, by contrast, must treat more than two-thirds of the population but with roughly the same resources as the private sector

The health policy challenges for South African governments, then, are daunting. The immediate task is to contain infectious diseases, particularly AIDS and the TB that often accompanies it. The second task is to construct a health care system that will provide quality care to all citizens, not just to the privileged few, when they need it. Failure to address the second task ensures failure in the first. In the case of AIDS, South African governments initially made disastrous policy choices and ignored the recommendations of the international scientific community and development agencies. This policy of denial allowed the disease to spread unchecked and led to avoidable suffering and death. The policy response since 2009, however, has embraced the mainstream scientific consensus on best practices and welcomed foreign assistance. Now, two-thirds of the population is on antiretroviral drug therapy. The result has been significant gains in treatment and life expectancy of those with HIV. Still, the sheer numbers of South Africans living with HIV—over six million persons, or roughly 12 percent of the population—will place a heavy burden on the health care system for years to come.

The policy response to the second challenge of constructing a health care system that meets the needs of all South Africans remains unsettled. In 1994, the African National Congress (ANC) committed itself to create a primary care led health care system in the public sector, but the job remains unfinished. In 2010, the ANC government released a policy paper that proposed a radical solution of single-payer national health insurance to bring more resources into the public sector health system. The proposal has sparked a vigorous debate pitting the ANC and its allies against those groups with a stake in the private health care system. The policy process has been marked by several delays and the government has yet to release its final legislative proposal for NHI.

The particular configuration of politics has shaped policy responses in South Africa. The first factor is the long shadow cast by the history of colonialism and apartheid, which has created widespread inequality and poverty responsible for infectious disease and a public health care system unable to cope with the challenges. Apartheid also sowed deep mistrust among the races, which initially hampered an appropriate response toward AIDS. Corrosive electoral politics in this new democracy has also seeped into health policy. The ANC still garners the loyalty and votes of the black majority on the basis of its legacy as the force that defeated apartheid and ushered in democracy. But two decades of one-party rule have fostered corruption and incompetence. Too often, the ANC government has placed party loyalty ahead of competence as the basis for public sector employment. This has made it difficult to improve the caliber of health sector administration.

Interest groups, both domestic and international, have also been key players in South Africa's policy struggles over AIDS and national health insurance. Moreover, international forces have played a bigger role in South Africa's health policies than they have in the United States or Germany. The government has pursued an economic strategy to woo foreign investors. But the policies have failed to delivered economic growth rates and tax revenues sufficient to address the country's pressing health care needs. Structural adjustment has also had the unintended effect of exacerbating unemployment, poverty, inequality, and consequently, the disease burden on the poor. Another important international actor in South Africa's AIDS story has been global pharmaceutical companies that hold patents on antiretroviral therapies and that long resisted efforts of AIDS activists and governments to make these medicines more affordable to the Global South. Global business, and not simply poor policy choices, hampered the South African government's response to AIDS. On the other hand, international NGOs and development agencies have partnered with local human rights and health groups, and have provided partnership, resources, and technical assistance to help the country address its AIDS crisis and strengthen its public health care system.

The Nature of Health Policy Change: Layering, Conversion, and Arresting Drift

Having sketched the particular interplay of politics and health policy in each country, we can draw some conclusions about the nature of policy change. Thinking of the health care system as a neighborhood can give us a visual image of what such policy change looks like.

The first conclusion is that sweeping aside the old health care system and constructing an entirely new one from scratch—i.e., *revision, or displacement*—is a rare occurrence. Such opportunities present themselves only in the midst of a cataclysmic event or when long-simmering demands from civil society boil over. A critical election or change in political regime (say, the replacement of dictatorship with democracy) occurs that sweeps into power a party and supporting constituencies that had long been excluded from governing. Those new groups in power may abolish older programs and replace them with fundamentally different ones in an exercise of radical policy change.[4]

But significant reform does not always require a rare cataclysmic event to precipitate it. Major policy change can occur in less obvious ways. Seemingly small changes over time can add up to big transformation short of destroying the existing health care system. Recall the less visible processes of policy change presented in Chapter One. *Layering* is the addition of new programs or institutions on top of older ones, in a form of sedimentation. *Conversion* is the transformation of an existing program to new purposes. *Drift* occurs when policymakers fail to update a program to meet changing social risks. These subtle processes of policy change have been at work in the German and American health care reforms. Policymakers opted to not raze entire blocks and erect brand new buildings in their stead. They have collaborated existing businesses and neighbors in a project of layering. They have made renovations to existing buildings to arrest drift, and have converted others to new uses. In this way, the neighborhood meets the needs of longtime residents and newer arrivals. We will look first at Germany and then the United States.

Germany's social health insurance system resembles the middle-class neighborhood of Friedenau in Berlin. Tall, stately trees line the side streets. Apartment buildings offer comfortable, affordable housing to young and old. Families are small and there are many senior citizens. The streets are bustling with activity. People are drawn to a variety of restaurants and stores that cater to their everyday needs. Every few blocks there is a small public park with children playing on the playgrounds and adults strolling in the lanes. The public transportation network of buses, subway, commuter trains, and bike paths makes it easy to get around the rest of the city. A few modest new buildings have gone up, but they fit the neighborhood's ambiance. Most buildings are older and some have been converted to new uses, such as the stately century-old home that is now a daycare center run by a local nonprofit group.

Likewise, the basic structures of German SHI that were in place by the early 1930s remain. Rather than replace the system with a single-payer scheme compulsory individual coverage, governments have created new structures alongside the old to meet new needs. The introduction of managed competition mechanisms among insurers in the 1990 and the creation of the Health Fund in 2009 to operate the risk adjustment scheme, constitute change by accretion or layering. German policymakers have also converted existing institutions to serve new purposes, for example, by transforming an advisory roundtable into the powerful Federal Joint Committee and by placing new regulations on for-profit private insurers to bring their closer to the SHI funds. Governments have been quick to counter early signs of drift that new forms of flexible employment posed to job-based insurance. An individual mandate and income-related premium subsidies for those in atypical employment have prevented the small number of uninsured from growing into a major problem.

The health care system in the United States resembles two adjacent but very distinct neighborhoods in a city undergoing a wrenching transformation from heavy industry to the new knowledge-based economy. The first neighborhood, East Towne, has been solidly middle class for generations. Well-tended single-family homes predominate and a variety of small businesses line the main street. For decades, life had been comfortable and secure. Yet the Great Recession of 2008 made the future uncertain. A number of residents lost their jobs and their homes; several small businesses failed and closed their doors. A feeling of uneasiness hangs over the residents as they ponder the future of their neighborhood: will it survive, or will it go the way of the Sherman Gardens neighborhood just across the line? The latter was once a vibrant working-class enclave, but two decades of deindustrialization have battered it. Factories have long since left, jobs are scarce, the public schools are cash-starved and troubled, and most residents must rely on public assistance. Many homes and storefronts are vacant.

A newly elected reform-minded mayor wants to revitalize both neighborhoods as part of a larger vision to turn around the city. Even though she has a majority on the city council, her party is badly divided on how to move forward. The progressive wing of her party has embraced a plan that would absorb both neighborhoods into a larger metropolitan region. A new public authority would be established that would spearhead an ambitious urban renewal project for the entire region. Traditionalists in her party have balked at such sweeping change. Seeking to find a consensus solution that can unite both wings of her party, the mayor has opted for a more modest proposal. Instead of creating a new regional entity, she has assured each neighborhood that they will retain their autonomy and has offered generous public stimulus money for revitalization. Activists and residents in East Towne have welcomed the money and are using it to restore foreclosed homes and woo new businesses to the main street. The area is now undergoing a renaissance, with young families moving in and smart new bistros and theaters injecting new vitality into the main street. Sherman Gardens, however, presents a mixed picture. One part of the neighborhood is represented by a city councilor who is a close ally of the mayor. He has forged partnerships with residents, local businesses, and community activists and together, they have welcomed the new funds and have used it to refurbish foreclosed homes and attract new shops to the moribund main street. The other part of Sherman Gardens is represented by a city councilor from the opposition party. Suspecting a power grab by the mayor and viewing community activists who favor the public money, in his neighborhood as upstarts, he has declined the funds. Not surprisingly, that part of Sherman Gardens has continued to deteriorate.

This tale of two neighborhoods is a parable of health care reform in the United States. The East Towne neighborhood is akin to employment-based private insurance available to many working Americans, while the adjacent Sherman Gardens neighborhood represents those dependent on the Medicaid program. The mayor and city council are President Obama and Congress, respectively. The president and congressional Democrats declined a radical alternative like single-payer NHI. Even a more modest public option government insurance they would have competed alongside private insurance they deemed beyond the pale. Instead, they have built upon the existing dual system of private and public insurance while correcting its weaknesses. The Affordable Care Act shores up private employment-based insurance by adding new institutions onto the old. The online health insurance exchanges in the states are a clear example of institutional layering. So, too, are the premium subsidies, individual and employer mandates, and the new regulations on private insurers. Likewise, the Medicaid expansion adds new segments of the population (low-income adults without children) to the existing beneficiaries (poor families and the disabled), but stops well short of transforming the program into a universal social insurance program. And the Medicaid renovations are incomplete: as of this writing, 20 states have chosen to not expand Medicaid or accept the federal money accompanying it. The 30 states (plus the District of Columbia) that have done so have seen a greater decline in the number of uninsured, particularly among those on lower incomes, while the states declining the Medicaid expansion and funding have not.[5] In short, both the United States and Germany have chosen to modernize their preexisting health care system arrangements to meet new challenges. In doing so they are constructing new hybrid models, even as much of the basic framework of their older systems endures.[6]

South Africa's quest to create a health care system for all its citizens is a different story in which the ANC is attempting to replace existing structures. Its ending has yet to be written. If we apply the neighborhood analogy to South Africa, we can think of its health care system as two buildings in a derelict neighborhood that has been gentrifying. The private health care system is like a trendy new condominium development, with spacious units, modern appliances, and a private gym. But it is open only to those who can afford to buy in. The public sector health care system is akin to a century-old, rundown tenement block around the corner. The poor can afford the low rents, but it is overcrowded, with an average of ten persons crammed into two tiny rooms. And there is only one communal lavatory for each floor. Single-payer NHI would be like a brand new mixed-income high-rise tower with a community center open to all residents in the neighborhood. Under this proposal, the city would demolish the tenement. But the building plans are not finished because of technical problems and political opposition from the condominium associations. The condominium residents fear that the new building will drive down property values and increase their taxes to pay for the underlying infrastructure needed to support it. But a wide array of local community organizations representing the neighborhood's poorer residents favor the new building. An alternative proposal calls for a neighborhood development consisting of a number of smaller mixed-income residences, from apartments to townhouses to single-family dwellings. These would primarily cater to the working and middle classes as well as the poor, although even the wealthy could live there if they chose. Those on lower incomes would receive rent subsidies from the government. All residents in the neighborhood would have access to a range of public amenities, such as community gardens, a library, and park. This alternative resembles something like the social health insurance proposals that would achieve universal coverage through a variety of private (for-profit and non-profit) insurers and a government plan for the very poorest who are not employed in the formal sector. It remains to be seen whether the city council will enact this high-rise building, retain the tenement and try to make repairs to it, or go with the alternative mixed-development proposal. Or, to use the language of policy change, will South Africa displace the dual system of public and private health care and replace it with a single-payer NHI system? Or will it try to achieve universal coverage by layering new insurance schemes onto the current public and private arrangements? Thus far, nothing is settled.

Naturally, the opponents of NHI are the medical associations and the private insurance industry in South Africa, fearing a loss of income and independence, oppose single-payer NHI. But without addressing the financial and personnel imbalances between the private and public sectors, it is difficult to see how South Africa will be able to meet the health care needs of the majority of its citizens. The question is whether a single-payer NHI is the solution, or whether a social health insurance model could achieve the same goal of universal coverage. SHI could consist of compulsory private insurance for those in formal sector employment, plus public insurance for the poor and those in informal work. Alternatively, SHI could consist of private coverage for all South Africans, with government subsidizing all or part of the premium for those with low incomes. This would preserve private insurance but bring it under tight regulation, as in the United States since PPACA or Germany's model of SHI with regulated insurers. Under SHI, providers could choose to work in public or private settings and receive income from a variety of insurers. The government could go so far as to mandate that all providers accept those covered by public insurance.

We have traversed three continents to explore in depth the health care reform projects in the United States, Germany, and South Africa and the nature of policy change. Let us now go beyond the specifics of each case to discover broader lessons for health policy.

Broader Lessons for Health Care

The World Health Organization (WHO) has taken the lead in exhorting all nations—rich and poor alike—to pursue equitable access to quality care that is affordable. The global community issued its first public commitment to achieving *universal primary care* with the Alma Ata Declaration of 1978. The signatories pledged to establish universal health care systems that would achieve a balance between primary care and acute care and rural and urban areas by the year 2000. Most nations have not achieved the goal, but remain committed to it, and the WHO reissued the call with the document, *Primary Health Care (Now More than Ever)* in 2008.[7] Three years earlier, WHO member states also adopted a resolution to achieve universal coverage, defined as everyone having access to health care when needed without incurring financial hardship. The 2010 WHO Report, *The Path to Universal Coverage*, laid out the basic minimum mechanisms to realize universal coverage and an agenda to meet them, but stopped short of listing specific deadlines:[8]

1. Raising sufficient resources for health
2. Removing financial risks and barriers to access
3. Promoting efficiency and eliminating waste
4. Addressing inequalities in coverage

The first two are largely problems of financing, the third is largely one of health care delivery, while the fourth extends to both financing and provision of services. Finding adequate resources is a much bigger challenge for the poor nations of the Global South. The rich nations arguably spend too much on health, but even they must ensure that they have the resources to meet the health needs of their aging populations. Dismantling barriers to access applies to rich and poor nations alike. We have seen how millions of Americans go uninsured or have insufficient coverage and high cost sharing at the time of care. Indeed, medical debt is the leading cause of bankruptcy in the United States. Likewise, the quest to achieve more efficient use of resources has been a challenge for all three of our countries. Finally, health equity requires all nations to ensure that the health needs of their most vulnerable populations, particularly women, minorities, and those on low incomes, are met.

Keeping the WHO's minimum conditions in mind and linking them to our three case studies, we can derive five broader lessons for health policy and health care reform.

Lesson 1. Risk pooling, compulsory contributions, and government assistance for the poor are key to realizing equitable access to affordable care.[9] *Risk pooling* is fundamental to the proper working of any kind of insurance. Health insurance markets work as they should when they pool risks associated with age, health status, and income. This makes coverage more affordable for everyone. Insurance pools must be large and diverse enough so that the younger, healthier, and wealthier cross-subsidize the health care of the older, sicker, and poorer. If these conditions do not hold, those who are most in need of health insurance will not be able to afford it. In markets with multiple insurers, we have seen that private for-profit and non-profit insurers have proven unable to pool risks on their own. Government has had to step in and regulate insurance markets to ensure that they do so. Government must also regulate individuals and firms. For adequate risk pooling, *everyone must contribute*, either through an individual or employer mandate or both. To ensure adequate risk pooling, *everyone must pay into the system.* If people are not required to carry insurance coverage, the younger and healthier, and perhaps the wealthier, may opt out, leaving the older, sicker, and poorer behind. But if everyone is mandated to have coverage, then it must be affordable. Even when insurance markets pool health and age risks, coverage may still cost too much for those on low incomes. Thus, *government must subsidize* insurance to make it affordable, especially for the poorest.

As we have seen, and as the work of the WHO makes clear, there are different paths to universal coverage. Where the government is the single payer, as in Britain and Canada, the entire nation or province constitutes the risk pool and all pay taxes into the system, even the minority of the population with additional private insurance. The more progressive the tax structure, the rich will pay proportionately more than the poor. In practice, these countries rely on a mix of progressive taxes on different types of income as well as less progressive sales taxes on purchased goods. In social health insurance models like Germany's, health insurance is compulsory for those below a certain income, but coverage is obtained from a number of different nonprofit insurers. Risk pooling typically extended only to the membership of the particular insurance fund. But as the Germans discovered, the existence of too many smaller funds can undermine the sharing of risks, even where insurers are nonprofit entities, coverage is compulsory, and insurance contributions are calculated as a percentage of wages and salaries to cover the health costs of the members of that particular insurance fund. Some funds had sicker and poorer members and therefore levied higher contribution rates than funds with healthier and wealthier members. To address this problem, the government now requires all SHI funds to participate in a risk-adjustment payment scheme that pools risks across different insurers. In the United States, the situation prior to the Affordable Care Act was even worse, since insurers could levy experience-rated premiums that made health insurance unaffordable for those with expensive medical conditions, or could simply deny them coverage altogether. Reforms in both Germany and the United States have addressed the need for risk pooling and fairness in contributions by requiring most if not all citizens to have insurance banning experience rating, and providing tax subsidies for those who cannot afford to pay. In Germany, the new individual mandate rounds out the long-standing employer mandate and local governments subsidize or pay the full insurance contributions for the poor and unemployed. In the United States, PPACA requires most individuals to carry insurance and, save for small businesses, most employers to offer it or else face a fine. Tax-financed subsidies for premiums and cost sharing are available for those on lower incomes. Taxpayers continue to finance Medicare for seniors and an expanded Medicaid program covers more of the poor.

However, in the United States not everyone has accepted the new reforms. Opinion polls show that the public remains almost equally divided on PPACA, with Democrats holding a favorable view of the law and Republicans a negative view.[10] Congressional Republicans continue their efforts to alter if not repeal the law.[11] Opponents of the law do not acknowledge the indivisibility of barring insurers from excluding the sick and charging experience-rated premiums, compulsory coverage to achieve risk pooling, and government subsidies to make coverage affordable.

The insurance reforms without an individual mandate will set in motion a classic death spiral. The healthier will opt out of coverage, the sickest will remain in the insurance pool as long as they can afford to, insurers will raise premiums to cover their care, and insurance will become increasingly unaffordable or the insurer will go broke. Republican alternatives to PPACA would repeal the individual mandate and, under some scenarios, would eliminate premium subsidies for insurance and allow insurers to levy experience rated premiums under certain conditions. They would also segregate the sickest persons into state high-risk pools. This would most certainly require significant taxpayer support to make premiums affordable and to cover the health care costs of the members of the pools. Republican proposals fail to specify how much these risk pools will cost state and federal taxpayers.

Where people can freely choose their health plan, risk-adjustment payment schemes are crucial to ensure that competition is fair. Even where insurers must accept all applicants and cannot levy premiums based on health status, they may still try to engage in subtle yet legal ways of cream skimming, such as targeted marketing or additional perks attractive to healthier people, to maintain market share or simply survive. This has been the case whether insurers are nonprofit entities as in Germany or for-profit concerns, as in the United States. So it is no accident that both countries have introduced risk-adjustment schemes alongside competition. In the United States, risk adjustment operates on the state marketplaces for individual and small business coverage. In Germany, there is one risk-adjustment program for all health funds under SHI, and a separate program for private insurers who offer coverage to high-risk persons who cannot afford the basic premium.[12] The key issue is whether the risk adjustment mechanisms are sophisticated enough to capture the costs associated with the care of sicker patients. Germany has had nearly twenty years of experience while the United States is a relative latecomer. Still, with all the resources that insurers have devoted to medical underwriting and experience rating, it seems plausible that the United States has ample brainpower and actuarial tools to put such knowledge to use in designing sophisticated risk-adjustment systems.

Despite their reforms, differences in access to care still persist in both countries depending on the type of coverage one has. Studies have documented that those with private insurance in Germany tend to get appointments with specialists more quickly and have longer consultations when they do see a doctor than those with SHI. The higher reimbursements under private insurance encourage doctors to provide such preferential treatment.[13] In the United States, the disparities are more marked. Many physicians do not accept Medicaid patients because the reimbursement is so low. In some areas there may be a shortage of providers for these patients. But the general trend of reform in both nations has been to expand insurance coverage and devise reimbursement systems that encourage providers to treat those with chronic medical conditions.

South Africa has yet to decide on a system that adequately pools health and income risks across the entire population. Private insurance for the wealthy and small middle class consumes a disproportionate share of national income, leaving the underfinanced public sector to deal with far more numerous sicker and poorer patients. Even within the private sector, the absence of risk adjustment among funds leads to wide variations in premiums and coverage. The ANC maintains that single-payer NHI is the best if not only solution to pool risks among the entire population and within the private sector insurance, although private sector stakeholders disagree. Yet, as the WHO has emphasized, there is no single path to universal coverage. If single-payer NHI is not the route that South Africa takes, the country has to find a different way to address the resource imbalance between the public and private sectors. This could involve some form of SHI consisting of compulsory coverage for formal sector workers through a multitude of insurers and financed by contributions or premiums, and separate insurance schemes for the poor or those in rural areas that rely on a mix of member contributions and different tax revenues. Perhaps not ideal, such models may be more practical, at least initially, in countries with limited national income and many workers in informal employment whose income is not subject to payroll taxes. Developing countries may also need to rely on overseas development aid to finance these insurance schemes and build administrative capability.[14]

Lesson 2. The respective roles of the government, the market, the individual, and community vary across nations. But even universal systems that have embraced competition and choice require government to set limits to the market to preserve solidarity. This is because they view health care as more than just a commodity. If health care is a commodity just like any other good, then market forces of supply and demand should determine access to it. Countries with universal coverage have decidedly rejected this view. Now it is coming under question in the United States, despite a political culture that elevates free market, individual liberty, and self-sufficiency, and that views government with suspicion. There, a consensus appears to be emerging that everyone should have access to some basic level of health care and that this requires that insurers should not be allowed to deny coverage to the sick or charge them premiums based on health status. All major Republican proposals offered since the enactment of the Affordable Care Act now contain such provisions.

Yet, the role of government and the market in the United States remains contested. The Affordable Care Act combines market and state through *managed competition*. This approach sees benefits in competition. Consumer choice may act as an powerful incentive for insurers and providers to be more responsive to their clients. Competition may also spur providers and insurers to be more efficient.[15] But managed competition also recognizes that *all markets need rules* and that the government must set them. Without such rules, competition will produce market failures that are unacceptably high, such as early death, disability, and bankruptcy due to illness. Germany has also adopted managed competition. The government has embedded competition to advance equity and efficiency by granting blue collar workers the same choice of insurer that white collar workers long enjoyed. The government has also embedded competition within the framework of universal coverage and rules that preserve solidarity and ensure that the most vulnerable are not left behind.

Not all countries that accept the idea that health care is a universal human right have answered the question of the role of government in the same way. National Health Service systems put the obligation on the government to directly finance and provide health care for all. Single-payer national health insurance systems require the government to finance health care but allow private entities to provide care. Under social health insurance systems, the government has more of an arm's-length relationship to the health care system. The government ensures that all citizens have access to medically necessary care, by setting rules on insurers and health care providers through laws or administrative regulations. But private and public entities may provide insurance and health care services. In all of these countries, the government guarantees that everyone has access to a minimal set of comprehensive benefits, even if it does not directly finance or provide health care. The United States has stopped short of universal coverage, but the role of government as guarantor and regulator is becoming more similar to that in social health insurance models.

In sum, countries with universal coverage view health care as a public good, if not a human right. Hence, making it available to everyone based on their need, not on their ability to pay, is a collective responsibility. However, not all countries require the government to finance or provide health care directly. Nor do they regulate the health sector in the same way. And some of them find room for some degree of competition and individual choice, as long as they include rules to safeguard solidarity.

Lesson 3. The drive toward evidence-based medicine and comparative effectiveness research is inexorable. Once a society accepts that everyone should have access to basic health care, new questions follow. Chief among them are: what is considered basic care, who should decide, and how? No country covers everything. Instead, most nations decide on a basic floor and ceiling setting the lower and upper limits of coverage. The minimum coverage, or floor, usually consists of access to medically necessary preventive, curative, and rehabilitative services. The maximum, or ceiling, sets an upper limit on what insurance will cover and normally excludes cosmetic or experimental treatments. Both the floor and ceiling will usually be more generous in wealthier nations that can devote more resources to health care and more austere in poorer nations.[16]

As governments come up against finite resources for health care, they are under pressure to ensure that the money spent on health care is put to the best possible uses. This is the impetus behind the quest for evidence-based medicine that has taken off in the new millennium. The health sector also possesses more sophisticated analytical and data instruments to make this possible. For instance, electronic medical records allow for better tracking of patient data and make more feasible better coordination of care than in the past. They also reduce medical errors and duplication of services that were characteristic of fragmented delivery systems and paper patient records. Governments are encouraging or mandating health care providers and insurers to adopt these improvements. Better data are also critical to developing payment systems that relate treatments to health outcomes. In addition, health economists have devised tools to under-take comparative effectiveness research, such as quality adjusted life years (QALYs), which calculate not only the additional years but also quality of life gained by a particular treatment. QALYs and other analytical tools face criticism that they are value judgments dressed up as statistics and that they bring cost considerations into clinical decisions. Nevertheless, national health ministries and international development organizations are increasingly relying on these analytical tools to guide their decisions on allocating health care resources.[17]

Such trends are a break with the practices of the last century. Under the old arrangements, governments set the budgets of their public health care systems but left the task of determining what constituted medically necessary care to the medical profession to decide. This often meant that individual doctors relied on their own clinical expertise, unencumbered by oversight, to diagnose and determine the appropriate treatment for patients. But with governments seeking to rein in health expenditures, such arrangements have come under increasing scrutiny. After all, physicians' treatment decisions determine most of the volume of health care resources and how they are used, which in turn contribute to the overall costs of the health care system.[18] Yet according to a study in the *British Medical Journal*, the effectiveness of nearly half of all medical treatments is unknown, and a mere 13 percent are of unequivocal benefit.[19] As governments have increasingly called into question the autonomy of the medical profession, they have turned to comparative effectiveness research and evidence-based medicine as a way to assure both quality and affordability of care.

Some countries have moved further along the path of comparative effectiveness research than others. Comparative effectiveness analysis can be limited to measures of clinical efficacy. But it can also extend to cost effectiveness. When properly used, it does not mean that the cheaper of the two procedures will be adopted regardless of its clinical efficacy. Rather, the less expensive procedure should be adopted if it yields the same clinical benefit as the more costly one.

Britain and Germany have instituted national level bodies to assess which treatments work and decide which should be covered by their universal health care systems. Britain's National Institute for Health and Care Excellence (NICE) and Germany's FJC bring together major health care stakeholders to devise clinical guidelines that will inform treatment decisions, and to determine which treatments should be covered under their national health care systems. Both of these national bodies exert significant power, since their decisions on coverage are binding on all health care system actors. However, NICE's remit goes further than the FJC: NICE weighs both cost and clinical effectiveness while the FJC confines itself to the latter.

The United States is taking small steps to bring systematic evidence-based medicine to bear on treatment decisions, but it is not as far along as other countries. The Patient-Centered Outcomes Research Institute (PCORI) disseminates the findings of scientific studies on clinical effectiveness, but its power is limited: it cannot issue binding treatment decisions for providers and insurers, nor can it consider the cost effectiveness of various treatments. Policymakers hope that furnishing clinicians and insurers with information on best practices will be enough to get them to adopt these voluntarily. Unlike PCORI, the Independent Payment Advisory Board (IPAB) for Medicare can make binding recommendations on provider reimbursement to keep Medicare expenditures below a specified target. But the Affordable Care Act expressly prohibits it from making decisions on treatments, coverage, benefits, or eligibility for the Medicare program. The Obama administration's cautious approach toward comparative effectiveness research likely reflects a broader public aversion to having a serious debate about rationing.[20]

The process of deciding what to cover can be controversial because it makes rationing scarce resources explicit. Moreover, some of the analytical tools such as QALYs contain value judgments about what constitutes quality of life that may differ from one person to the next. Applying value judgments to coverage decisions may therefore spark a public outcry, as was the case when Britain's NICE decided that the National Health Service (NHS) should not pay for certain expensive end-of-life cancer drugs. But policymakers have put their faith in such formalized, evidence-based, transparent, and inclusive decision-making structures for a number of reasons. One is the hope that incorporating rigorous scientific evidence into clinical guidelines and coverage decisions will reduce variations in clinical practice that cannot be explained by patients' health status, and thereby improve the quality of care.[21] A second rationale is that grounding coverage decisions in scientific evidence and making these decisions apply to all health care system actors is a fairer way to ration care than by arbitrary decisions of different insurers. As we saw in the era of managed care in the 1990s, the fragmented and largely unregulated insurance market in the United States allowed each insurer to decide whether to cover or deny specific treatments. In a setting of intense competition without adequate rules, some insurers put the bottom line ahead of quality and denied some patients medically necessary care. This provoked a public backlash against managed care.

An inclusive and transparent decision process can lend legitimacy to difficult rationing decisions. The public will have more confidence in the outcome if they believe the decision process is fair, that is, if all interests are represented in such deliberations, if the process is transparent, and if the decisions apply to everyone equally.[22] If public confidence erodes, then governments could develop new rules for these bodies such as mandating outside appeals, or requiring them to improve the evaluative tools they use. Alternatively, the public may judge that the decision making process is sound, but that more resources should be devoted to health care. If so, citizens can use democratic processes like elections, referenda, or other actions to pressure policymakers to spend more on health. Public pressure might prompt governments to create special funds earmarked for certain diseases, as Britain has done with its Cancer Drugs Fund, which provides public financing for expensive chemotherapy at the end of life.[23] As long as resources are finite and becoming increasingly so, however, the search for evidence-based medicine and the use of comparative effectiveness research will continue.

Lesson 4. Efforts to improve quality of care are also occurring on the ground. Thus far we have been discussing efforts to introduce evidence-based medicine at the national level. But there is also a clear trend to improve quality and efficiency of care at the point of patient contact. This requires that providers and insurers adopt clinical guidelines based on scientific evidence in their treatment of patients. Policymakers, insurers, and practitioners also recognize that quality and efficiency require better coordination of care between different providers, particularly between primary and specialty care. The US and German governments are funding innovative practice arrangements that coordinate care among these and other types of providers. While the United States is further along in integrated delivery systems that link ambulatory physicians, hospitals, and nursing care, even the German government now allows multispecialty group practices, or polyclinics. Both countries are also promoting collaborative practices for the care of patients with chronic diseases (such as accountable care organizations in the United States and disease management programs in Germany). Both governments are funding new forms of reimbursement that reward practitioners for meeting good health outcomes. The success of these innovations rests not only on the buy-in by providers and insurers, but also on the technical capability afforded by electronic medical records, and the systematic dissemination and application of scientific knowledge demonstrating which treatments work.

Health policymakers in all three countries in this book are also realizing that primary care deserves greater emphasis. Germany now requires all insurers to offer gatekeeper primary care plans even though patient participation is voluntary. The US government is encouraging the creation of patient-centered medical homes rooted in primary care teams and is also funding the education of more primary care providers. Since 1994, the South African government has worked to construct a primary care led health care system based on community clinics staffed by nurses. It is also establishing integrated clinical specialist support teams and placing them in the communities where they are most needed, rather than siting in urban hospitals. The government is also training more community health workers to address the shortage of primary care providers.

If we try to assess which of our three countries is furthest along in the system-wide diffusion of best practices, in both clinical and cost effective terms, Germany may have an advantage. The scope of the corporatist framework extends to all subsectors of the health care system and the directives that emanate from the FJC and the federal ministry of health are binding on all SHI actors. Corporatism operates at all levels of the health care system: in the FJC at national level, in the fee negotiations between insurers and provider associations at state level, and at the level of the individual doctor whose fees and treatment decisions can be reviewed by the state medical association. These institutional linkages could therefore facilitate the diffusion of best practices. But the diffusion of best practices and new forms of care will not become reality unless providers and insurers actually implement them on the ground. In the United States, by contrast, decision-making is more fragmented and takes place at the local level between provider groups (or individual practitioners) and insurers. System-wide decision-making like corporatism has no parallel in the American health care system. Moreover, the Affordable Care Act deliberately limits the decision-making authority of bodies like PCORI, instead hoping that providers and insurers will voluntarily adopt innovations in reimbursement and clinical treatments. In the United States, then, best practices—whether clinical guidelines, new forms of care, or provider reimbursement—are more likely to emanate from local experiments between private providers and insurers. Alternatively, Medicare may take the lead in piloting innovations that private payers subsequently adopt.[24]

South Africa is on the same path to improve quality and efficiency as Germany and the United States are on, but it has much further to go. The ANC government continues to construct a comprehensive delivery system centered in primary care and coordinates it with specialty care through district clinical teams. However, skilled managers and health care providers in the public sector still remain in short supply. And the government has limited leverage over the actions of the private sector, which suffers from serious inefficiencies and high costs of its own. Both sectors need to collaborate with each other and share best practices, and the broader education system must do a better job in preparing future health care workers with the necessary skills.

Lesson 5. Ensuring adequate resources for universal coverage requires new funding sources that raise controversial questions over redistribution. This observation applies not just to the poorer nations of the Global South, but also the richer countries of the West. In addressing the question of funding sources, the WHO suggests mainstream taxes like general revenues, payroll taxes, and premiums paid into voluntary community-based insurance schemes. But it also considers more novel sources, such as a tax on high-risk global financial transactions, or the so-called Robin Hood tax. This tax would redistribute resources from wealthy Western nations and financial institutions to poor nations of the Global South that are building up their health care systems. It could also fund health and social programs in the rich nations that underwent austerity during the Great Recession. The logic is as follows: The global financial sector's irresponsible speculative practices caused the Great Recession, and massive taxpayer bailouts were needed to rescue the banks in several rich Western countries. The cost of these bailouts, and the mass unemployment that the recession caused, forced governments to incur massive public debts or to slash public spending on health care and other social programs. The financial transaction tax would be a way for global banks to make amends for their bad behavior.[25] The WHO considers other revenues sources such as solidarity surcharges on goods and services and taxes on the biggest corporations. It also calls upon nations, especially those subject to widespread tax evasion, to improve their tax collection capacity with measures to combat corruption and improve information systems. At the same time, the WHO acknowledges that funding from rich donor countries and organizations will be necessary to finance the development of health care systems in developing nations, at least initially. Moreover, if wealthy nations were to make good on their past pledges of aid, it could more than double the amount that poor nations currently receive.[26]

Governments in all three of our case studies have sought out new sources of revenue for health care. In the United States, the Affordable Care Act introduced taxes on higher income earners as well as on the health care industry itself to underwrite premium subsidies on the exchanges and the expansion of Medicaid. To ensure SHI is solvent in the future Germany, too, has come up with its own recipe. It has added new ingredients to the payroll tax base, such as taxes on nonwage sources of income like dividends and real estate. And to relieve pressure on payroll contributions, the federal government has assumed responsibility to finance children's health care from general tax revenues. South Africa has yet to find an answer to the question of ensuring adequate revenues for health care. The government devotes 11 percent of its budget to health, but that is below the 15 percent target agreed by African nations and less than the 16 to 18 percent spent by some of its poorer neighbors.[27] And health spending is skewed so that the private sector serving a minority of the population consumes nearly the same amount of resources as the public sector that cares for the vast majority of citizens. As we have seen, the financing debate has been fierce and centers on the following questions:

- Will a transfer of resources from the private sector health care system to the public sector be enough to meet the health needs of the population? The advocates of NHI think so; some health policy experts as well as private sector interests are less certain. The WHO suggests that a variety of taxes can be raised from different sources and has cautioned against a one-size-fits-all system of health care financing for every country, such as single-payer NHI. Some health policy experts in South Africa have suggested imaginative public-private partnerships beyond financial transfers from the private sector to improve health care for all. Through such collaborations, the private sector could offer the public sector much-needed administrative expertise and health care providers.[28]
- Is South Africa too poor to rely only on domestic taxpayers to finance the nation's health care needs? If so, it will have to augment its own revenue raising efforts with assistance from external donors. Or it may have to find more creative revenue sources, such as the financial transaction tax, which is not infeasible given the size of the country's financial sector. Alternatively, the government have to adjust its economic strategy and relax its commitment to a balanced budget. This would allow it to devote more resources to much-needed social investments in health and education.
- Is the problem not that the public health care system receives too little funding, but that the money is not spent wisely? If so, then the answer is to halt the widespread corruption and patronage in the ANC that siphons off public health care resources and contributes to incompetent health care administration. Even if the government can halt corruption, it is unlikely to be sufficient to address the imbalance in resources between the public and private sectors.

More likely, the government will have to address all three questions with a variety of measures to find the resources necessary to construct a health care system that meets the needs of all citizens.

The Future

Great strides have been made in improving the health of the citizens of nearly all nations and most governments now recognize the principal tasks that remain to be tackled. They must assure adequate and equitable financing and improve the actual delivery of health care. This requires greater emphasis on primary care, better coordination between different health care providers, and systematically bringing scientific evidence on best practices to the development of clinical guidelines on care and to coverage decisions. But more needs to be done. If countries really want to ensure that their populations are healthy, then they must move beyond the biomedical model of disease and address the broader social determinants of health. This compels broader policy changes and interventions.[29]

Ample evidence demonstrates that those with lower incomes have poorer health outcomes than those who are wealthy. This holds not only between rich and poor nations but also between rich and poor within a nation. Low-income populations as well as minorities in the wealthy industrialized nations have higher mortality and morbidity rates for noncommunicable ailments such as heart disease, stroke, and cancer.[30] The question is why this is so and what health policy can do to change this. Those who subscribe to individual freedom and responsibility attribute poor health to either a person's genetic inheritance or to unwise lifestyle choices. They may acknowledge that the poor have difficult lives, which understandably leads them to take up unhealthy behaviors, such as smoking or substance abuse, in order to cope. We cannot do much to change our genes, so the argument goes, but we can decide to eat better, exercise regularly, and avoid drugs, alcohol, and cigarettes. So the correct policy response is for health care providers to give patients information on healthy diet and exercise, so that they will make the right choices. They can do this during patient office visits or through public health education campaigns.

Such information is certainly important. But to focus only on individual patient choices and doctors overlooks the larger environment that structures choices. It is harder to choose to live a healthy lifestyle when the only place to exercise is a park with a decrepit basketball court that has become the contested turf of rival gangs, when the nearest grocery store is more than a mile away and one does not have a car, and the only neighborhood fare is high-fat food from fare served by fast-food restaurants, or junk food from corner stores. This goes well beyond a doctor giving patient information on diet and exercise. It means upgrading public parks, or placing community gardens and grocery stores offering fresh produce in low-income neighborhoods to allow residents to make healthy choices.

But is bad health only due to poor lifestyle choices or inherited genes? What about those individuals living in poor neighborhoods who do not smoke or drink, who exercise regularly and eat healthy foods, but still have a higher incidence of heart disease or cancer even though there is no family history of such illnesses? In fact, the new field of *epigenetics* is discovering that adverse environmental factors can actually alter gene expression, which, in turn, leads one to contract noncommunicable diseases like cancer and heart disease. Epigenetics and neuroscience are discovering important links between genetic expression, brain development, illness, and the environment. A stressful environment can cause the body to release toxic levels of cortisol or can impair the immune system, leading to illnesses. Moreover, the diseases may not become manifest until well into adulthood.[31] In other words, the cause of illness is not a question of nature or nurture, but the interaction of *both*.

What's more, there is strong evidence that ill health is not confined to the poorest in society, but becomes successively worse as one goes down the income ladder. Those at the top of the social ladder, such as CEOs or doctors or lawyers, tend to be healthier and live longer than those at the next lowest rung, and this finding is repeated all the way down the entire ladder. People at the top are healthier not simply because they have more resources available to make healthy lifestyle choices, but also because they enjoy greater autonomy in their jobs and in their lives more generally. Those in successively lower occupations have less control over their work and their lives, experience more stress, and have worse health outcomes.[32] As Paul Farmer has succinctly stated, "Thus do fundamentally social forces and processes come to be embodied as biological events."[33] This means that if policymakers want to have a healthy nation, they need to do more than just target those at the bottom of the socioeconomic hierarchy.

The good news is that the processes of gene expression and brain development are dynamic, not fixed. The brain displays a remarkable degree of plasticity, and can rewire itself and form new neurons and pathways, and reverse or mitigate diseases or harmful behaviors. While there may be critical windows in human development that make interventions more effective, particularly in the early and adolescent years, the brain continues to develop well into early adulthood.[34] This finding suggests that the right kind of policy interventions informed by life sciences and social sciences, not to mention social justice, can make a positive difference for the individuals concerned as well as for the broader society.

This understanding of how the broader social environment affects health outcomes has profound implications for health policy and broader public policy throughout the globe. It requires a radical revision of the dominant model of disease and treatment that has driven health policy for the last hundred years in Western nations. Most health care systems in the industrialized world follow a biomedical model of disease and treatment rooted in Western allopathic medicine. In this model, the physician's sole concern is with the individual patient who comes to the clinic. The doctor's task is to diagnose the patient's condition and prescribe a medical procedure that will hopefully cure the patient's disease. This model also holds complex technological procedures of specialist physicians in much higher regard than primary and preventive care, as manifested by the social prestige and incomes of specialists. But the biomedical model must be paired with a model that understands how broader sociodemographic conditions contribute to health and illness, and that and focuses not simply on the individual patient but also on broader populations. Often termed a public health approach, it gives priority to prevention and primary care as a way to reduce the need for curative, high-tech medicine to treat conditions later on.

To fully address health needs of individuals and populations, communities and governments must combine these two approaches into a holistic model. This requires the following policies. First, it requires a health care system that provides the whole array of treatments to patients, including preventive, primary, and acute care and high-tech medicine when needed. Second, it requires better coordination of care between medical practitioners and those in other fields, such as behavioral mental health and social services. Finally, this multifaceted approach to health requires policy interventions that address the broader structural causes of illness. Such policies should seek to prevent, not simply ameliorate, the poverty and inequality that cause illness. These kinds of policy interventions would encompass educational policies to produce good schools, job training programs, and taxation and minimum wage policies, which together would help people to find employment at living wages. They would require community development initiatives to provide decent housing, good recreational facilities, and healthy foods.[35] Such a multipronged approach would be more effective on both cost and clinical grounds in keeping people healthy than the current reactive approach that waits until individuals fall ill and then relies almost entirely on the health care system to make them well. In short, healthy individuals require healthy communities.

The neighborhood analogy again serves to illustrate these points. Thus far, I have applied the analogy only to the financing of health care, but here I extend it to the provision of health and related services. Good health requires that everyone has access to necessary medical services, that is, a comprehensive and coordinated health care system. Like a vibrant neighborhood, a well-functioning health care system should link providers to social services as well as education, employment, and recreational services.

A neighborhood zoned for exclusively residential purposes and miles from the nearest shop or grocery store would be akin to a health care system having only primary care doctors but lacking a hospital. Likewise, an area zoned exclusively for commercial purposes, with only big box stores that are miles from residences and accessible only by car, would be like a health care system with only hospitals and no primary care doctors or mental health providers. But a health care system that is integrated with these broader community services is like a neighborhood zoned for mixed use, which offers a range of services and amenities (parks, theatres, shops, restaurants, and housing) vital to the quality of life of its residents, as well as a well-developed transportation system that connects residents to these amenities.

Policymakers in different nations are coming to accept the need for a broad-based understanding of health and are beginning to implement policies consistent with this way of thinking. As early as 1978, national governments and global health organizations signed on to the Alma Ata Declaration, which called for health care systems rooted in primary care and linked to the local community. Admittedly, progress on the ground has been slow, prompting the WHO to issue its 2008 annual report urging nations to make good on their commitment. And in that same year, the WHO published a landmark report calling on nations to address the social determinants of health and to adopt a broad range of multisectoral policy interventions to do so.[36]

The three countries in this book are taking up the call to establish a strong foundation in primary health care and to link the health care system to other types of health services. Patient-centered medical homes that consist of primary care teams of physicians, nurses, and other professions and that involve patients in decisions about their care are gaining traction in the United States. But researchers and policymakers there have gone further, calling for a "medical neighborhood" in which medical homes or accountable care organizations coordinate the care of patients and populations across a range of services and over the life-course. These services would encompass hospital care, dental care, behavioral health, and community care.[37] Germany's moves to introduce gatekeeper family doctors, integrated forms of care, and disease management programs are similar examples of the growing emphasis on primary care that is linked to other providers. Similar trends are at work in South Africa, whose government is establishing clinical specialist support teams at the district level and training and deploying community health workers at the local level. All of these innovations in health care delivery go in the same direction of improving coordination of care within their health care systems and with external community services providers.

But as we have seen, policymakers must go even further if they wish to achieve good health for all. Institutions and actors that make up a medical neighborhood gorge partnerships with those in other policy domains, such as education, employment, housing, food security, and safety, because all have a bearing on health. Healthy neighborhoods foster healthy individuals. This is because inequality and poverty, then, are not only social or political issues; they are also are health issues.[38] We can see this not only in the health disparities between the rich and poor nations but also within a nation, even a wealthy one, South Africa, one of the most unequal societies in the world, can attest to the devastating effect of inequality on the health and well-being of citizens. Its experience should be a wake-up call to the United States, which has the dubious distinction of having the greatest wealth disparity among all industrialized nations, a gap which gap continues to widen.[39] Indeed, the health problems of the poor in the richest nation on earth are strikingly similar to those in South Africa. The mediocre health outcome indicators in the United States reflect and are rooted in socioeconomic disparities based on race, gender, and income. Although Germany can claim a more even distribution of wealth than the other two countries, complacency is not in order: there, too, an underclass has emerged and poverty and inequality are growing in the new century.

Good health is vital to human life in so many ways. It not only promotes human survival but also improves the quality of life. Good health is also essential for human beings to reach their potential and to participate fully in the life of their society.[40] And it is a necessary input to a nation's economic productivity. These realities should motivate citizens and their governments to establish and maintain a robust health care system that provides quality care to all in an efficient manner. But an exclusive focus on the health care system, narrowly conceived, is not enough. Simply put, inequality and poverty make people sick. This means that governments and citizens must also synchronize health policy with other policy domains, such as education, employment, and housing, to tackle the broader social determinants of health. All of these, in a broad sense, are health policies. Health equity requires nothing less.[41] This is the challenge of our time, not only within each country but also across all nations, to achieve a healthy global neighborhood. Whether or how we decide to take up this challenge depends on the political and policy choices we make.

NOTES

One   The Intersection of Health and Politics

1. OECD (2013) *Health at a Glance 2013: OECD Indicators*, OECD Publishing. http://dx.doi.org/10.1787/health_glance-2013-en; US Census Bureau, *Income, Poverty, Health Insurance Coverage 2011, Highlights*, 2011; Thomas Bodenheimer and Kevin Grumbach, *Understanding Health Policy: A Clinical Approach*, 6th ed. (New York: McGraw Hill Lange, 2012), p. 17.
2. OECD, *Health at a Glance, 2013*; *Five Family Facts*, OECD, n.d.; www.oecd.org/social/family/doingbetter.
3. UNAIDS, South Africa, 2015. http://aidsinfo.unaids.org.
4. In 2013, tuberculosis was the leading cause of death in South Africa, followed by pneumonia and influenza, and HIV in third place. While deaths from TB and pneumonia and flu are declining, HIV has moved up in the mortality rankings since 2009. Noncommunicable diseases like stroke, diabetes, and heart disease rank next. See Statistics South Africa, *Mortality and Causes of Death in South Africa, 2013: Findings from Death Notifications*. Stat release P0309.3 December 2, 2014, pp. 24–27. The rise in HIV deaths is due to a change in reporting by medical personnel ("Statistics South Africa on Mortality and Causes of Death 2013," South African Government, December 2, 2014. http://www.gov.za/mortality-and-causes-death-2013.) On the growth of the noncommunicable disease burden in South Africa, see also Bongani M. Mayosi,, Alan J. Flisher, Umesh G. Lalloo, Freddy Sitas, Stephen M. Tollman, and Debbie Bradshaw, "The Burden of Non-communicable Diseases in South Africa," *The Lancet* 374 (September 12, 2009): 934–947.
5. See the discussion of Adam Przeworski and Henry Teune's most similar systems and most different systems approaches to comparative analysis in B. Guy Peters, *Comparative Politics: Theory and Methods* (New York: New York University Press, 1998), pp. 37–41.
6. *South Africa Economic Update: Fiscal Policy and Redistribution in an Unequal Society*, 6 (November 2014), no. 92167, World Bank: Washington DC, p. 43.
7. UNAIDS 2015; World Bank, "Incidence of Tuberculosis (per 100,000 People)," 2015.

8. Deborah A. Stone, "The Struggle for the Soul of Health Insurance," *Journal of Health Politics, Policy and Law* (Summer 1993): 286–317.

9. For a concise and illuminating discussion of such measures, see T. R. Reid, *The Healing of America: A Global Quest for Better, Cheaper, and Fairer Health Care* (New York: Penguin 2010), "Appendix: The Best Health Care System in the World," pp. 252–268; and Tsung-Mei Cheng, "NICE Approach," *Financial Times, Health* (3) Sept. 16, 2009, pp. 12–13.

10. *OECD Health at a Glance 2013*, pp. 36–37, 59.

11. Some researchers have hypothesized that institutionalized racism, which affects blacks rather than whites, may produce toxic levels of chronic stress in African-American women, leading to higher rates of preterm birth and infant mortality, regardless of income. See *Unnatural Causes: Is Inequality Making Us Sick?* esp. "When the Bough Breaks" segment, California Newsreel, 2008, www.unnaturalcauses.org; and Mark Johnson and Tia Ghose, "Is Stress Related to Preterm Birth?" *Milwaukee Journal Sentinel*, April 17, 2011. On the link between race, stress, and low birth rate, see Clayton J. Hilmert, Christine Dunkel Schetter, Tyan Parker Dominguez, Cleopatra Abdou, Calvin J. Hobel, Laura Glynn, and Curt Sandman, "Stress and Blood Pressure During Pregnancy: Racial Differences and Associations With Birthweight," *Psychosomatic Medicine* 70 (57) (2008): 57–64.

12. For the importance of linking the sector to the political system, see Kenneth Dyson, ed., *The Politics of German Regulation* (Aldershot, England: Dartmouth, 1992); and Susan Giaimo and Philip Manow, "Adapting the Welfare State: The Case of Health Care Reform in Britain, Germany, and the United States," *Comparative Political Studies* 32 (8) (December 1999): 967–1000.

13. James G. March and Johan P. Olsen, 1984, "The New Institutionalism: Organizational Factors In Political Life," *American Political Science Review* 78 (3): 734–749.

14. For example, the centralized British political system also pushes blame upwards to national government officials. See Rudolf Klein, *The Politics of the National Health Service*, 2nd ed. (London: Longman, 1989); and Susan Giaimo, *Markets and Medicine: The Politics of Health Care Reform in Britain, Germany, and the United States* (Ann Arbor: University of Michigan Press, 2002), pp. 38–42 and chap. 2.

15. Ellen M. Immergut, *Health Politics: Interests and Institutions in Western Europe* (Cambridge and New York: Cambridge University Press, 1992). A classic example of an argument that stresses the primacy of political institutions over other political factors in explaining health policy is Sven Steinmo and Jon Watts, "It's the Institutions Stupid! Why Comprehensive National Health Insurance Always Fails in North America," *Journal of Health Politics, Policy and Law* 20 (2) (Summer 1995): 329–372.

16. Immergut, *Health Politics*, pp. 28–32.

17. On the ways in which party systems freeze social cleavages born from past political struggles, see the classic study by Seymour M. Lipset and Stein Rokkan, "Cleavage Structures, Party Systems, and Voter Alignments; An Introduction,"

in *Party Systems and Voter Alignments* (New York: Free Press, 1967), pp. 1–64. For more general works on the functions of parties, see Maurice Duverger, *Political Parties*, trans. Barbara and Robert North (London: Methuen, 1954); Giovanni Sartori, *Parties and Party Systems* (New York: Cambridge University Press, 1976), esp. Chaps. 3 and 5; and Leon D. Epstein, *Political Parties in the American Mold* (Madison and London: University of Wisconsin Press, 1986).

18. Gøsta Esping-Andersen, *The Three Worlds of Welfare Capitalism* (Princeton: Princeton University Press, 1990), esp. Chap. 1.

19. On European Christian Democracy, see Kees van Kersbergen, *Social Capitalism: A Study of Christian Democracy and the Welfare State* (London and New York: Routledge, 1995).

20. David Vogel, "Why Businessmen Distrust their State," *British Journal of Political Science* 8 (1) (1978): 45–78; Stephen Skowronek, *Building a New American State: The Expansion of National Administrative Capacities, 1877–1920* (Cambridge: Cambridge University Press, 1982).

21. France's National Front is the oldest contemporary Far Right party in Western Europe. But such parties have seen electoral success in recent years in a number of countries, including Sweden, Finland, and Greece, as well as in the European Parliament. Anti-immigrant sentiment and economic insecurity have fueled their rise. Green parties have also become a more permanent feature of the electoral landscape in a number of European countries. See www.elections2014.eu/en.

22. For a good discussion of different health care system models and their organization principles, see Reid, *Healing of America*, Chap. 2.

23. WHO, *Achieving Universal Coverage* (Geneva 2012).

24. The power resources school explained universal welfare states and full employment in terms of the organizational characteristics of labor unions and their links to social democratic parties that governed for long periods of time. See Walter Korpi, *The Democratic Class Struggle* (London: Routledge and Kegan Paul, 1983), Chap. 3; John D. Stephens, *The Transition from Capitalism to Socialism* (London: Macmillan Press, Ltd., 1979). But the analytical framework can also be applied to business associations and their links to parties of the Right, or conservative religious parties and cross-class alliances. See Gøsta Esping-Andersen and Walter Korpi, "Social Policy as Class Politics in Post-War Capitalism: Scandinavia, Austria, and Germany," in *Order and Conflict in Contemporary Capitalism: Studies in the Political Economy of Western European Nations*, ed. John D. Goldthorpe (Oxford: Clarendon Press, 1984), pp. 179–209; and Gøsta Esping-Andersen, *The Three Worlds of Welfare Capitalism* (Princeton: Princeton University Press, 1990) and *Social Foundations of Postindustrial Economies* (Oxford and New York: Oxford University Press, 1999); Cathie Jo Martin and Duane Swank, *The Political Construction of Business Interests: Coordination, Growth, and Equality* (Cambridge: Cambridge University Press, 2012).

25. On the differences between pluralism and corporatism, see Philippe C. Schmitter, "Still the Century of Corporatism?" in *Trends toward Corporatist Intermediation*, ed. Philippe C. Schmitter and Gerhard Lehmbruch (Beverly Hills: Sage, 1979), pp. 7–52.

26. For an analysis of interest group politics and shifting alliances in health care, see Jill Quadagno, *One Nation Uninsured: Why the U.S. Has No National Health Insurance* (Oxford and New York: Oxford University Press, 2005).

27. Hugh Heclo and Henrik Madsen, *Policy and Politics in Sweden: Principled Pragmatism* (Philadelphia: Temple University Press, 1987), p. 23.

28. Ibid. p. 24. See also pp. 23–31 for a more detailed discussion of ideological hegemony.

29. For a definition of ideology and analysis of how ideology shapes policy proposals, see Sidney Verba and Gary R. Orren, *Equality in America* (Cambridge: Harvard University Press, 1985), Chap. 1; and Tim Tilton, *The Political Theory of Swedish Social Democracy* (Oxford: Clarendon Press, 1990), Chaps. 1 and 11.

30. Paul Pierson, "When Effect Becomes Cause: Policy Feedback and Political Change," *World Politics* 45 (1993): 595–628.

31. Paul Pierson, "Increasing Returns, Path Dependence, and the Study of Politics," *American Political Science* Review 94 (2) (June 2000): 251–267; Jacob S. Hacker, *The Divided Welfare State: The Battle over Public and Private Social Benefits in the United States* (Cambridge and New York: Cambridge University Press, 2002), pp. 51–62.

32. On path dependence and critical junctures, see Hacker, *Divided Welfare State*, pp. 51–62. On critical elections, see Walter Dean Burnham, *Critical Elections and the Mainspring of American Politics* (New York: Norton, 1970).

33. Ashley M. Fox and Michael R. Reich, "The Politics of Universal Health Coverage in Low- and Middle-Income Countries: A Framework for Evaluation and Action," *Journal of Health Politics Policy and Law* 40 (5) (October 2015): 1024.

34. Kathleen Thelen, "How Institutions Evolve: Insights from Comparative Historical Analysis," in *Comparative Historical Analysis in the Social Sciences*, ed. James Mahoney and Dietrich Rueschemeyer (New York: Cambridge University Press, 2003), pp. 208–240; Jacob S. Hacker, "Privatizing Risk without Privatizing the Welfare State: The Hidden Politics of Social Policy Retrenchment in the United States," *American Political Science Review* 98 (2) (May 2004): 243–260.

35. Hacker, Privatizing Risk, pp. 243–260.

36. Care of patients with chronic illnesses in the last two years of life accounts for 32 percent of Medicare spending, with average spending between $40,000 and $50,000 per beneficiary. Much of that amount is to reimburse physicians and hospitals as a result of repeat hospital admissions. See "Care of Chronic Illness in Last Two Years of Life," *The Dartmouth Atlas of Health Care*, http://www.dartmouthatlas.org/data/topic/topic.aspx?cat=1. Sixty percent of Medicare spending goes to the care of only ten percent of Medicare beneficiaries. See Juliette Cubanski, Christina Swoope, Cristina Boccuti, Gretchen Jacobson, Giselle Casillas, Shannon Griffin, and Tricia Neuman, *A Primer on Medicare*, Kaiser Family Foundation (March 2015), p. 30.

37. Obesity is rising among adults in all OECD countries, but the United States ranks first, with 36.5 percent of the population age 15 and older measured as obese. Among children, obesity is generally increasing, though the data are

mixed for some OECD countries. The United States ranks fifth among OECD countries, with 30 percent of children measuring as obese. Obesity is defined in terms of body mass index. *OECD Health Statistics 2013* (Paris, 2013), pp. 48–49, 58–59.

38. Gøsta Esping-Andersen, *Social Foundations*; Paul Pierson, "Post Industrial Pressures on Mature Welfare States," in *The New Politic of the Welfare State* (New York: Oxford University Press, 2000), pp. 80–106.

39. Bodenheimer and Grumbach, *Understanding Health Policy*, Chap. 3.

40. Medical Group Management Association, *MGMA Physician Compensation and Production Survey: 2014 Report Based on 2013 Data: Key Findings Summary Report*. Physician incomes also vary by type of specialty and region of the country. Physicians in the Midwest tend to have higher incomes than elsewhere in the United States. In the Midwest, an orthopedist specializing in spinal treatments earned $777,988 but a family practitioner only $189,912 in 2012 (Guy Boulton, "Efforts to Boost Number of Primary Care Physicians Face Pay Gap Hurdles," *Milwaukee Journal Sentinel*, December 1, 2012). For cross-national income comparisons, see Miriam J. Laugesen and Sherry A. Glied, "Higher Fees Paid to US Physicians Drive Higher Spending for Physician Services Compared to Other Countries," *Health Affairs* 30 (9) (September 2011): 1652.

41. See Paul Starr, *The Social Transformation of American Medicine* (New York: Basic Books, 1982) for an excellent treatment of the cultural authority that physicians gained as a result of the scientific revolution in medicine. By contrast, one of the most popular shows in Britain (and on US public television) in recent years has been *Call the Midwife*, which depicts nurse midwives delivering babies in the home and providing a range of primary care services to residents of the impoverished East End in London.

42. For a portal into this burgeoning field of study on the social determinants of health, see James S. House, "Relating Social Inequalities in Health and Income," *Journal of Health Politics, Policy and Law* 26 (3) (June 2001): 523–532; The Center on the Developing Child at Harvard University website (www.developingchild. harvard.edu); and the documentary, *Unnatural Causes: Is Inequality Making Us Sick?* California Newsreel, 2008, www.unnaturalcauses.org.

43. Jeffrey Sachs, *The End of Poverty: Economic Possibilities for Our Time* (New York: Penguin, 2005), maps 1 and 2.

44. The debate is more nuanced and complex than this. Jeffrey Sachs, for example, argues that single cause explanations of poverty in the developing world are incomplete and inaccurate. He points out to seven different causes, ranging from cultural practices that deny groups opportunity, poor governance, and bad geography, to an unfair trade regime imposed by the Western powers. His solution likewise rejects a one-size-fits-all approach and instead urges interventions that are tailored to local needs, developed by the recipient country, and that are constantly evaluated and modified if found to be failing. He also advocates a "global compact" that specifies the obligations of both donor countries and agencies and receiving countries. See Sachs, *End of Poverty*.

45. Robin Harding, Joseph Leahy, and Lucy Hornby, "Taking a Stand," *Financial Times,* July 16, 2014.

46. The major variants of this interpretation of international political economy are dependency theory and world systems analysis, with Andre Gunder Frank exemplifying the former and Immanuel Wallerstein the latter. See Andre Gunder Frank, "The Development of Underdevelopment," *Monthly Review,* 18 (4) (September 1966): 17–31; and Immanuel Wallerstein, *World Systems Analysis: An Introduction* (Durham: Duke University Press, 2004), esp. Chaps. 2 and 3.

47. Jeremy Greene, Marguerite Thorp Basilico, Heidi Kim, and Paul Farmer, "Colonial Medicine and its Legacies," in *Reimagining Global Health: An Introduction,* ed. Paul Farmer, Jim Yong Kim, Arthur Kleinman, and Matthew Basilico (Berkeley: University of California Press, 2013), pp. 34–49.

48. Reid, *Healing of America,* Chap. 9.

49. World Health Organization, "The Top 10 Causes of Death, Fact Sheet no. 310," updated May 2014, http://www.who.int/mediacentre/factsheets/fs310/en/; Mark W. Zacher and Tania J. Keefe, *The Politics of Global Health Governance: United by Contagion* (New York: Palgrave Macmillan, 2008), Appendix A, Tables 3 and 4.

50. Paul Farmer, "On Suffering and Structural Violence," in *Partner to the Poor: A Paul Farmer Reader,* ed. Hain Saussy (Berkeley: University of California Press, 2010), p. 335.

51. Ibid. Also see Paul Farmer, *Infections and Inequalities: The Modern Plagues* (Berkeley: University of California Press, 2001).

52. Paul Farmer, "Inequality and Poverty," in *Infections and Inequalities,* p. 14.

53. Varun Gauri and Evan S. Lieberman, "Boundary Institutions and HIV/AIDS Policy in Brazil and South Africa," *Studies in Comparative International Development* 41 (3) (Fall 2006): 63–66.

54. For critiques of structural adjustment see Guillermo O'Donnell, *Modernization and Bureaucratic-Authoritarianism* (Berkeley: University of California Press, 1973); Juan J. Linz, in J. Linz and A. Stepan, eds. *The Breakdown of Democratic Regimes* (Baltimore and London: Johns Hopkins Press, 1978); Sachs, *End of Poverty,* esp. Chaps. 3 and 4.

55. Greene et al. "Colonial Medicine," pp. 63–67.

56. Anne Becker, Anjali Motgi, Jonathan Weigel, Giuseppe Raviola, Salmaan Keshavjee, and Arthur Kleinman, "The Unique Challenges of Mental Health and MDRTB: Critical Perspectives on Metrics of Disease," in *Reimagining Global Health: An Introduction,* ed. Paul Farmer, Jim Yong Kim, Arthur Kleinman, and Matthew Basilico (Berkeley: University of California Press, 2013) esp. pp. 225–243.

57. Jane Galvão, "Brazil and Access to HIV/AIDS Drugs: A Question of Human Rights and Public Health," *American Journal of Public Health* 95 (7) (July 2005): 1110–1116; Jon Cohen, "Brazil: Ten Years After," *Science* 313 (5786) (July 28, 2006): 484–487; Luke Messac and Krishna Prabhu, "Redefining the Possible: The Global AIDS Response," in *Reimagining Global Health: An Introduction,* ed.

Paul Farmer, Jim Yong Kim, Arthur Kleinman, and Matthew Basilico (Berkeley: University of California Press, 2013), pp. 111–132.

58. Greene et al. "Colonial Medicine," pp. 67–70.

59. World Health Organization, *Health Systems Financing: The Path to Universal Coverage* (Geneva: WHO, 2010); and *Health Systems Financing: The Path to Universal Health Coverage. Plan of Action* (Geneva: WHO, 2012); Commission on the Social Determinants of Health, *Closing the Gap in a Generation: Health Equity through Action on the Social Determinants of Health. Final Report of the Commission on the Social Determinants of Health.* (Geneva: WHO, 2008); *World Health Report 2008: Primary Health Care (Now More than Ever)* (Geneva: WHO, 2008).

60. Matthew Basilico, Jonathan Weigel, Anjali Motgi, Jacob Bor, and Salmaan Keshavjee, "Health for All? Competing Theories and Geopolitics," in *Reimagining Global Health: An Introduction*, ed. Paul Farmer, Jim Yong Kim, Arthur Kleinman, and Matthew Basilico (Berkeley: University of California Press, 2013), pp. Chap. 4, pp. 74–110. On the progress and challenges of the MDGs, see "Global Targets, Local Ingenuity," *The Economist*, September 25, 2010, pp. 34–35; the World Health Organization website (www.who.org); and Paul Farmer, Matthew Basilico, Vanessa Kerry, Madeleine Ballard, Anne Becker, Gene Bukhman, Ophelia Dahl, Andy Ellner, Louise Ivers, David Jones, John Meara, Joia Mukherjee, Amy Sievers, and Alyssa Yamamoto, "Global Health Priorities for the Early Twenty-First Century," in *Reimagining Global Health: An Introduction*, ed. Paul Farmer, Jim Yong Kim, Arthur Kleinman, and Matthew Basilico (Berkeley: University of California Press, 2013), pp. 302–339.

61. Zacher and Keefe, *Global Health Governance*, Chap. 2 esp. pp. 15–18.

62. I am indebted to Jeffrey Drope for this observation.

63. Jeffrey Drope and Raphael Lencucha, "Evolving Norms at the Intersection of Health and Trade," *Journal of Health Politics, Policy and Law* 39 (3) (June 2014): 591–631.

64. For example, the biggest emerging market economies (Brazil, Russia, India, China, and South Africa, or BRICS), still wield only 10.3 percent of the votes on the governing board of the International Monetary Fund, even though they comprise 24.5 percent of the world economy. Harding et al. "Taking a Stand."

65. Ibid.

66. Debra L. DeLaet and David E. DeLaet, *Global Health in the 21st Century: The Globalization of Disease and Wellness* (Boulder and London: Paradigm Publishers, 2012), Chap. 11; Zacher and Keefe, *Global Health Governance*, p. 138.

67. For an excellent overview of the work of NGOs in global health policy, see Zacher and Keefe, *Global Health Governance*, Chaps. 5–7; and Paul Farmer, Jim Yong Kim, Arthur Kleinman, and Matthew Basilico, eds. *Reimagining Global Health: An Introduction* (Berkeley: University of California Press, 2013), Chap. 5 (Luke Messac and Krishna Prabhu, "Redefining the Possible: The Global AIDS Response) and Chap. 12 (Matthew Basilico, Vanessa Kerry, Luke Messac, Arjun Suri, Jonathan Weigel, Marguerite Thorp Basilico, Joia Mukherjee, and Paul Farmer, "A Movement for Global Health Equity? A Closing Reflection").

Two   The United States: An Ambivalent
Journey toward Universal Coverage

1. Donald L. Madison, "From Bismarck to Medicare—A Brief History of Medical Care Payment in America," in *The Social Medicine Reader: Health Policy, Markets and Medicine*, 2nd ed., ed. Jonathan Oberlander, Larry R. Churchill, Sue E. Estroff, Gail E. Henderson, Nancy M. P. King, and Ronald P. Strauss (Durham and London: Duke University Press, 2005), pp. 54–59.

2. Deborah A. Stone, "The Struggle for the Soul of Health Insurance," *Journal of Health Politics, Policy and Law* (Summer 1993): 286–317; Thomas S. Bodenheimer and Kevin Grumbach, *Understanding Health Policy: A Clinical Approach*, 6th ed. (Lange Medical Books/McGraw-Hill, 2012), Chap. 2.

3. Susan Starr Sered and Rushika Fernandopulle, *Uninsured in America: Life and Death in the Land of Opportunity*, updated edition (Berkeley: University of California Press, 2007), p. 114; *Employer Health Benefits Survey 2011* (Kaiser Family Foundation and Health Research and Educational Trust, September 27, 2011). www.kff.org.

4. Gregory Acs, Stephen H. Long, M. Susan Marquis, and Pamela Farley Short, "Self-Insured Employer Health Plans: Prevalence, Profile, Provisions, and Premiums," *Health Affairs* 15 (2) (Summer 1996): 266–278.

5. Steve Jagler, "But Will It Work?" *BizTimes Milwaukee*, March 19–April 1, 2012. For example, Anthem Blue Cross of California announced in 2010 a 39 percent rate increase for individual and small group insurance. See Lawrence R. Jacobs and Theda Skocpol, *Health Care Reform and American Politics: What Everyone Needs to Know* (Oxford and New York: Oxford University Press, 2012), p. 111.

6. Bodenheimer and Grumbach, *Understanding Health Policy*, pp. 10–13; Jonathan Blum, "What Is the Donut Hole?" HealthCare Bog, HealthCare.gov, August 9, 2010. www.healthcare.gov/blog/2010/08/donuthole.html.

7. The pay-as-you-go aspect of the program, in which current workers' payroll taxes contribute to the health care of current beneficiaries, is not well understood by the general public. If Medicare financing strictly followed the contributions of current beneficiaries, the benefits would be very meager and fall well short of the cost of their actual health care, the latter of which reflects inflation, longer life expectancy, and new technologies prolonging such lives.

8. William G. Weissert and Carol S. Weissert, *Governing Health: The Politics of Health Policy*, 4th ed. (Baltimore: Johns Hopkins University Press, 2012), pp. 264–268; Bodenheimer and Grumbach, *Understanding Health Policy*, p. 13.

9. Bodenheimer and Grumbach, *Understanding Health Policy*, p. 17 and Chap. 3.

10. Kaiser Commission on Medicaid and the Uninsured and U.S. Census Bureau Current Population Survey, March 2010. www.kff.org.

11. Kaiser Family Foundation and Health Research and Educational Trust Survey of Employer-sponsored Health Benefits, 1999–2012. www.kff.org.

12. "Hospitals by Ownership Type, 2013," *State Health Facts*, Kaiser Family Foundation, http://kff.org/other/state-indicator/hospitals-by-ownership/

13. Bodenheimer and Grumbach, *Understanding Health Policy*, pp. 53–55.
14. Paul Starr, *The Social Transformation of American Medicine* (New York: Basic Books, 1982).
15. Jill S. Quadagno, *One Nation Uninsured: Why the U.S. Has No National Health Insurance* (Oxford and New York: Oxford University Press, 2005).
16. Starr, *Social Transformation*; Susan Giaimo, *Markets and Medicine: The Politics of Health Care Reform in Britain, Germany, and the United States* (Ann Arbor: University of Michigan Press, 2002), chaps. 6–7.
17. Rick Romell, "Hospital Losses Hit City Heart," *Milwaukee Journal Sentinel*, May 14, 2006.
18. Bodenheimer and Grumbach, *Understanding Health Policy*, p. 135 and chaps 4–5; Atul Gawande, "The Cost Conundrum," *The New Yorker*, June 1, 2009; Miriam J. Laugesen and Sherry A. Glied, "Higher Fees Paid to US Physicians Drive Higher Spending for Physician Services Compared to Other Countries," *Health Affairs* 30(9) (September 2011): 1647–1656; Gerald F. Anderson, Uwe E. Reinhardt, Peter S. Hussey, and Varduhi Petrosyan, "It's the Prices, Stupid: Why the United States Is So Different from Other Countries," *Health Affairs* 22(3) (May/June 2003): 89–105. Within the federal Department of Health and Human Services, the Centers for Medicare and Medicaid Services claimed the largest budget at $808 billion in 2011, whereas the Centers for Disease Control had only $6.3 billion (Weissert and Weissert, *Governing Health*, pp. 225–226).
19. On political institutions as veto points, see Ellen M. Immergut, *Health Politics: Interests and Institutions in Western Europe* (Cambridge: Cambridge University Press, 1992), esp. pp. 21–33.
20. For example, Senator John McCain (R-AZ) has crossed party lines to pass legislation. His independent spirit has long been regarded positively and rewarded by Arizona voters.
21. Weissert and Weissert, *Governing Health*, Chap. 1.
22. In November 2013, the Senate agreed to ban the use of a filibuster in the cases of consideration of presidential nominees to the executive and judicial branches. The vote to limit the use of the filibuster fell largely along party lines, with no Republican support and only three Democrats defecting. Jeremy W. Peters, "In Landmark Vote, Senate Limits Use of Filibuster," *New York Times*, November 21, 2013.
23. Allan J. Cigler and Burdett A. Loomis. *Interest Group Politics* (Washington DC: CQ Press, 2002), chap 1; Leon D. Epstein, *Political Parties in the American Mold* (Madison and London: University of Wisconsin Press, 1986); Weissert and Weissert, *Governing Health*, pp. 174, 177–179.
24. Weissert and Weissert, *Governing Health*, pp. 172–179.
25. Ibid. p. 135.
26. David Vogel, "Why Businessmen Distrust Their State: The Political Consciousness of American Corporate Executives," *British Journal of Political Science* 8 (January 1978): 45–78.
27. Quadagno, *One Nation Uninsured*.
28. Vogel, "Why businessmen."

29. To be sure, the Founding Fathers conducted a lively debate on the permissible reach of national government and executive power, as the *Federalist Papers* make clear. Nevertheless, the Constitution established a separation of powers system with checks and balances to prevent tyranny by any one branch over the others. As with political liberalism, American history contains periods of reformist movements—such as Jacksonian democracy in the nineteenth century, the Populist and Progressive movements in the early twentieth century and the varied social movements of the 1960s and 1970s—that have challenged the economic and political power of private capital (Vogel, "Why businessmen.").

30. See Steven Vogel, *Freer Markets, More Rules* (Ithaca and London: Cornell University Press, 1996) on the neoliberal realignment. For a discussion and examples of neoliberal critiques of education and social welfare policies, see John E. Chubb and Terry M. Moe, *Politics, Markets, and America's Schools* (Washington DC: Brookings Institution, 1990); Charles Murray, *Losing Ground: American Social Policy, 1950–1980* (New York: Basic Books, 1984); and Jason DeParle, *American Dream: Three Women, Ten Kids, and a Nation's Drive to End Welfare* (New York: Viking, 2004), esp. Chap. 5.

31. Paul Pierson, "When Effect Becomes Cause: Policy Feedback and Political Change," *World Politics* 45 (1993): 595–628.

32. Mollyann Brody and Robert J. Blendon, "Public Opinion and Health Policy," in *Health Politics and Policy*, 4th ed., ed. James A. Morone, Theodore A. Litman, and Leonard S. Robins (Clifton Park, NY: Delmar Cengage, 2008), pp. 249–270; Madison, "From Bismarck to Medicare."

33. Theodore R. Marmor, *The Politics of Medicare.* 2nd ed. (New York: Aldine de Gruyter, 2000); Quadagno, *One Nation Uninsured.*

34. Milt Freudenheim, "A Health Care Taboo is Broken," *New York Times.* May 8, 1989.

35. Jacob S. Hacker, *The Road to Nowhere: The Genesis of President Clinton's Plan for Health Security* (Princeton: Princeton University Press, 1997), pp. 17–20; Theda Skocpol, *Boomerang: Clinton's Health Security Effort and the Turn against Government in U.S. Politics* (New York and London: W. W. Norton, 1996). Skocpol, *Boomerang*, pp. 13, 21–23.

36. Hacker, *Road to Nowhere*, pp. 16–17.

37. Alain C. Enthoven, *Health Plan: The Only Practical Solution to the Soaring Cost of Medical Care* (Boston: Addison-Wesley, 1980); "Managed Competition: An Agenda for Action," *Health Affairs* 7 (3) (1988): 25–47.

38. Weissert and Weissert, *Governing Health*, p. 132.

39. Skocpol, *Boomerang.*

40. Mark A. Peterson, "From Trust to Political Power: Interest Groups, Public Choice, and Health Care," *Journal of Health Politics, Policy and Law* 26 (5): 1145–1163.

41. Skocpol, *Boomerang*, p. 75.

42. Robert J. Blendon, Mollyann Brodie, John M. Benson, Drew E. Altman, Larry Levitt, Tina Hoff, and Larry Hugick, "Understanding the Managed Care Backlash," *Health Affairs* 17 (4) (1998): pp. 80–94.

43. Kaiser Family Foundation and Health Research and Educational Trust, *Employer Health Benefits Survey, 2012.* www.kff.org.

44. Milliman Medical Index, 2011, 2014.www.milliman.com/mmi/

45. OECD (2013) *Health at a Glance 2013: OECD Indicators,* OECD Publishing. http://dx.doi.org/10.1787/health_glance-2013-en, pp. 155, 157.

46. Robert L. Bennefield, "Health Insurance Coverage: 1995," *U.S. Census Bureau Current Population Reports, P60–195.* September 1996, p. 1; Kaiser Family Foundation, *Key Facts about the Uninsured Population,* September 2013.

47. This section draws on Susan Giaimo, "Interest Groups, Think Tanks, and Health Care Policy, 1960s-present," in *The CQ Guide to U.S. Health and Health Care Policy,* ed. Thomas Oliver (New York: DWJ Books, 2014), pp. 384–389; *Summary of New Health Reform Law,* Kaiser Family Foundation, April 15, 2011, www.kff.org; *Summary of Coverage Provisions in the Patient Protection and Affordable Care Act,* Kaiser Family Foundation, July 17, 2012, www.kff.org; and Jacobs and Skocpol, *Health Care Reform,* chap. 4. On the origins of the individual mandate, see Paul Starr, *Remedy and Reaction: The Peculiar American Struggle over Health Care Reform,* New Haven and London: Yale University Press, 2011, p. 81; and Skocpol, *Boomerang,* pp. 98, 105, 163.

48. Bureau of Labor Statistics, *Labor Force Statistics from the Current Population Survey,* http://data.bls.gov/timeseries/LNS14000000.

49. US Census Bureau, *Income Poverty and Health Insurance, Highlights: 2011.* https://www.census.gov/hhes/www/hlthins/data/incpovhlth/2011/highlights.html

50. The Children's Health Insurance Program is the current name of the Medicaid expansion program for children of the working poor. It was originally enacted in 1997 as the State Children's Health Insurance Program.

51. On the Massachusetts Health plan, see Kaiser Family Foundation, *Massachusetts Health Care Reform: Six Years Later,* no. 8321, May 2012. www.kff.org

52. Jacobs and Skocpol, *Health Care Reform,* Chap. 4 and p. 171.

53. Atul Gawande nicely captures the nature of experimentation in delivery system reform in "Testing Testing," *The New Yorker,* December 14, 2009, pp. 34–41.

54. "Health Policy Brief: The Independent Payment Advisory Board," *Health Affairs* (December 15, 2011); Sarah Kliff, "As Health-Care Costs Slow, IPAB's Launch Is Delayed," *Wonkblog, Washington Post,* May 3, 2013.

55. See *Summary of New Health Reform Law,* April 15, 2011, Kaiser Family Foundation, p. 9. www.kff.org

56. Alan Maynard, "Health Care Rationing: Doing It Better in Public and Private Health Care Systems," *Journal of Health Politics, Policy and Law,* 38 (6) (December 2013): 1119–1121.

57. Susan Giaimo, "Behind the Scenes of the Patient Protection and Affordable Care Act: The Making of a Health Care Co-op," *Journal of Health Politics, Policy and Law* 38 (3) (June 2013): 599–610. Congress cut co-op funding in 2012, so that only 23 cooperatives were actually established. "Your Health Plan Will Now Self-Destruct," *Businessweek,* November 2–8, 2015, pp. 28–29.

58. On abortion coverage in PPACA, see Alina Salganicoff, Adara Beamesderfer, Nisdha Kurani, and Laurie Sobel, "Coverage for Abortion Services and the ACA,"

Kaiser Family Foundation, September 2014; "Health Reform: Implications for Women's Access to Coverage and Care," Issue Brief, Kaiser Family Foundation, August 2013; Jacobs and Skocpol, *Health Care Reform*, pp. 118–119. With the Hobby Lobby ruling in summer 2014, the Supreme Court also permits for-profit companies, whose owners object to contraceptive coverage on religious grounds, to not offer such benefits. See Adam Liptak, "Supreme Court Rejects Contraceptives Mandate for Some Corporations," *New York Times*, June 30, 2014.

59. Stuart Altman and David Shactman, *Power, Politics, and Universal Health Care: The Inside Story of a Century-Long Battle* (Amherst, NY: Prometheus Books, 2011), Chap. 12, esp. 254–255.

60. Steven Greenhouse, "Dennis Rivera Leads Labor Charge for Health Reform," *New York Times*, August 27, 2009; Robert Pear, "Industry Pledges to Control Health Care Costs," *New York Times*. May 11, 2009.

61. Pear, "Industry pledges."

62. Greenhouse, "Dennis Rivera leads."

63. AHIP was now the single trade association for the insurance industry, the result of the merger between American Association of Health Plans (AAHP), whose members were larger companies, and Health Insurance Association of America (HIAA) representing small insurers.

64. Altman and Shactman, *Power, Politics*, Chap. 12.

65. Edward Luce and Alexandra Ulmer, "Obama Foes Turn to '60s Radical for Tactical Tips," *Financial Times*. August 17, 2009, p. 2; Kate Zernike and Megan Thee-Brenan, "Poll Finds Tea Party Backers Wealthier and More Educated," *New York Times*, April 14, 2010.

66. Jacob S. Hacker, "Putting Politics First," *Health Affairs* 27 (3) (May/June 2008): 718–723; "The Case for Public Plan Choice in National Health Reform: Key to Cost Control and Quality Coverage," Berkeley, CA: Center on Health, Economic and Family Security, University of California School of Law, and Institute for America's Future. n.d. www.law.berkeley.edu/chefs.htm. Downloaded May 2009.

67. Richard Cauchi, "State Actions to Address Health Insurance Exchanges," Oct. 16, 2014, National Conference of State Legislatures, www.ncsl.org. Accessed 10/17/14; State Decisions on Health Insurance Marketplaces and the Medicaid Expansion, KFF State Health Facts, updated July 20, 2015. http://kff.org/health-reform/state-indicator/state-decisions-for-creating-health-insurance-exchanges-and-expanding-medicaid/.

68. *New York Times*, "Is the Affordable Care Act Working?" October 27, 2014. http://nyti.ms/1tuklhM.

69. Jackie Calmes and Robert Pear, "Crucial Rule Is Delayed a Year for Obama's Health Law," *New York Times*, July 2, 2013; Robert Pear, "Further Delays for Employers in Health Law," *New York Times*, February 10, 2014.

70. Gardiner Harris and Robert Pear, "Still No Relief in Sight for Long-Term Needs," *New York Times*, October 24, 2011.

71. Julia Paradise, "Medicaid Moving Forward," Issue Brief, Kaiser Family Foundation, March 9, 2015, p. 9.

72. Adam Liptak, "Justices by 5–4, Uphold Health Care Law," *New York Times*, June 29, 2012; MaryBeth Musumeci, "A Guide to the Supreme Court's Review of

the 2010 Health Care Reform Law," Kaiser Family Foundation Focus on Health Reform, (Jan. 2012, pub. #8270) www.kff.org.

73. "Status of State Action on the Medicaid Expansion Decision," KFF State Health Facts, updated July 20, 2015. http://kff.org/health-reform/state-indicator/state-activity-around-expanding-medicaid-under-the-affordable-care-act/; Section 1115 Medicaid waivers allow states flexibility to test innovations as long as they are consistent with the goals of the Medicaid program. The innovations are also subject to evaluation for their continuation. See Robin Rudowitz, Samantha Artiga, and MaryBeth Musumeci, "The ACA and Medicaid Expansion Waivers," Issue Brief, Kaiser Family Foundation, February 2015.

74. Rachel Garfield, Anthony Damico, Jessica Stephens, and Saman Rouhani, "The Coverage Gap: Uninsured Poor Adults in States that Do Not Expand Medicaid—An Update," Issue Brief, Kaiser Family Foundation, April 2015. This publication estimates the coverage gap at over 3.7 million persons in 22 states rejecting Medicaid expansion money. Since then, two more states have accepted Medicaid money, so that figure is lower. But in 2014, with more states opting out of the Medicaid expansion, the number in the coverage gap was 5 million persons ("The Coverage Gap: Uninsured Poor Adults in States that Do Not Expand Medicaid," Issue Brief, Kaiser Family Foundation, March 2014).

75. See "Coverage gap," 2014. Wisconsin is the only state not accepting federal Medicaid money that does not have the coverage gap. This is because the state has extended Medicaid to all adults up to the poverty line, but expects those above the poverty line to purchase subsidized insurance on the exchange. There are concerns, however, that those on very low incomes may still find insurance unaffordable, even after taking account of the subsidies for premiums and cost sharing expenses. Indeed, 26,000 Wisconsinites with incomes between 100 and 138 percent of the poverty line had declined to buy coverage on the exchange in September 2014. Guy Boulton, "Gov. Scott Walker, Mary Burke and the Affordable Care Act," *Milwaukee Journal Sentinel*, September 26, 2014.

76. Ibid; Robert Pear and Michael Cooper, "Reluctance in Some States over Medicaid Expansion," *New York Times*, June 30, 2012.

77. Jonathan Weisman and Jeremy W. Peters, "Government Shuts Down in Budget Impasse," *New York Times*, September 30, 2013; "Republicans Back Down, Ending Crisis on Shutdown and Debt Limit," Jonathan Weisman and Ashley Parker, *New York Times*, October 16, 2013.

78. The medical device manufacturers failed to obtain repeal of their tax in 2013 during the government shutdown episode, but have continued to lobby the Republican controlled Congress for repeal. See Jason Millman, "How Killing the Medical Device Tax Became One of Washington's Top Priorities," Wonkblog, *Washington Post*, November 7, 2014. Medicare Advantage Plans, private plans that serve Medicare beneficiaries, have seen reductions from the federal government, but in the last year actually saw an increase as health care costs slowed. See Jay Hancock, "Decoding the High-Stakes Debate Over Medicare Advantage Cuts," *Kaiser Health News*, April 7, 2014 and Caroline Humer, "Government Payments for Medicare Advantage Plans to Rise in 2016," Reuters, *New York Times*, April 6, 2015.

79. Ryan originally laid out his reform vision for employment-based insurance, Medicare, and Medicaid in *A Roadmap for America's Future* in 2008; *A Roadmap to America's Future Version 2.0: A Plan to Solve America's Long-Term Economic and Fiscal Crisis,* January 2010; and House Budget Committee, *The Path to Prosperity: Restoring America's Promise, Fiscal Year 2012 Budget Resolution,* House Committee on the Budget, April 5, 2011, budget.GOP.gov; *The Path to Prosperity: A Blueprint for American Renewal, Fiscal Year 2013 Budget Resolution,* March 20, 2012, prosperity.budget.house.gov; *The Path to Prosperity: A Responsible, Balanced Budget, Fiscal Year 2014 Budget Resolution,* March 2013, budget.house.gov; Congressional Budget Office, *Analysis of Paul Ryan's Roadmap for America's Future Act of 2010,* January 27, 2010. www.cbo.gov.

80. Ryan's plan for Medicare vouchers was far more radical in his earlier 2008 and 2010 Roadmaps. Premium support (vouchers) would begin in 2021 and could only go toward the purchase of private insurance on the Medicare exchange. The average voucher would be $5,900 for a person aged 65 but would be risk adjusted by age and health status. If older and sicker beneficiaries were taken into account, the average voucher would be $11,000 (figures are in 2010 dollars). He has subsequently reformulated this voucher to set it at the equivalent of the second-cheapest plan on the exchange and has allowed the government fee-for-service Medicare plan to compete with private plans.

81. Congressman Ryan made a speech to this effect to the Milwaukee Press Club. See "The Future of US Healthcare: Is Rationing Inevitable?" Milwaukee Press Club, Milwaukee, Wisconsin, March 2, 2012.

82. Bob Moffit, "Ryan-Wyden: The Basic Ingredients of Structural Medicare Reform," *The Foundry: Conservative Policy News Blog from The Heritage Foundation,* December 16, 2011.http://blog.heritage.org. Moffit was referring to the Ryan-Wyden plan, which was another iteration of Ryan's premiums support proposal, this time teaming up with Democratic senator Ron Wyden. The Ryan Wyden plan, see Ron Wyden and Paul Ryan, *Guaranteed Choices to Strengthen Medicare and Health Security for All: Bipartisan Options for the Future,* December 15, 2011. www.budget.house.gov/bipartisanhealthoptions; www.wyden.senate.gov/bipartisonhealthoptions. For a detailed outline of the Heritage Foundation's proposals for Medicare premium support, see Heritage Foundation, *Saving the American Dream: The Heritage Plan to Fix the Debt, Cut Spending, and Restore Prosperity,* Washington DC: 2011.

83. Uwe E. Reinhardt, "The Wyden-Ryan Plan: Déjà vu All Over Again," *New York Times* December 23, 2011. The nonpartisan *CBO* expressed similar reservations on Ryan's 2010 voucher proposal, which was far more stringent than his subsequent proposals. See CBO, Roadmap 2010 and n. 80 above.

84. Sarah Kliff, "As Health-Care Costs Slow, IPAB's Launch is Delayed," *Washington Post,* May 3, 2013.

85. Laura D'Andrea Tyson, "Wyden-Ryan's Unrealistic Assumptions," *New York Times,* December 30, 2011.

86. Ryan, *Path to Prosperity,* 2012.

87. Ryan, *Path to Prosperity*, 2012; *The Long-Term Budgetary Impact of Paths for Federal Revenues and Spending Specified by Chairman Ryan*, Congressional Budget Office, March 2012.

88. CBO, *Long Term Impacts*, 2012.

89. John Holahan, Matthew Buettgens, Caitlin Carroll, and Vicki Chen, "National and State-by-State Impact of the 2012 House Republican Budget Plan for Medicaid," Kaiser Family Foundation, October 2012.

90. This section draws on the summary of the CARE Act (*The Patient Choice, Affordability, Responsibility, and Empowerment Act: A Legislative Proposal* January 2014); and Timothy Stoltzfus Jost, "Beyond Repeal-A Republican Proposal for Health Care Reform," *New England Journal of Medicine*, 370 (10) (March 6, 2014): 894–896.

91. Ryan, *Roadmap*, 2008, 2010; *Path to Prosperity, FY 2013*.

92. Karen Pollitz, "State High-Risk Health Insurance Pools," *Expert Voices*, NIHCM Foundation, April 2009. www.nihcm.org

93. Jost, "Beyond Repeal."

94. The CARE Act borrows some of Paul Ryan's earlier proposals for insurance for those under age 65. For example, Ryan's 2008 and 2010 *Roadmaps* call for an end to the tax exemption for employment-based insurance and offered instead each American a tax subsidy for individual and family coverage at $2,300 and $5,700 respectively. The amount of these vouchers represented less than half the actual average premiums for employment-based insurance at the time. Similarly, the CARE Act's premium subsidies are far less than the actual value of an average health plan today. But unlike Ryan, the Care Act preserves the health insurance tax deduction for employers while capping it for employees. See CARE Act summary, esp. p. 3.

95. CBO, *Long Term Impacts*.

96. Ibid; Martin Wolf, "Paul Ryan's Plan for America Is Not Credible," *Financial Times,* August 20, 2012.

97. On the effects of the first open enrollment period, see "Is the Affordable Care Act Working?" *New York Times,* October 27, 2014, http://nyti.ms/1tuklhM; Gary Claxon, Larry Levitt, Mollyann Brodie, Rachel Garfield, and Anthony Damico, "Measuring Changes in Insurance Coverage Under the Affordable Care Act," April 2014, Kaiser Family Foundation. By April 2015, 16.4 million uninsured persons had obtained insurance, with 14 million of them obtaining coverage on the exchanges and 2.3 million adult children remaining on their parents' insurance. An additional 13.6 million persons had enrolled in Medicaid.

98. *Key Facts about the Uninsured Population*, Kaiser Family Foundation, October 2015, www.kfff.org; Department of Health and Human Services, U.S. Center for Medicare and Medicaid Services, and Medicaid.gov, *Medicaid and CHIP: August 2015 Monthly Applications, Eligibility Determinations and Enrollment Report,* October 26, 2015, http://medicaid.gov/medicaid-chip-program-information/program-information/medicaid-and-chip-enrollment-data/medicaid-and-chip-application-eligibility-determination-and-enrollment-data.html.

99. Kaiser Family Foundation, *Key Facts*, 2015, p. 2, 4.

100. Jenna Levy, "In U.S., Uninsured Rate Dips to 11.9% in First Quarter," *Gallup Well-Being*, April 13, 2015. www.gallup.com/poll/182348/uninsured-rate-dips-first-quarter.aspx. An analysis in May 2015 by the Department of Health and Human Services Office of the Assistant Secretary for Planning and Evaluation found similar trends but with slightly higher numbers. That analysis calculated the uninsured rate in March 2015 at 13.2 percent, but also recorded a higher rate of uninsured in 2013 at 20.3 percent. "Health Insurance Coverage and the Affordable Care Act," May 5, 2015. aspe.hhs.gov/health/reports/2015/uninsured.../ib_uninsured_change.pdf. For an in-depth overview of the uninsured and the effects of the ACA, see Melissa Majerol, Vann Newkirk, and Rachel Farfield, *The Uninsured: A Primer*, Kaiser Family Foundation, January 2015.

101. Buettgens and his colleagues estimate that if states were to take up the Medicaid expansion, there would be a 40 percent increase in enrollment, or seven million people by 2016, and the number of uninsured would decline by more than four million persons. States would also receive $472 billion in federal funding between 2015 and 2024. See Matthew Buettgens, John Holahan, and Hannah Recht, "Medicaid Expansion, Health Coverage, and Spending: An Update for the 21 States that Have Not Expanded Eligibility," Issue Brief, Kaiser Family Foundation, April 2015.

102. "CMS Proposes Major Initiative for Hip and Knee Replacements," News release, U.S. Department of Health and Human Services, July 9, 2015, hhs.gov; Robert E Mechanic, "Mandatory Medicare Bundled Payment—Is It Ready for Prime Time?" *The New England Journal of Medicine*, nejom.org, August 26, 2015.

103. On delivery system reform, see Health Policy Brief, "Next Steps for ACOs," *Health Affairs* (January 31, 2012); Atul Gawande, "Testing, Testing," *The New Yorker*, December 14, 2009, pp. 34–41 and "Overkill," The New Yorker, May 8, 2015, pp. 42–53; and "Health Policy Brief, Pay for Performance," *Health Affairs* (October 11, 2012). For evaluations of Medicare and private insurance ACOs, see Lawrence P. Casalino. 2015. "Pioneer Accountable Care Organizations: Traversing Rough Country," *Journal of the American Medical Association*, 313 (21) June 2: 2126–27; David J. Nyweide, Woulton Lee, Timothy T. Cuerdon, Hoangmai H. Pham, Megan Cox, Rahul Rajkumar, and Patrick H. Conway. 2015. "Association of Pioneer Accountable Care Organizations vs Traditional Medicare Fee For Service with Spending, Utilization, and Patient Experience," *Journal of the American Medical Association* 313 (21): 2152–2161; and J. Michael McWilliams, Bruce E. Landon, and Michael E. Chernew. 2013. "Changes in Health Care Spending and Quality for Medicare Beneficiaries Associated with a Commercial ACO Contract." *Journal of the American Medical Association* 310 (8): 829–836.

104. For a comprehensive review of medical homes, see Patient Centered Primary Care Collaborative and Milbank Memorial Fund, *The Patient-Centered Medical Home's Impact on Cost and Quality: Annual Review of the Evidence, 2013–2014*, January 2015. That report makes specific recommendations for further improvements. Likewise, the Agency for Healthcare Research and Quality, "Ensuring that Patient-Centered Medical Homes Effectively Serve Patients with Complex Health Needs," (2011) highlights the need to design effective risk-adjusted payment systems.

105. Craig Gilbert," "Ryan Blasts Obama's Immigration Plan," *Milwaukee Journal Sentinel*, November 20, 2014, p. 8A.
106. Adam Liptak, "Justices to Hear New Challenge to Health Law," *New York Times*, November 7, 2014. The high court's decision to take the case was unusual, since the lower appeals court had ruled against the plaintiffs. In a similar case, an appeals court in a different district had not yet settled the matter. Thus, the lower courts had not finished their deliberations on the question.
107. Two analyses of a related appeals court case offer estimates of the effects on the uninsured. Larry Levitt and Gary Claxton in "The Potential Side Effects of Halbig" (Kaiser Family Foundation, July 31, 2014) estimate 9.5 million people will not be eligible for subsidies. A second study estimates that over 11 million individuals will enroll in the 34 exchanges in 2016, yet 7.3 million of them will see a loss of subsidies totaling $36.1 billion. See Linda J. Blumberg, John Holahan, and Matthew Buettgens in "Halbig v Burwell: Potential Implications for ACA Coverage and Subsidies," Robert Wood Johnson Foundation and Urban Institute, July 2014.
108. Blumberg et al. "Halbig v Burwell," p. 1.
109. Adam Liptak, "Supreme Court Allows Nationwide Health Care Subsidies," *New York Times*, June 25, 2015.
110. The Republicans are pursuing the strategy to repeal the PPACA in 2015. See Andrew Raylor, "Senate Adopts GOP Budget Targeting 'Obamacare,'" *Washington Post*, May 5, 2015. The reconciliation procedure applies to fiscal items only.
111. Edward Luce, "Obamacare's Drip-fed Success," *Financial Times*, October 26, 2014.

Three   Germany: Modernizing Social Health Insurance to Meet New Challenges

1. This book refers to Germany's variant of national health insurance as social health insurance (SHI) to distinguish it from single-payer government insurance. However, I will sometimes refer to Germany as having NHI because that is how it is commonly referred to in some of the literature. Japan has modeled its health care system on the German model of SHI (T. R. Reid, *The Healing of America: A Global Quest for Better, Cheaper, and Fairer Health Care* [New York: Penguin Books, 2010], chap. 6). Switzerland's variant of NHI removes employers from financing and mandates all individuals to purchase coverage from a number of nonprofit insurers. The government subsidizes premiums for those on low incomes. See Uwe E. Reinhardt, "The Swiss Health System: Regulated Competition without Managed Care," *Journal of the American Medical Association* 292 (10) (September 8, 2004): 1227–1231; Reid, *Healing of America*, pp. 176–182.
2. I will more fully describe corporatism as the chapter proceeds.
3. Peter J. Katzenstein, *Policy and Politics in West Germany: The Growth of a Semi-Sovereign State* (Philadelphia: Temple University Press, 1987).
4. This is the German designation for health insurance funds.

5. Kees van Kersbergen, *Social Capitalism: A Study of Christian Democracy and the Welfare State* (London and New York: Routledge, 1995); Susan Giaimo, *Markets and Medicine: The Politics of Health Care Reform in Britain, Germany, and the United States* (Ann Arbor: University of Michigan Press, 2002), pp. 89–91.
6. Deborah A. Stone, *The Limits of Professional Power* (Chicago: University of Chicago Press, 1980), Chap. 1; Marian Döhler, "The State as Architect of Political Order: Policy Dynamics of German Health Care," *Governance* 8:3 (1995): 380–404; Katzenstein, *Policy and Politics*, pp. 172–173.
7. Stephan Leibfried and Florian Tennstedt, "Health-Insurance Policy and Berufsverbote in the Nazi Takeover," in *Political Values and Health Care: The German Experience*, ed. Donald W. Light and Alexander Schuller (Cambridge and London: MIT Press, 1986), pp. 127–184.
8. Giaimo, *Markets and Medicine*, pp. 89–91; Katzenstein, *Policy and Politics*, Chap. 1, esp. pp. 67–68 and 172–176.
9. Heinz Rothgang, Achim Schmid, and Claus Wendt, "The Self-Regulatory German Healthcare System Between Growing Competition and State Hierarchy," in *The State and Heatlhcare: Comparing OECD Countries*. Heinz Rothgang, Mirella Cacace, Lorraine Frisina, Simone Grimmeisen, Achim Schmid, and Claus Wendt (London and New York: Palgrave Macmillan, 2010), pp. 119–120.
10. Reinhard Busse and Miriam Blümel, *Germany: Health System Review*, vol. 16, issue 2, *Health Systems in Transition* (European Observatory on Health Systems and Policies, 2014), pp. 24–25. The German Democratic Republic (communist East Germany) had 100 percent of its population covered under the government health care system during its existence (1949–1990). Jens Martin Hoyer, *Social Health Insurance in Germany and the Market Position of the TK: Current Changes and Future Challenges*, May 10, 2009; Katzenstein, *Policy and Politics*, p. 172.
11. Busse and Blümel, *Germany*, p. 25; Miriam Blümel and Reinhard Busse, "The German Health Care System, 2014," in *2014 International Profiles of Health Care Systems*, ed. Elias Mossialos, Martin Wenzl, Robin Osborn, and Chloe Anderson (New York and Washington DC: The Commonwealth Fund, January 2015), p. 63.
12. Busse and Blümel, *Germany*, pp. 45–46, 121–122, 251.
13. Melanie Lisac, Lutz Reimers, Klaus-Dirk Henke, and Sophia Schlette, "Access and Choice–Competition under the Roof of Solidarity in German Health Care: An Analysis of Health Policy Reforms Since 2004," *Health Economics, Policy and Law* (2010) 5, pp. 38–39.
14. Ibid. pp. 38–39.
15. Blümel and Busse, "German Health Care System," p. 63; Busse and Blümel, *Germany*, pp. 121, 137–138; Lisac et al., "Access and choice," pp. 38–39.
16. Lisac et al., "Access and Choice," pp. 38–39.
17. Ibid, p. 41.
18. Ibid. pp. 35–36.
19. Busse and Blümel, *Germany*, p. 169.
20. Interview with Franz Knieps, June 13, 2009.
21. Busse and Blümel, *Germany*, pp. 161–162.

22. The government announced its intention to develop a DRG system that began with the 1993 Health Care Structural Act. The 2003 Case Fees Act legislated the current DRG system, but DRGs were only fully implemented in 2010. See Giaimo, *Markets and Medicine*, Chap. 4; Rothgang et al., "Self-Regulatory German Healthcare," pp. 124–125; 161–162.
23. Busse and Blümel, *Germany*, pp. 205–219.
24. This type of welfare state, which is based on payroll contributions to compulsory employment-based social insurance and administration by corporatist interest associations, is a model that other nations have adopted, such as France, the Netherlands (up to 2006), and Japan, as well as some former communist countries of Eastern and Central Europe. This welfare state type goes by different names, depending on the analyst. Some term it the Bismarckian welfare state, owing to its origins. Others label it a Christian Democratic or conservative corporatist welfare state.
25. Corporatism has a long history in Germany and extends to the economy and other parts of the welfare state. Associational self-regulation of members of the professions dates from the guild tradition of the medieval era that survived into the industrial era. Corporatism is part of Germany's conservative tradition of ordered or organized capitalism, whereby state actors indirectly direct the economy and society through large associations representing major social groups. These large associations bring order to an otherwise chaotic sector by controlling their members and serving as the chief representative of interests in negotiations with the government. See Kenneth Dyson, ed. *The Politics of German Regulation* (Aldershot, England: Dartmouth, 1992), esp. Dyson, "Theories of Regulation and the Case of Germany: A Model of Regulatory Change," pp. 1–28; Katzenstein, *Policy and Politics*, 1987.
26. Separate from the KVs are professional physician chambers (Ärztekammern). The chambers at state level determine medical education and practice standards for all doctors, while their peak association represents the profession in scientific matters and on matters of national policy. Purely private organizations representing physician interests also exist. But they do not enjoy the privileged access to government in formulating or implementing health policy that the KVs do. Such organizations also tend to be more strident in their defense of physician interests than the KVs. As public-law associations, the KVs are constrained and sometimes conflicted by their need to balance the private interests of physicians with the broader public interest. See Webber, "Die KVs," and Giaimo, *Markets and Medicine*, chap. 3.
27. Hoyer, *Social Health Insurance in Germany*, 2009; Rothgang et al. "Self-Regulatory German Healthcare," chap. 6.
28. Busse and Blümel, *Germany*, pp. 44–45.
29. Dirk Sauerland, "The Legal Framework for Health Care Quality Assurance in Germany," *Health Economics, Policy and Law* 4 (2009): 79–98; Tsung-Mei Cheng and Uwe E. Reinhardt, "Shepherding Major Health System Reforms: A Conversation with German Health Minister Ulla Schmidt," *Health Affairs* 27(3) (2008): w204–2213, esp. pp. 210.

30. For an excellent description of corporatist regulation see Wolfgang Streeck and Philippe C. Schmitter, "Community, Market, State-and Associations? The Prospective Contribution of Interest Governance to Social Order," *European Sociological Review* 1(2) (1985): 119–138. In the health sector, see Katzenstein, *Policy and Politics*, chaps. 1 and 4; Marion Döhler, "The State as Architect of Political Order: Policy Dynamics in German Health Care," *Governance* 8(3) (1995): 380–404; Douglas Webber, "Die Kassenärztlichen Vereinigungen zwischen Mitgliederinteressen und Gemeinwohl," in *Verbände zwischen Mitgliederinteressen und Gemeinwohl*, ed. Renate Mayntz (Gütersloh: Verlag Bertelsmann Stiftung); Giaimo, *Markets and Medicine*, pp. 91–93 and chaps. 3 and 4; Giaimo, "Health Care Reform in Britain and Germany: Recasting the Political Bargain with the Medical Profession." *Governance* 8 (3) (July 1995): 354–379.

31. Giaimo, *Markets and Medicine*, chap. 4; Heinz Rothgang, "The Converging Role of the State in OECD Healthcare Systems," in *The State and Healthcare: Comparing OECD Countries*, Heinz Rothgang, Mirella Cacace, Lorraine Frisina, Simone Grimmeisen, Achim Schmid, and Claus Wendt (London and New York: Palgrave Macmillan, 2010), pp. 237–247.

32. The mixed electoral system actually gives Germans two votes in Bundestag elections. Under the first vote, roughly half the seats in the Bundestag on the basis of single-member district simple plurality rules. The remaining seats are allocated on the basis of the percentage of the national vote that each party wins in the second vote. The seats won under the single-member district vote are deducted from the party's percentage of the vote won in the second ballot. The overall effect, then, is proportional. There are threshold rules to prevent extremely small splinter parties from winning seats. For a good description of how the mixed electoral system works, see David P. Conradt, *The German Polity,* 9th ed. (Boston and New York: Houghton Mifflin Harcourt, 2009), chap. 6.

33. German corporatism does not operate uniformly across all sectors of the economy and society. Interest groups possess greater autonomy from government in some sectors rather than in others. In industrial relations, for example, the constitution guarantees free collective bargaining among unions and employers associations and forbids the government from intervening directly. Even so, unions and employers operate under a strong legal framework that governs their activities. In social policy, by contrast, government supervision of and intervention in the activities of key interest groups is more direct. Their designation as public-law bodies grants the government such authority.

34. Kenneth Dyson. "Theories of Regulation and the Case of Germany: A Model of Regulatory Change," in *The Politics of German Regulation*, ed. Kenneth Dyson (Aldershot: England: Dartmouth, 1992). van Kersbergen, *Social Capitalism*, 1995, chaps. 4 and 8.

35. The social market economy was largely a creation of conservatives, especially the CDU and its predecessors. However, the Social Democrats and the trade unions were reformist and came to accept the market economy as long as it had state oversight and generous social provision. See Gaston V. Rimlinger, *Welfare*

Policy and Industrialization in Europe, America, and Russia (New York: John Wiley and Sons, 1971), pp. 138–148; van Kersbergen, *Social Capitalism*, chaps. 4, 8, and 10. The FDP is the strongest champion of the free market, yet liberalism has not been the dominant force in German politics as it has been in the United States.

36. van Kersbergen, *Social Capitalism*, esp. chaps. 4, 8, and 10.

37. OECD, *Health at a Glance 2011: OECD Indicators*, pp. 25, 149, 150. With an extensive public transportation network, shops in close proximity to where people live, and ample bike paths and green spaces even in urban areas, Germans are also arguably less sedentary than Americans who commonly rely on cars to reach distant supermarkets. The exercise built into the average German's daily regimen may partially offset their intake of beer and chocolate.

38. Stephanie Stock, Marcus Redaelli, and Karl Wilhelm Lauterbach, "The Influence of the Labor Market on German Health Care Reforms," *Health Affairs* 25(4) (2006): 1145.

39. Philip Manow and Eric Seils, "Adjusting Badly: The German Welfare State, Structural Change, and the Open Economy," in *Welfare and Work in the Open Economy, Vol. II: Diverse Responses to Common Challenges*, ed. Fritz W. Scharpf and Vivien A. Schmidt (Oxford and New York: Oxford University Press, 2000), pp. 264–307; Stock et al., "The Influence of the Labor Market on German Health Care Reforms," pp. 1146–1147.

40. Manow and Seils, "Adjusting Badly," pp. 292–293; Susan Giaimo, "Who Pays for Health Care Reform?" in *The New Politics of the Welfare State*, ed. Paul Pierson (Oxford and New York: Oxford University Press, 2000), p. 352. Some of the increase in contribution rates was due to an aging population, but using the welfare state to absorb unemployment in the East was also a significant factor.

41. Bertrand Benoit, "A Temporary Solution? Germany's Labour Market Develops a Second Tier," *Financial Times*, October 27, 2006.

42. Anke Hassel, "Twenty Years after German Unification: The Restructuring of the German Welfare and Employment Regime," *German Politics and Society*, 28(2) (Summer 2010), pp. 109–115.

43. Cheng and Reinhardt, "Shepherding Major Health," pp. w208.

44. This section draws on Giaimo, *Markets and Medicine*, pp. 93–105; Rothgang, "Converging Role of the State," pp. 157–160.

45. Stone, *Limits of Professional Power*, pp. 17–18.

46. Marian Döhler, "Regulating the Medical Profession in Germany: The Politics of Efficiency Review," Berlin: Social Science Research Center, Research Unit Market Processes and Corporate Development, May 1987, typescript; Stone, *Limits of Professional Power*, chap. 7

47. Giaimo, *Markets and Medicine*, p. 105.

48. Ibid. p. 100; Philip Manow, "Social Insurance the German Political Economy," *MPIFG Discussion Paper* 97:2 (Cologne: Max Planck Institute for the Study of Societies, 1997).

49. The 1993 law followed the 1989 Health Care Reform Act, which had relied on corporatist processes for implementation. When providers and insurers refused

to negotiate those provisions, policymakers responded with the 1993 law, which constituted a more forceful intrusion of government power into health care administration.

50. There were some exceptions, however. While most sickness funds now had to accept all applicants regardless of occupation, company funds could choose to remain closed to those were not employees of that particular firm.

51. Giaimo, *Markets and Medicine*, p. 247, n. 11.

52. For a detailed account of the content and politics of the 1993 law, see Giaimo, *Markets and Medicine*, chap. 4.

53. This section draws on Dirk Sauerland, "The Legal framework for Health Care Quality Assurance in Germany," *Health Economics, Policy and Law* 4 (2009): 79–98 and Busse and Blümel, *Germany*, esp. pp. 61–63, 239–243.

54. Busse and Blümel, *Germany*, 2014, pp. 63–68.

55. Ibid. p. 64.

56. Tsung-Mei Cheng and Uwe E. Reinhardt, "Shepherding Major Health System Reforms" p. w210.

57. This section draws on Busse and Blümel, *Germany*, 2014, esp. Chap. 6, and Melanie Lisac, Kerstin Blum and Sophia Schlette, "Changing Long-Established Structures for More Competition and Stronger Coordination—Health Care Reform in Germany in the New Millennium," *Intereconomics* (July/August 2008): 184–189.

58. The law's intent was for ICCs to provide more encompassing population-based care. See Lisac et al. "Changing Long-Established Structures."

59. Ibid. p. 187; Kerstin Blum, "Care Coordination Gaining Momentum in Germany," *Health Policy Monitor Survey* (9) 2007, Bertelsmann Stiftung, Gütersloh, Germany.

60. Blümel and Busse, "German Health Care System," p. 65; Lisac et al. "Changing Long-Established Structures," p. 187; Lisac et al, "Access and Choice," p. 47.

61. Blümel and Busse, "German Health Care System," p. 69.

62. Ibid. p. 65, 69; Rothgang et al., "Self-Regulatory German Healthcare," and Rothgang, "Converging Role of the State."

63. Lisac et al., "Access and Choice," pp. 44, 48.

64. The surcharge was a compromise that followed from an earlier scheme to introduce supplemental dental coverage financed solely by patients. The government settled for the surcharge after analysis indicated that the supplemental insurance would have entailed high administrative costs and hurt the more vulnerable. See Busse and Blümel, *Germany*, pp. 239–241.

65. Ibid. p. 239.

66. The description of the 2007 law relies on Busse and Blümel, *Germany*, chap. 6, esp. pp. 247–252, and Lisac et al., "Access and Choice."

67. Public pensions already followed this model of mixed financing, relying on payroll contributions as well as on federal government tax revenues. The income ceiling limit subject to payroll taxes for pensions is also higher than it is for health insurance.

68. Lisac et al., "Access and Choice," p. 39.

69. Ibid. pp. 43–44.
70. Lisac et al., "Access and Choice," pp. 39–42.
71. See Busse and Blümel, *Germany*, pp. 124–127; 260–261.
72. Interview with Franz Knieps, Director-General, Public Health Care, Health Insurance, Long-term Care Insurance, German Federal Ministry of Health, Berlin, Germany, June 13, 2009.
73. Busse and Blümel, *Germany,* pp. 149–154; Rothgang et al., *State and Healthcare,* pp. 157–161.
74. Busse and Blümel, *Germany*, pp. 122, 249.
75. Bundesministerium für Gesundheit, *Willkommen in der Solidarität! Informationen zur Gesundheitsreform 2007*, March 2007; Lisac et al., "Access and Choice," p. 37. Blümel and Busse, "German Health Care System," p. 65.
76. Some of the reform ideas, such as managed competition had been gestating since the mid-1990s. For example, the economists at the apex of the Concerted Action in Health Care had called for sickness fund competition on additional benefits and new forms of insurance contracts in 1995. Along with major employers' associations, they had proposed that the employers' share of the premium be fixed while letting employees shoulder the higher premiums. But at the time they were proposed, they were viewed as too controversial to be enacted into law. Giaimo, *Markets and Medicine*, pp. 145–147.
77. Busse and Blümel, *Germany*, pp. 243–245; Susanne Weinbrenner and Reinhard Busse, "Proposals for SHI Reform," *Health Policy Monitor* (2) (November 2003), http://www.hpm.org/survey/de/a2/2; and Melanie Zimmermann, "Health Financing Reform Idea: Health Fund," *Health Policy Monitor* (7) (June 2006), http://www.hpm.org/survey/de/b7/1.,
78. A minority group on the commission, consisting largely of Social Democrats, Greens, unions and consumer associations, rejected both proposals. It offered its own alternative, which closely resembled the proposal for citizens' insurance (Weinbrenner and Busse, "Proposals for SHI Reform," 2003). For an analysis of the underlying rationale for citizen's insurance, see Simone Leiber, Stefan Greß, and Maral-Sonja Manouguian, "Health Care System Change and the Cross-Border Transfer of Ideas: Influence of the Dutch Model on the 2007 German Health Reform," *Journal of Health Politics, Policy and Law* 35 (4) August 2010, esp. pp. 553–554.
79. The CDU, which, as the opposition party, was excluded from the Rürup commission, formed its own commission. Like the Rürup Commission, the CDU commission included major health care stakeholders. It recommended flat-rate premiums and compulsory individual insurance, with additional contributions of the insured to build up the reserves and make it self-funded. See Zimmermann, "Health Fund," 2006.
80. Jost Müller-Neuhof, "Sozialfall Gesundheit," *Der Tagesspiegel*, June 11, 2009, p. 4.
81. Busse and Blümel, *Germany,* pp. 252–254, 260–261; Miriam Blümel, "Changes in Contribution Rate Setting from 2015," *Health Policy Monitor* site. Accessed 12/28/14; Blümel and Busse, "German Health Care System," p. 71.
82. Rothgang, "Converging Role of the State."

83. Busse and Blümel, *Germany*, pp. 124–127, 260–261, 265; Blümel and Busse, "German Health Care System," p. 71.
84. Rothgang, "Converging Role of the State."

Four South Africa: Confronting the Legacies of Apartheid

1. Numerous groups in civil society (human rights groups, political parties, trade unions, and religious denominations) fought for full democratization and coalesced into the antiapartheid movement. These groups engaged in largely peaceful protest but were often met with brutal repression by the white security forces. The African National Congress (ANC), the political party leading the antiapartheid movement, also supported a guerilla wing that engaged in violent acts against the white minority government. So there was significant violence in the struggle to end apartheid. Nonetheless, both sides recognized that they were at a stalemate. Wishing to avoid an all-out civil war, the ANC and the ruling National Party (NP) engaged initially in behind the scenes and later, open talks, to come to a negotiated settlement. For an account of these difficult negotiations, see Allister Sparks, *Tomorrow is Another Country: The Inside Story of South Africa's Road to Change* (New York: Hill and Wang, 1995). Sparks also provides an excellent analysis of the myriad challenges facing governments in the first decade following the end of apartheid in *Beyond the Miracle: Inside the New South Africa* (London: Profile Books, 2003).
2. Mia Malan, "South Africa Has Highest Number of New HIV Infections Worldwide – Survey," *Mail and Guardian*, April 4, 2014. South Africa had the fourth largest TB incidence rate in the world in 2006. See Salim S. Abdool Karim, Gavin J. Churchyard, Quarraisa Abdool Karim and Stephen D. Lawn, "HIV Infection and Tuberculosis in South Africa: An Urgent Need to Escalate the Public Health Response," *Lancet* 374 (September 12, 2009): 924; World Bank statistics, Incidence of Tuberculosis, 2015.
3. Varun Gauri and Even S. Lieberman, "Boundary Institutions and HIV/AIDS Policy in Brazil and South Africa," *Studies in Comparative International Development* 41 (3) (Fall 2006): 47–73. The authors note that apartheid's legal prohibition of sexual relations among different races sought to reverse the miscegenation that had occurred since imperialism.
4. "South Africa Lifts 3.6 Million out of Poverty Thanks to its Fiscal Policies," World Bank press release no. 2015/179/AFR, November 4, 2014.
5. In 2013, tuberculosis was the leading cause of death in South Africa, followed by pneumonia and influenza, and HIV in third place. While deaths from TB and pneumonia and flu are declining, HIV has moved up in the mortality rankings since 2009. Noncommunicable diseases like stroke, diabetes, and heart disease rank next. See Statistics South Africa, *Mortality and Causes of Death in South Africa, 2013: Findings from Death Notifications*. Stat release P0309.3 December

2, 2014, pp. 24–27. The rise in HIV deaths is due to a change in reporting by medical personnel (Statistics South Africa on "Mortality and Causes of Death 2013," South African Government, December 2, 2014. http://www.gov.za/mortality-and-causes-death-2013. For an overview of the growing burden of noncommunicable disease in South Africa, see Bongani M. Mayosi, Alan J. Flisher, Umesh G. Lalloo, Freddy Sitas, Stephen M. Tollman, and Debbie Bradshaw,"The Burden of Non-communicable Diseases in South Africa," *The Lancet* 374 (September 12, 2009): 934–947;.

6. See World Health Organization, *Health Systems Financing: The Path to Universal Health Coverage* (Geneva: WHO, 2010).

7. For a highly readable description of health care provision in developing nations, see T. R. Reid, *The Healing of America: A Global Quest for Better, Cheaper, and Fairer Health Care* (New York: Penguin, 2010), Chap. 9.

8. *Health at a Glance 2013: OECD Indicators*, OECD: Paris, 2013, pp. 155, 157.

9. Hoosen Coovadia, Rachel Jewkes, Peter Barron, David Sanders, and Diane McIntyre, "The Health and Health System of South Africa: Historical Roots of Current Public Health Challenges," *The Lancet* 374 (September 5, 2009): 828–829; Yogan Pillay, "The Impact of South Africa's New Constitution on the Organization of Health Services in the Post-Apartheid Era," *Journal of Health Politics, Policy and Law* 26 (4) (August 2001): 756–759.

10. Pillay, "South Africa's New Constitution," pp. 753, 755.

11. The figures for public and private spending are 2013 data from the World Bank, *World Development Indicators: Health Systems*, 2015. See Coovadia et al., "Health and Health System," p. 830 for the figures on physicians.

11. Coovadia et al., "Health and Health System," pp. 826–830. Roughly 20 percent of South Africans migrate between the private and public systems, paying out of pocket for primary care from private providers, but then relying on the public system for expensive hospital care. Nearly two-thirds of South Africans rely entirely on the public health care system. Taking these last two groups together, the public health care system cares for 84 percent of the population.

13. Ibid. p. 828. (Ten rand is roughly equivalent to one US dollar.)

14. Ibid., pp. 824–828. The number of health insurance funds declined from over 180 in 2001 to 102 at the end of the decade. See Department of Health, Republic of South Africa, *National Health Insurance in South Africa: Policy Paper* (August 12, 2011), p. 11.

15. This section draws on Coovadia et al., "Health and Health System," pp. 817–834.

16. Sparks, *Beyond the Miracle*, pp. 48–49. The bantustans, or tribal reserves, that whites created in South Africa were similar to the reservations for Native Americans in the United States. In both cases, white settlers forcibly removed indigenous peoples to some of the least inhabitable areas of the country.

17. For example, in 1960, the wages of black miners in the gold mines were 20 percent lower than in 1911. Though the gap had narrowed by 1972, black miners' wages were still 8 percent less than in 1911. Coovadia et al. "Health and Health System," p. 823.

18. Ibid., 819–820. The number of miners soared from 10,000 in 1889 to 400,000 in 1940.

19. Ibid., p. 825.

20. Abdool Karim et al. "HIV Infection and Tuberculosis," p. 923.

21. Ibid., pp. 921–923; Coovadia et al. "Health and Health System," pp. 822–283.

22. O. Shisana, T. Rehle, LC. Simbaayi, K. Zuma, S. Jooste, N. Zungu, D. Labadarios, D. Onoya et al. *South African National HIV Prevalence, Incidence and Behaviour Survey, 2012* (Cape Town: HSRC Press, 2014), pp. xxvi, 50.

23. Salim S. Abdool Karim et al.,, "HIV Infection and Tuberculosis," pp. 922–923.

24. Coovadia et al., "Health and Health System," pp. 819–823.

25. Nicoli Nattrass, "Meeting the Challenge of Unemployment?" Annals of the American Academy of Political and Social Science 652 (March 2014), pp. 89-90; *World Development Indicators: Health Systems*, World Bank, 2015, http://data.worldbank.org/data-catalog/world-development-indicators.

26. Coovadia, "Health and Health System," p. 824; Mickey Chopra, Joy E. Lawn, David Sanders, Peter Barron, Salim s. Abdool Karim, Debbie Bradshaw, Rachel Jewkes, Quarraisha Abdool Karim, Alan J. Flisher, Bongani M. Mayosi, Stephen M. Tollman, Gavin J. Churchyard, Hoosen Coovadia, "Achieving the Health Millennium Development Goals for South Africa: Challenges and Priorities," *Lancet* 374 (September 19, 2009): 835.

27. World Bank, 2015. The South African Medical Research Council's (SAMRC) life expectancy figures are slightly higher, at 62 years in 2013. See SAMRC, *Rapid Mortality Surveillance Report 2012*. There are also gender differences, with male life expectancy at 56 years and 62 years for females in 2012 (WHO, Statistics South Africa.).

28. "Don't Get Ill," The Price of Freedom: A Special Report on South Africa, *The Economist*, June 5, 2010, p. 15.

29. Abdool Karim et al., "HIV Infection and Tuberculosis," pp. 921–923; Chopra et al. "Achieving the MDGs," p. 1023; UNAIDS South Africa, 2015. http://aidsinfo.unaids.org

30. Shisana et al., *South African National HIV Prevalence*, p. 50.

31. Mohaded Seedat, Ashley Van Niekerk, Rachel Jewkes, Shahnaaz Fuffla, and Kopano Ratele, "Violence and Injuries in South Africa: Prioritising an Agenda for Prevention," *Annals of the American Academy of Political and Social Science* 652 (March 2014): 1011–1022.

32. Bongani M. Mayosi, Alan J. Flisher, Umesh G. Lalloo, Freddy Sitas, Stephen M. Tollman, and Debbie Bradshaw, "The Burden of Non-communicable Diseases in South Africa," *Annals of the American Academy of Political and Social Science* 652 (March 2014): 934–947.

33. There have been instances of government attempts to limit press freedom or influence judges, but thus far these have been isolated and unsuccessful.

34. Roger Southall, "Democracy at Risk? Politics and Governance under the ANC," *Annals of the American Academy of Political and Social Science* 652 (March 2014): 48–69.

35. Gauri and Lieberman, "Boundary Institutions."

36. Southall, "Democracy at Risk," pp. 52–54.

37. Mandela, along with Archbishop Desmond Tutu (who was not an ANC member), also sought to heal the wounds of apartheid through the Truth and Reconciliation Commission. That process granted amnesty to those who perpetrated human rights abuses during apartheid if they acknowledged their guilt and expressed remorse. The 1996 constitution recognizes 11 official languages, indicating a commitment to diversity.

38. For example, the ANC has whites on the national executive committee and appoints whites to cabinet and provincial government ministries. See "Your Friendly Monolith," The Price of Freedom: A Special Report on South Africa, *The Economist,* June 5, 2010.

39. The forceful ejection of a rival party led by Julius Malema during President Zuma's state of the nation speech in February 2015 illustrates this concern. Malema, who was expelled from the ANC following his radical views and inflammatory language, since formed his own party. Malema and his fellow MPs disrupted Zuma's state of the nation speech with questions about the president's involvement in a corruption scandal in which he allegedly used taxpayer funds to upgrade his home. Plainclothes police used force to eject Malema and his party from parliament. Journalists covering the proceedings also found that their cellphone connections had been jammed. The incident was not only an unprecedented incident of parliamentary violence; it also indicated that the government was willing to trample on the rights of press freedom. See Andrew England, "Parliamentary Punch-Up Bodes Ill for Zuma's South Africa," *Financial Times,* February 16, 2015 and "South Africa Parliament Erupts as Jacob Zuma is Grilled over Scandal," *Financial Times,* February 12, 2015.

40. Southall, "Democracy at Risk," pp. 52–54.

41. Pillay, "South Africa's New Constitution," p. 755.

42. Mickey Chopra, Emmauelle Daviaud, Robert Pattinson, Sharon Fonn, and Joy E. Lawn, "Saving the Lives of South Africa's Mothers, Babies, and Children: Can the Health System Deliver?" *Lancet* 374 (September 5, 2009): 835.

43. Coovadia et al., "Health and Health System," pp. 820, 825.

44. Chopra et al., "Saving the Lives," pp. 835–837.

45. Department of Health, Republic of South Africa, *National Health Insurance in South Africa,* August 12, 2011, pp. 1–8.

46. Abdool Karim et al., "HIV Infection and Tuberculosis," pp. 921–925.

47. Gauri and Lieberman, "Boundary Institutions," p. 65.

48. Abdool Karim et al., "HIV Infection and Tuberculosis," pp. 921–925.

49. WHO recommended DOTS (directly observed treatment, short course) regimen of antibiotics for TB. But this failed to combat multiple drug-resistant strains of the disease. What was needed was a supplemental regimen of additional drug therapy and monitoring (DOTS-Plus). However, the WHO has been slow to recognize the efficacy of DOTS-Plus on the grounds that it costs too much for poor countries. See Anne Becker, Anjali Motgi, Jonathan Weigel,

Giuseppe Raviola, Sahmaan Keshavjee, and Arthur Kleinman, "The Unique Challenges of Mental Health and MDRTB: Critical Perspectives on Metrics of Disease," in *Reimagining Global Health: An Introduction*, ed. Paul Farmer, Jim Yong Kim, Arthur Kleinman, and Matthew Basilico (Berkeley: University of California Press, 2013), pp. 234–243.

50. Michael Specter, "The Denialists," *The New Yorker*, March 12, 2007, pp. 31–38.
51. Ibid. p. 36.
52. Sparks, *Beyond the Miracle*, pp. 291–295; Gauri and Lieberman, "Boundary Institutions," pp. 65–66.
53. Gauri and Lieberman, "Boundary Institutions," p. 65.
54. See Jeremy Greene, Marguerite Thorp Basilico, Heidi Kim, and Paul Farmer, "Colonial Medicine and its Legacies," in *Reimagining Global Health: An Introduction*, ed. Paul Farmer, Jim Yong Kim, Arthur Kleinman, and Matthew Basilico (Berkeley: University of California Press, 2013), pp. 33–73.
55. Luke Messac and Krishna Prabhu, "Redefining the Possible: The Global AIDS Response," in *Reimagining Global Health: An Introduction*, ed. Paul Farmer, Jim Yong Kim, Arthur Kleinman, and Matthew Basilico (Berkeley: University of California Press, 2013), pp. pp. 111–132.
56. Government-owned labs in Brazil first began to manufacture older ARTs as generic drugs. The Brazilian government also negotiated price reductions with drug companies on newer patented drugs. In 2007, the government began to manufacture generic versions of newer HAARTs in 2007. See Jane Galvão, "Brazil and Access to HIV/AIDS Drugs: A Question of Human Rights and Public Health," *American Journal of Public Health* 95 (7) (July 2005): 1110–1116; Jon Cohen, "Brazil: Ten Years After," *Science* 313 (5786) (July 28, 2006): 484–487; and Eduardo J. Gomez, "How Brazil Outpaced the United States When It Came to AIDS: The Politics of Civic Infiltration, Reputation, and Strategic Internationalization," *Journal of Health Politics, Policy and Law* 36 (2) (April 2011): 317–352.
57. Specter, "The Denialists," p. 38.
58. Matthew Basilico, Vanessa Kerry, Luke Messac, Arjun Suri, Jonathan Weigel, Marguerite Thorp Basilico, Joia Mukherjee, and Paul Farmer, "A Movement for Global Health Equity? A Closing Reflection," in *Reimagining Global Health: An Introduction*, ed. Paul Farmer, Jim Yong Kim, Arthur Kleinman, and Matthew Basilico (Berkeley: University of California Press, 2013), p. 344.
59. 53 Ibid., pp. 343–347. For further reading on TAC, see Mark Heywood, "South Africa's Treatment Action Campaign: Combining Law and Social Mobilization to Realize the Right to Health," *Journal of Human Rights Practice* 1 (1) (2009): 14–36; Steven Friedman and Shauna Mottiar, "A Rewarding Engagement? The Treatment Action Campaign and the Politics of HIV/AIDS," *Politics and Society* 33 (4) (2005): 511–565; and Amy Nunn, Samuel Dickman, Nicoli Nattrass, Alexandra Cornwall, and Sofia Gruskin, "The Impacts of AIDS Movements on the Policy Responses to HIV/AIDS in Brazil and South Africa: A Comparative Analysis," *Global Public Health* 7 (10) (December 2012): 1031–1044. As Nunn et al. show, relations between government officials and civil society were very

different in Brazil and South Africa. In Brazil the government forged a partnership with AIDS activists and appointed them to key positions in the health ministry. In South Africa, Mbeki's government treated the AIDS movement with disdain until the president's second term.

60. Mark W. Zacher and Tania J. Keefe, *The Politics of Global Health Governance: United by Contagion* (New York: Palgrave Macmillan, 2008), chap. 5, esp. pp. 116–118.
61. Ibid. pp. 120–121.
62. Messac and Prabhu, "Redefining the Possible," p. 126.
63. Ibid. pp. 111–132.
64. UNAIDS Bulletin; Karim et al., HIV Infection and Tuberculosis," pp. 923–928.
65. Tabelo Timse, "Zuma Reveals His HIV Status," *Mail and Guardian*, April 26, 2010. While former Democratic Alliance leader Helen Zille went so far as to charge that his polygamy was far more harmful to the fight against AIDS than Mbeki's inaction, the Zuma government's record on combating AIDS does not bear this out. See Kate Wilkinson, "Has Jacob Zuma Hurt the Fight against AIDS More Than Thabo Mbeki?" *Africa Check*, September 23, 2014. http://africacheck.org/reports/has-jacob-zuma-hurt-the-fight-against-aids-more-than-mbeki/.
66. UNAIDS 2015; World Bank statistics, 2015.
67. UNAIDS, 2013 data; UNAIDS "Regional Fact Sheet 2012."
68. Pillay, "South Africa's New Constitution"; Coovadia et al., "Health and Health System," pp. 828–829.
69. Chopra et al., "Saving the Lives," esp. pp. 835–844.
70. Peter Drobac, Matthew Basilico, Luke Messac, David Walton, and Paul Farmer, "Building an Effective Rural Health Delivery Model in Haiti and Rwanda," pp. 133–183 and Jim Yong Kim, Michael Porter, Joseph Rhatigan, Rebecca Weintraub, Matthew Basilico, Cassia van der Hoof Holstein, and Paul Farmer, "Scaling Up Effective Delivery Models Worldwide," pp. 184–211 in *Reimagining Global Health: An Introduction*, ed. Paul Farmer, Jim Yong Kim, Arthur Kleinman, and Matthew Basilico (Berkeley: University of California Press, 2013).
71. Coovadia et al., "Health and Health System," p. 830.
72. Ibid. pp. 828–832.
73. Chopra et al., "Saving the Lives," pp. 843–846; Chopra et al., "Achieving the MDGs," pp. 1028–1030.
74. Some assert that GEAR's emphasis on fiscal discipline has been too harsh and done harm to social and health needs of the population. See Coovadia et al., "Health and Health Systems," pp. 824, 832; Chopra et al., "Achieving the MDGs," p. 1030. Others fault the government for rigid labor market protections and its unwillingness to allow private providers a greater role in education. See Ann Bernstein, "South Africa's Key Challenges: Tough Choices and New Directions," *Annals of the American Academy of Political and Social Science* 652 (March 2014): 20–47.

75. Health care researchers have been critical of government economic policies. See Coovadia et al., "Health and Health Systems," pp. 824, 832; Chopra et al., "Achieving the MDGs," p. 1030. Other observers, such as journalist and author Allister Sparks, have also voiced concern. See Sparks, *Beyond the Miracle*, chap. 16.

76. African National Congress with the technical support of WHO and UNICEF, *A National Health Plan for South Africa* (May 1994) p. 77.

77. Department of Health, Republic of South Africa, *National Health Insurance in South Africa*, August 12, 2011, pp. 12–15.

78. This section draws on the Department of Health, *National Health Insurance in South Africa*, August 12, 2011.

79. Ibid. pp. 16–18.

80. Ibid. pp. 23–31. The plans resemble the structures of the British NHS since 1990.

81. See also Department of Health, Republic of South Africa, National Health Insurance. www.health.gov.za/nhi.php. (accessed Jan. 24, 2015); Department of Health, Republic of South Africa, *National Health Insurance: Healthcare for All South Africans*, n. d. www.health.gov/za (accessed Jan. 24, 2015).

82. Department of Health, *NHI in South Africa*, 2011, pp. 34, 41–42.

83. *National Health Insurance: Healthcare For All South Africans*, n.d. www.health.gov/za (accessed Jan. 24, 2015).

84. If South Africa adopts single-payer, its health care system would resemble something like Britain or Canada's. If it requires all citizens to have coverage but permits multiple insurers alongside a government program for the poorest, it would look something like German SHI or the US system of private insurers and a public program for the poorest. In any case, it would be a hybrid model that borrows elements from other countries.

85. M. P. Matsoso and R. Fryatt, "National Health Insurance: The First 18 Months," *South African Medical Journal*, 103 (3) (2013).

86. Helen Suzman Foundation, *Submission to National Department of Health: National Health Insurance Green Paper*, December 2011.

87. Ibid.

88. Alex van den Heever, *Evaluation of the Green Paper on National Health Insurance*, Graduate School of Public and Development Management, Johannesburg, December 20, 2011.

89. South African Private Practitioner Forum, *National Health Insurance in South Africa: SAPPF Submission on the Green Paper on National Health Insurance*, December 2011.

90. South African Medical Association, *Submission of Comments on National Health Insurance (NHI) Green Paper*, December 2011.

91. Discovery Health (Pty) Ltd., and Discovery Health Medical Scheme, *Comments on Government Gazette No. 34523, on the National Health Act, 2003. Green Paper: Policy on National Health Insurance*, December 2011.

92. Shivani Ramjee, Tim Vieyra, Matan Abraham, Josh Kaplan, and Richard Taylor, "National Health Insurance and South Africa's Private Sector," *South*

African Health Review, 2013/14 (Durban: Health Systems Trust, September 2014): 93–103.

93. Matsoso and Fryatt, "NHI: The First 18 Months."

94. Anna Voce, Fiorenza Monticelli, Yogan Pillay, Shuaib Kauchali, Rakshika Bhana, Magalagadi Makua, and Gugulethu Ngubane, "District Clinical Specialist Teams," *South African Health Review, 2013/14* (Durban: Health Systems Trust, September 2014): 48.

95. Nattrass, "Meeting the Challenge," p. 89.

96. John Ele-Ojo Ataguba and James Akazili, "Health Care Financing in South Africa: Moving Towards Universal Coverage," CME 28 (2) (February 2010): 74–78; Rob Yates, "Only Public Funding Can Guarantee Universal Health Coverage," *The Guardian*, October 9, 2013. See also World Health Organization, *Health Systems Financing: The Path to Universal Coverage* (Geneva: WHO, 2010), chap. 3, which makes a case for prepayment and risk pooling and rejects direct payments at the time of service. The WHO also cautions against an exclusive reliance on payroll-based financing in developing nations.

97. Ataguba and Akazili, "Health Care Financing"; and *NHI for All South Africans*, Department of Health, p. 8.

98. WHO, *Achieving Universal Coverage*, 2012.

99. Sparks, *Beyond the Miracle*, chap. 2, pp. 15–28; Southall, "Democracy at Risk," p. 51.

100. Coovadia et al., "Health and Health System," p. 824.

101. World Bank, *South Africa Economic Update: Fiscal Policy and Redistribution in an Unequal Society* (Washington DC: November 2014). See esp. pp. 23–24 and pp. 42–45.

102. Ibid; Statistics South Africa, *Poverty Trends in South Africa: An Examination of Absolute Poverty between 2006 and 2011*, 2014.

103. World Bank, *South Africa Economic Update*, esp. pp. 2, 9–12, and 42–45.

104. "The Great Scourges," The Price of Freedom: A Special Report on South Africa, *The Economist*, June 5, 2010, pp. 11–12.

105. *Quarterly Labour Force Survey, Quarter 4, 2014*, Statistics South Africa, P0211 (February 10, 2015), pp. vi and viii.

106. Sparks, *Beyond the Miracle*, pp. 333–338.

107. Coovadia et al., "Health and Health Systems," pp. 830–831.

108. This is one of the key recommendations of academic health care researchers from the 2009 *Lancet* series on South African health care (see Chopra et al., "Achieving the MDGs," p. 1030). Sparks makes a case that policymakers must give up their single-minded pursuit of neoliberal structural adjustment and do more for the informal sector. This requires investment in education and also granting residents of informal settings legal title to their shanties. Legal title would allow them to access bank loans to start a business. He also calls for a massive program of public works employment to reduce unemployment and address the country's infrastructure deficiencies simultaneously (Sparks, *Beyond the Miracle*, Chap. 16, pp. 329–342. See "Cheerleaders and Naysayers," Emerging Africa: Special Report, *The Economist*, March 2, 2013 for additional arguments.

109. Southall, "Democracy at Risk," pp. 59–60.
110. Southall, "Democracy at Risk," pp. 63–64; Robert I. Rotberg, "Overcoming Difficult Challenges: Bolstering Good Governance," *Annals of the American Academy of Political and Social Science,* 652 (March 2014): 8–19.
111. Southall, "Democracy at Risk," pp. 54, 63.

Five   Conclusions and Prospects

1. Tyler Brûlé's column on urban neighborhood revitalization, "Some Neighbourhoods Are Streets Ahead," *Financial Times*, April 4, 2015, is the inspiration for the description and metaphor I develop here.
2. "Americans' Views on the Affordable Care Act Hold Steady, with 43% Now Viewing It Favorably and 42% Unfavorably," News Release, Kaiser Family Foundation, April 21, 2015. http://kff.org/health-reform/press-release/americans-views-on-the-affordable-care-act-hold-steady-with-43-now-viewing-it-favorably-and-42-unfavorably/
3. This seeming paradox of greater state intervention in creating and sustaining markets has been noted before. For a more general discussion of this relationship, see Steven Vogel, *Freer Markets, More Rules* (Ithaca and London: Cornell University Press, 1996). As applied to the case of German health care reform, see Heinz Rothgang, "The Converging Role of the State in OECD Healthcare Systems," in *The State and Healthcare: Comparing OECD Countries.* Heinz Rothgang, Mirella Cacace, Lorraine Frisina, Simone Grimmeisen, Achim Schmid, and Claus Wendt (London and New York: Palgrave Macmillan, 2010), pp. 237–247.
4. Walter Dean Burnham, *Critical Elections and the Mainspring of American Politics* (New York: Norton, 1970). In a similar vein, Britain enacted its landmark NHS scheme only in the wake of the upheaval of World War II and after an election that brought the Labor Party into a majority government for the first time in history.
5. "Health Insurance Coverage and the Affordable Care Act," Office of the Assistant Secretary for Planning and Evaluation, U.S. Department of Health and Human Services (May 8, 2015), http://aspe.hhs.gov/health/reports/2015/uninsured_change/ib_uninsured_change.pdf. Also see Matthew Buettgens, John Holahan, and Hannah Recht, "Medicaid Expansion, Health Coverage, and Spending: An Update for the 21 States that Have Not Expanded Eligibility," Issue Brief, Kaiser Family Foundation (April 29, 2015).
6. On the trend toward hybrid health care systems in the industrialized countries, see Heinz Rothgang, Mirella Cacace, Lorraine Frisina, Simone Grimmeisen, Achim Schmid, and Claus Wendt. *The State and Healthcare: Comparing OECD Countries* (London and New York: Palgrave Macmillan, 2010).
7. WHO, *World Health Report 2008: Primary Health Care (Now More than Ever)* (Geneva: World Health Organization, 2008).

8. WHO, *Health Systems Financing: The Path to Universal Coverage* (Geneva: World Health Organization, 2010), executive summary, pp. ix–xxii.

9. Ibid., pp. xiv–xvi and Chap. 3; T. R. Reid, *The Healing of America: A Global Quest for Better, Cheaper, and Fairer Health Care* (New York: Penguin, 2010), Chap. 13; Deborah A. Stone, "The Struggle for the Soul of Insurance," *Journal of Health Politics, Policy and Law* (Summer 1993): 286–317.

10. Bianca DiJulio, Jamie Firth, and Mollyann Brodie, "Kaiser Health Tracking Poll: April 2015," Kaiser Family Foundation, http://kff.org/health-reform/poll-finding/kaiser-health-tracking-poll-april-2015/; "Americans' views," Kaiser Family Foundation.

11. See *The Patient Choice, Affordability, Responsibility, and Empowerment Act: A Legislative Proposal,* January 2014.

12. Miriam Blümel and Reinhard Busse "The German Health Care System, 2014," in *2014 International Profiles of Health Care Systems,* ed. Elias Mossialos, Martin Wenzl, Robin Osborn, and Chloe Anderson (New York and Washington, DC: The Commonwealth Fund, 2015), p. 65.

13. Reinhard Busse and Miriam Blümell, *Germany: Health System Review,* vol. 16, issue 2, *Health Systems in Transition.* European Observatory on Health Systems and Policies, 2014, Chap. 7.

14. A number of developing nations, as economically diverse as China and Rwanda, have sought to achieve universal coverage through a mix of insurance schemes rather than a single payer. See WHO, *Health Systems Financing,* pp. xxi and 7.

15. That depends on the parameters of competition. If there are too many insurers, administrative costs may be high. If providers compete by offering the latest high-tech procedures or private hospital rooms with breathtaking views of nature, it may add to health care spending.

16. Reid, *Healing of America,* pp. 223–225; WHO, *Health Systems Financing,* p. xvi.

17. Reid, *Healing of America,* Appendix.

18. An "implicit concordat" between the government and doctors in Britain's NHS held until the 1990s. Under this unspoken agreement, doctors left decisions on the NHS budget to the government and rationed scarce resources on its behalf; in return, politicians let doctors decide how to use NHS resources and did not question their clinical freedom. Government austerity measures in the 1980s strained this settlement, leading to a very public confrontation between Conservative governments and the medical profession. See Rudolf Klein, *The Politics of the NHS,* 2nd ed. (London: Longman, 1989), Chap. 7 and p. 235. In Germany, peer review of individual doctors' treatment decisions began in the 1930s. Starting in the 1970s, insurers won representation on such review bodies. The clinical autonomy of the individual practitioner went furthest in the United States until the advent of managed care in the 1990s, when insurers increasingly decided whether a procedure was medically necessary and thus subject to coverage. PPACA limits insurers' infringement of doctors' clinical freedom by requiring an external appeals process for treatment denials. See www.healthcare.gov/https://www.healthcare.gov/search/?q=appeals&output=xml_no_dtd&site=healthcare&proxystylesheet=json&client=json&lr=lang_en&ie=UTF-

8&oe=UTF-8&access=p&sort=date%3AD%3AL%3Ad1&start=0&num=6&g
etfields=search-title.content-type.topics.bite.yturl.thumbnail&rc=1&filter=0.
On the question of limiting clinical freedom, see Susan Giaimo, *Markets and Medicine: The Politics of Health Care Reform in Britain, Germany, and the United States* (Ann Arbor: University of Michigan Press, 2002); Paul Starr, *The Social Transformation of American Medicine* (New York: Basic Books, 1982).

19. The BMJ study quoted is cited in Tsung-mei Cheng, "NICE Approach," Health (3), *Financial Times,* September 16, 2009, p. 12. Odin W. Anderson estimated that physician treatment decisions accounted for 80 percent of US health care spending (*Health Services in the United States: A Growth Enterprise Since 1875* [Ann Arbor, Health Administration Press, 1985], p. 36).

20. Republican Sarah Palin's infamous allegation that the Democrats health care reform law would introduce "death panels" into Medicare illustrates the character of the public debate, which had plenty of emotion but sometimes little basis in fact.

21. For evidence of geographical variations in medical practice in the United States, see *Dartmouth Atlas on the US*, www.dartmouthatlas.org. Even the British NHS, which guaranteed universal access, saw large regional differences in treatment protocols for the same disease. Observers termed this a "postal code lottery" in obtaining treatment for conditions like cancer. See Andrew Ward, "NHS to Stop Funding 16 Cancer Treatments," *Financial Times,* January 12, 2015

22. On controversies surrounding NICE, see Cheng, "NICE Approach," and Ward, "NHS to stop funding cancer." For a good overview of NICE, see *NICE Statement of Principles.* https://www.nice.org.uk/about/who-we-arewww.nice. co.uk. On procedural justice, see Bo Rothstein, *Just Institutions Matter: The Moral and Political Logic of the Universal Welfare States* (New York: Cambridge University Press, 1998), esp. chap. 5.

23. Andrew Ward, "NHS to Stop Funding 16 Cancer Treatments," *Financial Times,* January 12, 2015.

24. Integrated delivery systems gained significant ground in the United States. Between 2002 and 2008, the share of physician-owned practices declined from 70 percent to 48 percent while hospital-owned practices increased from 24 percent to 50 percent (Bodenheimer and Grumbach, *Understanding Health Policy,* p. 71). In Germany, by contrast, 60 percent of ambulatory care doctors were in solo practice and 25% in dual practice in 2013. Only 10 percent of physicians were in multispecialty polyclinics. (Blümel and Busse, "German Health Care System," p. 65; Lisac et al. "Changing Long-Established Structures," p. 187; Lisac et al, "Access and Choice," p. 47). In patient and physician surveys, Germany scores poorly relative to peer countries on measures of coordinated care, especially on communication among health care providers (Karen Davis, Kristof Stremikis, David Squires, and Cathy Schoen, *Mirror, Mirror on the Wall: How the Performance of the US Health Care System Compares Internationally,* [New York and Washington DC: Commonwealth Fund, 2014]). On the decentralized and piecemeal nature of delivery system

reform in the United States, see Atul Gawande, "Testing, Testing," *The New Yorker*, December 14, 2009, pp. 34–41. Medicare has also been a pioneer in payment reform, as its introduction of DRGs (a type of bundled payment) in 1983 attests.

25. See www.robinhoodtax.org.uk/
26. WHO, *Health Systems Financing*, pp. xii-xiii and Chap. 2.
27. Ibid., p. xii.
28. See Shivani Ramjee, Tim Vieyra, Matan Abraham, Josh Kaplan, and Richard Taylor, "National Health Insurance and South Africa's Private Sector," in *South African Health Review 2013/14* (Durban: Health Systems Trust, September 2014), pp. 93–103.
29. The University of Wisconsin Population Health Institute posits a model of population health that highlights the variety of factors responsible for good health outcomes. This model estimates that access to quality health care accounts for only 20 percent of health outcomes; individual behaviors (such as diet, exercise, and drug use) 30 percent; physical environment (clean air and water, good housing and transportation) 10 percent; with social and economic factors accounting for the largest share at 40 percent. University of Wisconsin Population Health Institute 2014, http://www.countyhealthrankings.org/our-approach.
30. Bodenheimer and Grumbach, *Understanding Health Policy: A Clinical Approach*, 6th ed. (New York: McGraw Hill Lange, 2012), Chap. 3.
31. For example, if people are unsure whether they will have enough money to put food on the table or pay their utility bills, if they are victims of domestic violence or live in a crime-ridden neighborhood where gunfire is normal, or experience unconscious yet institutionalized racism on a regular basis, they are living in a stressful situation that may trigger the body to release elevated levels of cortisol. This in turn causes plaque to build up in the arteries (hardening of the arteries), which can then trigger a heart attack or stroke. Other diseases linked to a stressful environment include depression, cancer, and preterm birth that result in infant mortality. National Scientific Council on the Developing Child (2005/2014), "Excessive Stress Disrupts the Architecture of the Developing Brain: Working Paper 3. Updated Edition," (2005/2014), http://www.developingchild.harvard. edu; National Scientific Council on the Developing Child, "Early Experiences Can Alter Gene Expression and Affect Long-Term Development, Working Paper No. 10" (2010), http://www.developingchild.net; National Scientific Council on the Developing Child, "The Timing and Quality of Early Experiences Combine to Shape Brain Architecture, Working Paper No. 5" (2007); National Scientific Council on the Developing Child "The Science of Neglect: The Persistent Absence of Responsive Care Disrupts the Developing Brain, (2012)," Jack P. Shonkoff and Deborah A. Phillips, eds., *From Neurons to Neighborhoods*, (Washington DC: National Academy Press, 2000). Evidence also shows that genes altered by the environment can be passed down from one generation to the next, but that these processes can also be reversed by specific interventions. See Tie Yuan Zhang, Benoit Labonte, Xiang Lan Wen, Gustavo Turecki,

and Michael J. Meaney, "Epigenetic Mechanisms for the Early Environmental Regulation of Hippocampal Glucocortioid Receptor Gene Expression in Rodents and Humans," *Neuropsychopharmacology Reviews* 8 (2013): 111–123; and Frank Masterpasqua, "Psychology and Epigenetics," *Review of General Psychology* 13 (3) (2009): 194–201.

32. M. G. Marmot, G. Davey Smith, S. Stansfeld, C. Patel, and A. Feeney, "Health Inequalities among British Civil Servants: The Whitehall II Study," *Lancet* 337 (8754) (1991): 1387–1393.

33. Paul Farmer, "Inequality and Poverty," in *Infections and Inequality* (Berkeley: University of California Press, 2001), p. 14.

34. Center on the Developing Child, Harvard University, "Building the Brain's 'Air Traffic Control' System: How Early Experiences Shape the Development of Executive Function, Working Paper 11." http://www.developingchild.harvard.edu.

35. Center on the Developing Child, Harvard University, *A Science-Based Framework for Early Childhood Policy* (2007). Also see James S. House, "Relating Social Inequalities in Health and Income," *Journal of Health Politics, Policy and Law* 26 (3) (June 2001): 523–532; *Unnatural Causes: Is Inequality Making Us Sick?* (DVD) California Newsreel, 2008; and WHO Commission on the Social Determinants of Health (CSDH), *Closing the Gap in a Generation: Health Equity through Action on the Social Determinants of Health. Final Report of the Commission on the Social Determinants of Health* (Geneva: World Health Organization, 2008).

36. See Matthew Basilico, Jonathan Weigel, Anjali Motgi, Jacob Bor, and Salmaan Keshavjee, "Health for All? Competing Theories and Geopolitics, " pp. 74–110, and "Declaration of Alma Ata: International Conference on Primary Health Care, Alma Ata, USSR, September 6–12, 1978," pp. 355–358, both in *Reimagining Global Health: An Introduction*, edited by Paul Farmer, Jim Yong Kim, Arthur, Kleinman, and Matthew Basilico, Berkeley: University of California Press, 2013; and WHO, *Primary Health Care*, 2008. The breakthrough report on the social determinants of health was the WHO's *Closing the Gap*, 2008.

37. Marci Nielsen, Amy Gibson, Lisabeth Buelt, Paul Grundy, and Kevin Grumbach, *The Patient-Centered Medical Home's Impact on Cost and Quality*, Annual Review of Evidence, 2013–2014, Milbank Memorial Fund, 2015, esp. pp. 29–32; Bodenheimer and Grumbach, Understanding Health Policy, pp. 51–52 and 71–72.

38. Concerns about inequality's corrosive effects on society and democracy are not new. But there is a renewed public debate on the question. For recent analyses, see Thomas Piketty, *Capital in the Twenty-First Century* (Boston: Harvard University Press, 2014); Robert D. Putnam, *Our Kids: The American Dream in Crisis* (New York: Simon and Schuster, 2015); and "An Hereditary Meritocracy," *The Economist,* January 24, 2015, pp. 17–20.

39. Using the GINI coefficient of income inequality after taxes and transfers, the United States ranks second in the OECD behind Chile. See Drew DeSilver, "Global Inequality: How the U.S. Compares," Pew Research Center, December 19, 2013. http://www.pewresearch.org/fact-tank/2013/12/19/global-inequality-how-the-u-s-compares/. There are other ways to measure inequality. Piketty

(*Capital*) uses a broader measure of wealth while other analysts examine wage data only. See David H. Autor, "Skills, Education, and the Rise of Earnings Inequality among the 'Other 99 Percent,'" *Science* 344 (6186) (May 23, 2014): 843–850; John Schmid, "Help Wanted: Most U.S. Job Openings Are for Low-skill, Low-pay workers," *Milwaukee Journal Sentinel*, April 4, 2015.

40. T. H. Marshall, "Citizenship and Social Class," in *Sociology at the Crossroads, and Other Essays* (London: Heinemann, 1963), pp. 67–127. Likewise, Sir William Beveridge, the middle-class reformer and architect of Britain's postwar welfare state, viewed social insurance as the weapon to slay the "five giant evils" of want, disease, ignorance, squalor, and idleness. See Nicholas Timmins, *The Five Giants: A Biography of the Welfare State* (London: HarperCollins Publishers, 1995), p. 24 and Chaps 1–3.

41. CSDH, *Closing the Gap; Unnatural Causes.*

BIBLIOGRAPHY

Abdool Karim, Salim S., Gavin J. Churchyard, Quarraisa Abdool Karim and Stephen D. Lawn. 2009. "HIV Infection and Tuberculosis in South Africa: An Urgent Need to Escalate the Public Health Response." *Lancet* 374 (September 12): 921–933.

Acs, Gregory, Stephen H. Long, M. Susan Marquis, and Pamela Farley Short. 1996. "Self-Insured Employer Health Plans: Prevalence, Profile, Provisions, and Premiums." *Health Affairs* 15 (2) (Summer): 266–278.

African National Congress with the technical support of WHO and UNICEF. 1994. *A National Health Plan for South Africa* (May).

Agency for Healthcare Research and Quality. 2011. "Ensuring that Patient-Centered Medical Homes Effectively Serve Patients with Complex Health Needs."

Altman Stuart and David Shactman. 2011. *Power, Politics, and Universal Health Care: The Inside Story of a Century-Long Battle*. Amherst, NY: Prometheus Books.

"Americans' Views on the Affordable Care Act Hold Steady, with 43% Now Viewing It Favorably and 42% Unfavorably," 2015. News Release, Kaiser Family Foundation, April 21. http://kff.org/health-reform/press-release/americans-views-on-the-affordable-care-act-hold-steady-with-43-now-viewing-it-favorably-and-42-unfavorably/

Anderson, Odin W. 1985. *Health Services in the United States: A Growth Enterprise Since 1875*. Ann Arbor, Health Administration Press.

Anderson, Gerald F., Uwe E. Reinhardt, Peter S. Hussey, and Varduhi Petrosyan. 2003. "It's the Prices, Stupid: Why the US Is So Different from Other Countries." *Health Affairs* 22 (3) (May/June): 89–105.

"An Hereditary Meritocracy." 2015. *The Economist,* January 24, pp. 17–20.

Ataguba, John Ele-Ojo and James Akazili. 2010. "Health Care Financing in South Africa: Moving Towards Universal Coverage." CME 28 (2) (February): 74–78.

Autor, David H. 2014. "Skills, Education, and the Rise of Earnings Inequality among the 'Other 99 Percent.'" *Science* 344 (6186) (May 23): 843–850.

Basilico, Matthew, Vanessa Kerry, Luke Messac, Arjun Suri, Jonathan Weigel, Marguerite Thorp Basilico, Joia Mukherjee, and Paul Farmer. 2013. "A Movement for Global Health Equity? A Closing Reflection." In *Reimagining Global Health: An Introduction*, edited by Paul Farmer, Jim Yong Kim, Arthur Kleinman, and Matthew Basilico, 340–353. Berkeley: University of California Press.

Basilico, Matthew, Vanessa Kerry, Luke Messac, Arjun Suri, Jonathan Weigel, Anjali Motgi, Jacob Bor, and Salmaan Keshavjee. 2013. "Health for All? Competing Theories and Geopolitics." In *Reimagining Global Health: An Introduction*, edited by Paul Farmer, Jim Yong Kim, Arthur Kleinman, and Matthew Basilico, 74–110. Berkeley: University of California Press.

Becker, Anne, Anjali Motgi, Jonathan Weigel, Giuseppe Raviola, Salmaan Keshavjee and Arthur Kleinman. 2013. "The Unique Challenges of Mental Health and MDRTB: Critical Perspectives on Metrics of Disease." In *Reimagining Global Health: An Introduction*, edited by Paul Farmer, Jim Yong Kim, Arthur Kleinman, and Matthew Basilico, 212–244. Berkeley: University of California Press.

Bennefield, Robert L. 1996. "Health Insurance Coverage: 1995." *U.S. Census Bureau Current Population Reports, P60–195.* (September).

Benoit, Bertrand. 2006. "A Temporary Solution? Germany's Labour Market Develops a Second Tier." *Financial Times*, October 27.

Bernstein, Ann. 2014. "South Africa's Key Challenges: Tough Choices and New Directions." *Annals of the American Academy of Political and Social Science* 652 (March): 20–47.

Blendon, Robert J., Mollyann Brodie, John M. Benson, Drew E. Altman, Larry Levitt, Tina Hoff, and Larry Hugick. 1998. "Understanding the Managed Care Backlash." *Health Affairs* 17 (4): 80–94.

Blum, Jonathan. 2010. "What Is the Donut Hole?" HealthCare Blog, HealthCare.gov. (August 9). www.heatlhcare.gov/blog/2010/08donuthole.html.

Blum, Kerstin. 2007. "Care Coordination Gaining Momentum in Germany." *Health Policy Monitor Survey* (9): Bertelsmann Stiftung, Gütersloh, Germany.

Blumberg, Linda J., John Holahan, and Matthew Buettgens. 2014. "Halbig v Burwell: Potential Implications for ACA Coverage and Subsidies." Robert Wood Johnson Foundation and Urban Institute (July).

Blümel, Miriam. 2014. "Changes in Contribution Rate Setting from 2015," *Health Policy Monitor* site. http://www.hpm.org/. Accessed 12/28/14.

Blümel, Miriam and Reinhard Busse. 2015. "The German Health Care System, 2014," in *2014 International Profiles of Health Care Systems*, edited by Elias Mossialos, Martin Wenzl, Robin Osborn, and Chloe Anderson, 63–71. New York and Washington, DC: The Commonwealth Fund.

Bodenheimer, Thomas and Kevin Grumbach. 2012. *Understanding Health Policy: A Clinical Approach*, 6th ed. New York: McGraw Hill Lange.

Boulton, Guy. 2012. "Efforts to Boost Number of Primary Care Physicians Face Pay Gap Hurdles." *Milwaukee Journal Sentinel*, December 1.

———. 2014. "Gov. Scott Walker, Mary Burke and the Affordable Care Act." *Milwaukee Journal Sentinel*, September 26.

Brodie, Mollyann and Robert J. Blendon. 2008. "Public Opinion and Health Policy." In *Health Politics and Policy*, 4th ed., edited by James A. Morone, Theodore A. Litman, and Leonard S. Robins, 249–270. Clifton Park, NY: Delmar Cengage.

Brûlé, Tyler. 2015. "Some Neighbourhoods are Streets Ahead." *Financial Times*, April 4.

Buettgens, Matthew, John Holahan, and Hannah Recht. 2015. "Medicaid expansion, Health Coverage, and Spending: An Update for the 21 States that Have Not Expanded Eligibility." Issue Brief. Kaiser Family Foundation. April 29.

Bundesministerium für Gesundheit (BMG). Federal Republic of Germany. 2007. *Willkommen in der Solidarität! Informationen zur Gesundheitsreform 2007* (Marsch).

Bureau of Labor Statistics, U.S. *Labor Force Statistics from the Current Population Survey,* http://data.bls.gov/timeseries/LNS14000000.

Burnham, Walter Dean. 1970. *Critical Elections and the Mainspring of American Politics.* New York: Norton.

Busse, Reinhard and Miriam Blümel. 2014. *Germany: Health System Review,* vol. 16, issue 2, *Health Systems in Transition.* European Observatory on Health Systems and Policies.

Call the Midwife. http://www.pbs.org/call-the-midwife/home/

Calmes, Jackie and Robert Pear. 2013. "Crucial Rule Is Delayed a Year for Obama's Health Law." *New York Times,* July 2.

"Care of Chronic Illness in Last Two Years of Life." *The Dartmouth Atlas of Health Care.* http://www.dartmouthatlas.org/data/topic/topic.aspx?cat=1.

Casalino, Lawrence P. 2015. "Pioneer Accountable Care Organizations: Traversing Rough Country." *Journal of the American Medical Association* 313 (21) 2126–27.

Cauchi, Richard. 2014. "State Actions to Address Health Insurance Exchanges." National Conference of State Legislatures. October 16. www.ncsl.org. Accessed October 17, 2014.

Census Bureau. U.S. 2011. *Income Poverty and Health Insurance, Highlights: 2011.* https://www.census.gov/hhes/www/hlthins/data/incpovhlth/2011/highlights.html.

Center on the Developing Child, Harvard University. 2007. *A Science-Based Framework for Early Childhood Policy.* August. www.developingchild.harvard.edu.

———. 2011. "Building the Brain's 'Air Traffic Control' System: How Early Experiences Shape the Development of Executive Function, Working Paper 11." http://www.developingchild.harvard.edu.

"Cheerleaders and Naysayers," Emerging Africa: Special Report. 2013. *The Economist,* March 2.

Cheng, Tsung-Mei. 2009. "NICE Approach." *Financial Times.* Health (3): September 16, pp. 12–13.

——— and Uwe E. Reinhardt. 2008. "Shepherding Major Health System Reforms: A Conversation with German Health Minister Ulla Schmidt." *Health Affairs* 27 (3): w204–w213.

Chopra, Mickey, Emmauelle Daviaud, Robert Pattinson, Sharon Fonn, and Joy E. Lawn. 2009. "Saving the Lives of South Africa's Mothers, Babies, and Children: Can the Health System Deliver?" *Lancet* 374 (September 5): 835–846.

———, Joy E. Lawn, David Sanders, Peter Barron, Salim S. Abdool Karim, Debbie Bradshaw, Rachel Jewkes, Quarraisha Abdool Karim, Alan J. Flisher, Bongani M. Mayosi, Stephen M. Tollman, Gavin J. Churchyard, Hoosen Coovadia. 2009. "Achieving the Health Millennium Development Goals for South Africa: Challenges and Priorities." *Lancet* 374 (September 19): 1023–1031.

Chubb, John E. and Terry M. Moe. 1990. *Politics, Markets, and America's Schools.* Washington DC: Brookings Institution.

Cigler, Allan J. and Burdett A. Loomis. 2002. *Interest Group Politics.* Washington DC: CQ Press.

Claxon, Gary, Larry Levitt, Mollyann Brodie, Rachel Garfield, and Anthony Damico. 2014. "Measuring Changes in Insurance Coverage Under the Affordable Care Act." (April), Kaiser Family Foundation.

Cohen, Jon. 2006. "Brazil: Ten Years After." *Science* 313 (5786) (July 28): 484–487.

Congressional Budget Office (CBO). *U.S.* 2010. *Analysis of Paul Ryan's Roadmap for America's Future Act of 2010.* (January 27). www.cbo.gov.

———. U.S. 2012. *The Long-Term Budgetary Impact of Paths for Federal Revenues and Spending Specified by Chairman Ryan* (March).

Conradt, David P. 2009. *The German Polity,* 9th ed. Boston and New York: Houghton Mifflin Harcourt.

Coovadia, Hoosen, Rachel Jewkes, Peter Barron, David Sanders, and Diane McIntyre. 2009. "The Health and Health System of South Africa: Historical Roots of Current Public Health Challenges." *Lancet* 374 (September 5): 817–834.

"County Health Rankings: Our Approach." 2015. University of Wisconsin Population Health Institute. http://www.countyhealthrankings.org/our-approach.

"The Coverage Gap: Uninsured Poor Adults in States that Do Not Expand Medicaid." 2014. Issue Brief. Kaiser Family Foundation (March).

Cubanski, Juliette, Christina Swoope, Cristina Boccuti, Gretchen Jacobson, Giselle Casillas, Shannon Griffin, and Tricia Neuman. 2015. *A Primer on Medicare.* Kaiser Family Foundation (March).

Current Population Survey. 2010. Kaiser Commission on Medicaid and the Uninsured and U.S. Census Bureau (March). www.kff.org.

Dartmouth Atlas on the US, www.dartmouthatlas.org.

Davis, Karen, Kristof Stremikis, David Squires, and Cathey Schoen, 2014. *Mirror, Mirror on the Wall: How the Performance of the US Health Care System Compares Internationally.* New York and Washginton DC: Commonwealth Fund, 2014.

"Declaration of Alma Ata: International Conference on Primary Health Care, Alma Ata, USSR, September 6–12, 1978," pp. 355–358, both in *Reimagining Global Health: An Introduction,* edited by Paul Farmer, Jim Yong Kim, Arthur, Kleinman, and Matthew Basilico, Berkeley: University of California Press, 2013.

DeLaet, Debra L. and David E. DeLaet, 2012. *Global Health in the 21st Century: The Globalization of Disease and Wellness.* Boulder and London: Paradigm Publishers.

DeParle, Jason. 2004. *American Dream: Three Women, Ten Kids, and a Nation's Drive to End Welfare.* New York: Viking.

Department of Health, Republic of South Africa. "National Health Insurance." n.d. www.health.gov.za/nhi.php. Accessed January 24, 2015.

———. n.d. *National Health Insurance: Healthcare for All South Africans.* www.health.gov/za. Accessed January 24, 2015.

———. 2011. *National Health Insurance in South Africa: Policy Paper* (August 12).

Department of Health and Human Services (DHHS) 2015. U.S. Office of the Assistant Secretary for Planning and Evaluation. 2015. *Health Insurance Coverage and the*

Affordable Care Act. May 5. aspe.hhs.gov/health/reports/2015/uninsured.../ib_uninsured_change.pdf.

Department of Health and Human Services, U.S. 2015, "CMS Proposes Major Initiative for Hip and Knee Replacements," News release, July 9, hhs.gov.

Department of Health and Human Services. U.S. Center for Medicare and Medicaid Services. Medicaid.gov. 2015. *Medicaid and CHIP: August 2015 Monthly Applications, Eligibility Determinations and Enrollment Report.* (October 26). http://medicaid.gov/medicaid-chip-program-information/program-information/medicaid-and-chip-enrollment-data/medicaid-and-chip-application-eligibility-determination-and-enrollment-data.html.

Department of Health and Humans Services, U.S. Centers for Disease Control and Prevention, and National Center for Health Statistics. 2015. *"Early Release of Selected Estimates Based on Data from the National Health Interview Survey, January – March 2015.* September.

DeSilver, Drew. 2013. "Global Inequality: How the U.S. Compares." Pew Research Center, December 19. http://www.pewresearch.org/fact-tank/2013/12/19/global-inequality-how-the-u-s-compares/.

DiJulio, Bianca, Jamie Firth, and Mollyann Brodie. 2015. "Kaiser Health Tracking Poll: April 2015." Kaiser Family Foundation, http://kff.org/health-reform/poll-finding/kaiser-health-tracking-poll-april-2015/.

Discovery Health (Pty) Ltd. and Discovery Health Medical Scheme. 2011. *Comments on Government Gazette No. 34523, on the National Health Act, 2003. Green Paper: Policy on National Health Insurance.* December.

Döhler, Marian. 1987. "Regulating the Medical Profession in Germany: The Politics of Efficiency Review." Berlin: Social Science Research Center, Research Unit Market Processes and Corporate Development (May). Typescript.

———. 1995. "The State as Architect of Political Order: Policy Dynamics in German Health Care." *Governance* 8(3): 380–404.

"Don't Get Ill." The Price of Freedom: A Special Report on South Africa. 2010. *The Economist,* June 5, pp. 14–15.

Drobac, Peter, Matthew Basilico, Luke Messac, David Walton, and Paul Farmer. 2013. "Building an Effective Rural Health Delivery Model in Haiti and Rwanda." In *Reimagining Global Health: An Introduction,* edited by Paul Farmer, Jim Yong Kim, Arthur Kleinman, and Matthew Basilico, 133–183. Berkeley: University of California Press.

Drope, Jeffrey and Raphael Lencucha. 2014. "Evolving Norms at the Intersection of Health and Trade." *Journal of Health Politics, Policy and Law* 39 (3) (June): 591–631.

Duverger, Maurice. 1954. *Political Parties,* trans. Barbara and Robert North. London: Methuen.

Dyson, Kenneth, ed. 1992. *The Politics of German Regulation.* Aldershot, England: Dartmouth.

———. 1992. "Theories of Regulation and the Case of Germany: A Model of Regulatory Change." *The Politics of German Regulation.* Aldershot, England: Dartmouth.

Employer Health Benefits Survey 2011. 2011. Kaiser Family Foundation and Health Research and Educational Trust. (September 27). www.kff.org.

———. 2012. Kaiser Family Foundation and Health Research and Educational Trust. www.kff.org.

England, Andrew. 2015. "South Africa Parliament Erupts as Jacob Zuma is Grilled over Scandal." *Financial Times*, February 12.

———. 2015. "Parliamentary Punch-Up Bodes Ill for Zuma's South Africa." *Financial Times*, February 16.

Enthoven, Alain C. 1980. *Health Plan: The Only Practical Solution to the Soaring Cost of Medical Care.* Boston: Addison-Wesley.

Enthoven, Alain C. 1980. "Managed Competition: An Agenda for Action." *Health Affairs* 7 (3) (1988): 25–47.

Epstein, Leon D. 1986. *Political Parties in the American Mold.* Madison and London: University of Wisconsin Press.

Esping-Andersen, Gøsta. 1990. *The Three Worlds of Welfare Capitalism.* Princeton: Princeton University Press.

———. 1999. *Social Foundations of Postindustrial Economies.* Oxford and New York: Oxford University Press.

——— and Walter Korpi. 1984. "Social Policy as Class Politics in Post-War Capitalism: Scandinavia, Austria, and Germany," In *Order and Conflict in Contemporary Capitalism: Studies in the Political Economy of Western European Nations,* edited by John D. Goldthorpe. Oxford: Clarendon Press.

European Union. 2014. "Results of the 2014 European Elections." www.elections2014.eu/en.

Farmer, Paul. 2001. *Infections and Inequalities: The Modern Plagues.* Berkeley: University of California Press.

———. 2001. "Inequality and Poverty." In *Infections and Inequalities: The Modern Plagues.* Berkeley: University of California Press, pp. 1–20.

———. 2010. "On Suffering and Structural Violence." In *Partner to the Poor: A Paul Farmer Reader,* edited by Hain Saussy. Berkeley: University of California Press, pp. 328–349.

———, Matthew Basilico, Vanessa Kerry, Madeleine Ballard, Anne Becker, Gene Bukhman, Ophelia Dahl, Andy Ellner, Louise Ivers, David Jones, John Meara, Joia Mukherjee, Amy Sievers, and Alyssa Yamamoto. 2013. "Global Health Priorities for the Early Twenty-First Century." In *Reimagining Global Health: An Introduction,* edited by Paul Farmer, Jim Yong Kim, Arthur Kleinman, and Matthew Basilico, 302–339. Berkeley: University of California Press.

Fox, Ashley M. and Michael R. Reich. 2015. "The Politics of Universal Health Coverage in Low- and Middle-Income Countries: A Framework for Evaluation and Action." *Journal of Health Politics Policy and Law* 40 (5) (October): 1019–1056.

Freudenheim, Milt. 1989. "A Health Care Taboo is Broken." *New York Times.* May 8.

Friedman, Steven and Shauna Mottiar. 2005. "A Rewarding Engagement? The Treatment Action Campaign and the Politics of HIV/AIDS." *Politics and Society* 33 (4): 511–565.

Galvão, Jane. 2005. "Brazil and Access to HIV/AIDS Drugs: A Question of Human Rights and Public Health." *American Journal of Public Health* 95 (7) (July): 1110–1116.

Garfield, Rachel, Anthony Damico, Jessica Stephens, and Saman Rouhani. 2015. "The Coverage Gap: Uninsured Poor Adults in States that Do Not Expand Medicaid – An Update." Issue Brief. Kaiser Family Foundation (April).

Gauri, Varun and Evan S. Lieberman. 2006. "Boundary Institutions and HIV/AIDS Policy in Brazil and South Africa." *Studies in Comparative International Development* 41 (3) (Fall): 47–73.

Gawande, Atul, 2009. "Testing, Testing." *The New Yorker,* December 14, pp. 34–41.

———. 2009. "The Cost Conundrum." *The New Yorker,* June 1.

———. 2015. "Overkill." *The New Yorker,* May 11, pp. 42–53.

Giaimo, Susan. 1995. "Health Care Reform in Britain and Germany: Recasting the Political Bargain with the Medical Profession." *Governance* 8 (3) (July) 354–379.

———. 2000. "Who Pays for Health Care Reform?" In *The New Politics of the Welfare State,* edited by Paul Pierson, 334–367. Oxford and New York: Oxford University Press.

———. 2002. *Markets and Medicine: The Politics of Health Care Reform in Britain, Germany, and the United States.* Ann Arbor: University of Michigan Press.

———. 2013. "Behind the Scenes of the Affordable Care Act: The Making of a Health Care Cooperative," *Journal of Health Politics, Policy and Law* 38 (3) (June): 599–610.

———. 2014. "Interest Groups, Think Tanks, and Health Care Policy, 1960s-present." In *The CQ Guide to U.S. Health and Health Care Policy,* edited by Thomas R. Oliver, 384–389. New York: DWJ Books.

——— and Philip Manow. 1999. "Adapting the Welfare State: The Case of Health Care Reform in Britain, Germany, and the United States." *Comparative Political Studies* 32:8 (December): 967–1000.

Gilbert, Craig. 2014. "Ryan Blasts Obama's Immigration Plan." *Milwaukee Journal Sentinel,* November 20, p. 8A.

"Global Targets, Local Ingenuity." 2010. *The Economist,* September 25, pp. 34–35.

Gomez, Eduardo J. 2011. "How Brazil Outpaced the United States When It Came to AIDS: The Politics of Civic Infiltration, Reputation, and Strategic Internationalization." *Journal of Health Politics, Policy and Law* 36 (2) (April): 317–352.

"The Great Scourges." The Price of Freedom: A Special Report on South Africa. 2010. *The Economist,* June 5, pp. 11–12.

Greene, Jeremy, Marguerite Thorp Basilico, Heidi Kim, and Paul Farmer. 2013. "Colonial Medicine and its Legacies. In. *Reimagining Global Health: An Introduction,* edited by Paul Farmer, Jim Yong Kim, Arthur Kleinman, and Matthew Basilico, 33–73. Berkeley: University of California Press.

Greenhouse, Steven. 2009. "Dennis Rivera Leads Labor Charge for Health Reform." *New York Times,* August 27.

Gunder Frank, Andre. 1966. "The Development of Underdevelopment." *Monthly Review* 18 (4) (September): 17–31.

Hacker, Jacob S. 1997. *The Road to Nowhere: The Genesis of President Clinton's Plan for Health Security.* Princeton: Princeton University Press.

———. 2002. *The Divided Welfare State: The Battle over Public and Private Social Benefits in the United States.* Cambridge and New York: Cambridge University Press.

———. 2004. "Privatizing Risk without Privatizing the Welfare State: The Hidden Politics of Social Policy Retrenchment in the United States." *American Political Science Review* 98 (2) (May): 243–260.

———. 2008. "Putting Politics First." *Health Affairs* 27 (3) (May/June): 718–723.

———. n.d. "The Case for Public Plan Choice in National Health Reform: Key to Cost Control and Quality Coverage," Berkeley, CA: Center on Health, Economic and Family Security, University of California School of Law, and Institute for America's Future. www.law.berkeley.edu/chefs.htm. Downloaded May 2009.

Hancock, Jay. 2014. "Decoding the High-Stakes Debate Over Medicare Advantage Cuts." *Kaiser Health News*, April 7.

Harding, Robin, Joseph Leahy, and Lucy Hornby. 2014. "Taking a Stand," *Financial Times* (July 16.).

Harris, Gardiner and Robert Pear. 2011. "Still No Relief in Sight for Long-Term Needs." *New York Times*, October 24.

Hassel, Anke. 2010. "Twenty Years after German Unification: The Restructuring of the German Welfare and Employment Regime." *German Politics and Society* 28 (2) (Summer): 102–115.

"Health Policy Brief: The Independent Payment Advisory Board." 2011. *Health Affairs* (December 15).

——— "Health Policy Brief: Next Steps for ACOs." 2012. *Health Affairs* (January 31).

——— "Health Policy Brief: Pay for Performance." 2012. *Health Affairs* (October 11).

——— "Health Reform: Implications for Women's Access to Coverage and Care." 2013. Issue Brief. Kaiser Family Foundation (August).

Healthcare.gov website. Appeals. www.healthcare.gov/https://www.healthcare.gov/search/?q=appeals&output=xml_no_dtd&site=healthcare&proxystylesheet=json&client=json&lr=lang_en&ie=UTF-8&oe=UTF-8&access=p&sort=date%3AD%3AL%3Ad1&start=0&num=6&getfields=search-title.content-type.topics.bite.yturl.thumbnail&rc=1&filter=0.

Heclo, Hugh and Henrik Madsen. 1987. *Policy and Politics in Sweden: Principled Pragmatism.* Philadelphia: Temple University Press.

Helen Suzman Foundation. 2011. *Submission to National Department of Health: National Health Insurance Green Paper.* December.

Heritage Foundation. 2011. *Saving the American Dream: The Heritage Plan to Fix the Debt, Cut Spending, and Restore Prosperity.* Washington DC.

Heywood, Mark. 2009. "South Africa's Treatment Action Campaign: Combining Law and Social Mobilization to Realize the Right to Health." *Journal of Human Rights Practice* 1 (1): 14–36.

Hilmert, Clayton J., Christine Dunkel Schetter, Tyan Parker Dominguez, Cleopatra Abdou, Calvin J. Hobel, Laura Glynn, and Curt Sandman. 2008. "Stress and Blood Pressure During Pregnancy: Racial Differences and Associations With Birthweight." *Psychosomatic Medicine* 70 (57) 57–64.

Holahan, John, Matthew Buettgens, Caitlin Carroll, and Vicki Chen. 2012. "National and State-by-State Impact of the 2012 House Republican Budget Plan for Medicaid." Kaiser Family Foundation (October).

"Hospitals by Ownership Type, 2013." 2013. *State Health Facts.* Kaiser Family Foundation, http://kff.org/other/state-indicator/hospitals-by-ownership/

House, James S. 2001. "Relating Social Inequalities in Health and Income." *Journal of Health Politics, Policy and Law* 26 (3) (June): 523–532.

Hoyer, Jens Martin. 2009. *Social Health Insurance in Germany and the Market Positon of the TK: Current Changes and Future Challenges* (May 10). PowerPoint.

Humer, Caroline. 2015. "Government Payments for Medicare Advantage Plans to Rise in 2016." *New York Times*, April 6.

Immergut, Ellen M. 1992. *Health Politics: Interests and Institutions in Western Europe.* Cambridge and New York: Cambridge University Press.

"Is the Affordable Care Act Working?" 2014. *New York Times*, October 27. http://nyti.ms/1tuklhM.

Jacobs, Lawrence R. and Theda Skocpol, 2012. *Health Care Reform and American Politics: What Everyone Needs to Know.* Oxford and New York: Oxford University Press.

Jagler, Steve. 2012. "But Will It Work?" *BizTimes Milwaukee.* (March 19–April 1).

Johnson, Mark and Tia Ghose. 2011. "Is Stress Related to Preterm Birth?" *Milwaukee Journal Sentinel*, April 17.

Jost, Timothy Stoltzfus. 2014. "Beyond Repeal – A Republican Proposal for Health Care Reform." *New England Journal of Medicine* 370 (10) (March 6): 894–896.

Katzenstein, Peter J. 1987. *Policy and Politics in West Germany: The Growth of a Semi-Sovereign State.* Philadelphia: Temple University Press.

Key Facts about the Uninsured Population. 2013. Kaiser Family Foundation (September).

———. 2015. Kaiser Family Foundation (October).

Kim, Jim Yong, Michael Porter, Joseph Rhatigan, Rebecca Weintraub, Matthew Basilico, Cassia van der Hoof Holstein, and Paul Farmer. 2013. "Scaling Up Effective Delivery Models Worldwide." In *Reimagining Global Health: An Introduction*, edited by Paul Farmer, Jim Yong Kim, Arthur Kleinman, and Matthew Basilico, 184–211. Berkeley: University of California Press.

Klein, Rudolf. 1989. *The Politics of the National Health Service*, 2nd ed. London: Longman.

Kliff, Sarah. 2013. "As Health-Care Costs Slow, IPAB's Launch Is Delayed." *Washington Post*, May 3.

Knieps, Franz. Director-General, Public Health Care, Health Insurance, Long-term Care Insurance, German Federal Ministry of Health. Interview by author, June 13, 2009, Berlin, Germany.

Korpi, Walter. 1983. *The Democratic Class Struggle.* London: Routledge and Kegan Paul.

Laugesen, Miriam J. and Sherry A. Glied. 2011. "Higher Fees Paid to US Physicians Drive Higher Spending for Physician Services Compared to Other Countries." *Health Affairs* 30 (9) (September): 1647–1656.

Leiber, Simone, Stefan Greß, and Maral-Sonja Manouguian. 2010. "Health Care System Change and the Cross-Border Transfer of Ideas: Influence of the Dutch Model on the 2007 German Health Reform." *Journal of Health Politics, Policy and Law* 35 (4) (August) 539–568.

Leibfried, Stephan and Florian Tennstedt. 1986. "Health-Insurance Policy and Berufsverbote in the Nazi Takeover." In *Political Values and Health Care: The German Experience*, edited by Donald W. Light and Alexander Schuller, 127–184. Cambridge and London: MIT Press.

Levitt, Larry and Gary Claxton. 2014. "The Potential Side Effects of Halbig." Kaiser Family Foundation (July 31).

Levy, Jenna. 2015. "In U.S., Uninsured Rate Dips to 11.9% in First Quarter." *Gallup Well-Being* (April 13). www.gallup.com/poll/182348/uninsured-rate-dips-first-quarter.aspx.

Linz, Juan J. and Alfred Stepan, eds. 1978. *The Breakdown of Democratic Regimes*, Vol. 1. Baltimore and London: Johns Hopkins Press.

Lipset, Seymour M. and Stein Rokkan. 1967. "Cleavage Structures, Party Systems, and Voter Alignments; An Introduction." In *Party Systems and Voter Alignments*. New York: Free Press, pp. 1–64.

Liptak, Adam. 2012. "Justices by 5–4, Uphold Health Care Law." *New York Times*, June 29.

———. 2014. "Supreme Court Rejects Contraceptives Mandate for Some Corporations." *New York Times*, June 30.

———. 2014. "Justices to Hear New Challenge to Health Law." *New York Times*, November 7.

———. 2015. "Supreme Court Allows Nationwide Health Care Subsidies." *New York Times*, June 25.

Lisac, Melanie, Kerstin Blum and Sophia Schlette. 2008. "Changing Long-Established Structures for More Competition and Stronger Coordination—Health Care Reform in Germany in the New Millennium." *Intereconomics* (July/August): 184–189.

———, Lutz Reimers, Klaus-Dirk Henke, and Sophia Schlette. 2010. "Access and Choice—Competition under the Roof of Solidarity in German Health Care: An Analysis of Health Policy Reforms Since 2004." *Health Economics, Policy and Law* 5 (1) (January): 31–52.

Luce, Edward. 2014. "Obamacare's Drip-fed Success." *Financial Times*, October 26.

——— and Alexandra Ulmer. 2009. "Obama Foes Turn to '60s Radical for Tactical Tips." *Financial Times*, August 17, p. 2.

Madison, Donald L. 2005. "From Bismarck to Medicare—A Brief History of Medical Care Payment in America." In *The Social Medicine Reader: Health Policy, Markets and Medicine*, 2nd ed., edited by Jonathan Oberlander, Larry R. Churchill, Sue E. Estroff, Gail E. Henderson, Nancy M. P. King, and Ronald P. Strauss, 54–59. Durham and London: Duke University Press.

Majerol, Melissa, Vann Newkirk, and Rachel Farfield. 2015. *The Uninsured: A Primer.* Kaiser Family Foundation (January).

Malan, Mia. 2014. "South Africa Has Highest Number of New HIV Infections Worldwide—Survey." *Mail and Guardian*, April 4.

Manow, Philip. 1997. "Social Insurance the German Political Economy." *MPIFG Discussion Paper* 97:2 (Cologne: Max Planck Institute for the Study of Societies).

——— and Eric Seils. 2000. "Adjusting Badly: The German Welfare State, Structural Change, and the Open Economy." In *Welfare and Work in the Open Economy, Vol. II: Diverse Responses to Common Challenges*, edited by Fritz W. Scharpf and Vivien A. Schmidt, 264–307. Oxford and New York: Oxford University Press.

March, James G. and John P. Olsen. 1984. "The New Institutionalism: Organizational Factors in Political Life." *American Political Science Review* 78 (3): 734–749.

Marmor, Theodore R. 2000. *The Politics of Medicare*. 2nd ed. New York: Aldine de Gruyter.

Marmot, M. G., G. Davey Smith, S. Stansfeld, C. Patel, and A. Feeney. 1991. "Health Inequalities among British Civil Servants: The Whitehall II Study." *Lancet* 337 (8754): 1387–1393.

Marshall, T. H. 1963. "Citizenship and Social Class," in *Sociology at the Crossroads, and Other Essays*. London: Heinemann, pp. 67–127.

"Massachusetts Health Care Reform: Six Years Later." 2012. no. 8321. Kaiser Family Foundation. (May). www.kff.org

Martin, Cathie Jo and Duane Swank. 2012. *The Political Construction of Business Interests: Coordination, Growth, and Equality*. Cambridge and New York: Cambridge University Press.

Masterpasqua, Frank. 2009. "Psychology and Epigenetics." *Review of General Psychology* 13 (3): 194–201.

Matsoso, M. P. and R. Fryatt. 2013. "National Health Insurance: The First 18 Months," *South African Medical Journal* 103 (3).

Maynard, Alan. 2013. "Health Care Rationing: Doing It Better in Public and Private Health Care Systems." *Journal of Health Politics, Policy and Law* 38 (6) (December): 1103–1127.

Mayosi, Bongani M., Alan J. Flisher, Umesh G. Lalloo, Freddy Sitas, Stephen M. Tollman, and Debbie Bradshaw. 2009. "The Burden of Non-communicable Diseases in South Africa." *The Lancet* 374 (September 12): 934–947.

McWilliams, J. Michael, Bruce E. Landon, and Michael E. Chernew. 2013. "Changes in Health Care Spending and Quality for Medicare Beneficiaries Associated with a Commercial ACO Contract." *Journal of the American Medical Association* 310 (8) 829–836.

Mechanic, Robert E. 2015. "Mandatory Medicare Bundled Payment—Is It Ready for Prime Time?" *The New England Journal of Medicine*, nejom.org, August 26.

Medical Group Management Association. 2014. *MGMA Physician Compensation and Production Survey: 2014 Report Based on 2013 Data: Key Findings Summary Report*.

Messac, Luke and Krishna Prabhu. 2013. "Redefining the Possible: The Global AIDS Response." In *Reimagining Global Health: An Introduction*, edited by Paul Farmer, Jim Yong Kim, Arthur Kleinman, and Matthew Basilico, 111–132. Berkeley: University of California Press.

Milliman Medical Index. 2011.www.milliman.com/mmi/

———. 2014. www.milliman.com/mmi/

Millman, Jason. 2014. "How Killing the Medical Device Tax Became One of Washington's Top Priorities." Wonkblog. *Washington Post*, November 7.

Moffit, Bob. 2011. "Ryan-Wyden: The Basic Ingredients of Structural Medicare Reform." *The Foundry: Conservative Policy News Blog from The Heritage Foundation*, December 16. http://blog.heritage.org.

Müller-Neuhof, Jost. 2009. "Sozialfall Gesundheit." *Der Tagesspiegel*, June 11, p. 4.

Murray, Charles. 1984. *Losing Ground: American Social Policy, 1950–1980*. New York: Basic Books.

Musumeci, MaryBeth. 2012. "A Guide to the Supreme Court's Review of the 2010 Health Care Reform Law." Pub. No. 8270. Kaiser Family Foundation, (January). www.kff.org.

National Institute for Care and Health Excellence. (United Kingdom). n.d. *NICE Statement of Principles*. https://www.nice.org.uk/about/who-we-arewww.nice.co.uk.

National Scientific Council on the Developing Child. 2007. "The Timing and Quality of Early Experiences Combine to Shape Brain Architecture: Working Paper No. 5."

———. 2010. "Early Experiences Can Alter Gene Expression and Affect Long-Term Development: Working Paper No. 10." http://www.developingchild.net.

National Scientific Council on the Developing Child. 2012. "The Science of Neglect: The Persistent Absence of Responsive Care Disrupts the Developing Brain."

———. 2005/2014. "Excessive Stress Disrupts the Architecture of the Developing Brain: Working Paper 3." Updated Edition. http://www.developingchild.harvard.edu.

Nattrass, Nicoli. 2014. "Meeting the Challenge of Unemployment? *Annals of the American Academy of Political and Social Science* 652 (March): 87–105.

Nielsen, Marci, Amy Gibson, Lisabeth Buelt, Paul Grundy, and Kevin Grumbach. 2015. *The Patient-Centered Medical Home's Impact on Cost and Quality*, Annual Review of Evidence, 2013–2014, Patient Centered Primary Care Colalborative and Milbank Memorial Fund.

Nunn, Amy, Samuel Dickman, Nicoli Nattrass, Alexandra Cornwall, and Sofia Gruskin. 2012. "The Impacts of AIDS Movements on the Policy Responses to HIV/AIDS in Brazil and South Africa: A Comparative Analysis." *Global Public Health* 7 (10) (December): 1031–1044.

Nyweide, David J., Woulton Lee, Timothy T. Cuerdon, Hoangmai H. Pham, Megan Cox, Rahul Rajkumar, and Patrick H. Conway. 2015. "Association of Pioneer Accountable Care Organizations vs Traditional Medicare Fee For Service with Spending, Utilization, and Patient Experience." *Journal of the American Medical Association* 313 (21) 2152–2161.

Obermann, Konrad, Peter Müller, Hans-Heiko Müller, Burkhard Schmidt, Bernd Glazinski. *Understanding the German Health Care System*, n.d.

O'Donnell, Guillermo. 1973. *Modernization and Bureaucratic-Authoritarianism*. Berkeley: University of California Press.

OECD. (Organization for Economic Cooperation and Development). 2011. *Health at a Glance 2011: OECD Indicators* (Paris).

———. n.d. *Five Family Facts.* www.oecd.org/social/family/doingbetter.

———. 2013. *Health at a Glance 2013: OECD Indicators.* OECD Publishing. http://dx.doi.org/10.1787/health_glance-2013-en.

———. 2013. *OECD Health Statistics 2013* (Paris).

Paradise, Julia. 2015. "Medicaid Moving Forward." Issue Brief. Kaiser Family Foundation. March 9.

The Patient Choice, Affordability, Responsibility, and Empowerment Act: A Legislative Proposal. 2014. (January).

Pear, Robert. 2009. "Industry Pledges to Control Health Care Costs." *New York Times*, May 11.

———. 2014. "Further Delays for Employers in Health Law." *New York Times*, February 10.

——— and Michael Cooper. 2012. "Reluctance in Some States over Medicaid Expansion." *New York Times*, June 30.

Peters, B. Guy. 1998. *Comparative Politics: Theory and Methods.* New York: New York University Press.

Peters, Jeremy W. 2013. "In Landmark Vote, Senate Limits Use of Filibuster." *New York Times*, November 21.

Peterson, Mark A. 2001. "From Trust to Political Power: Interest Groups, Public Choice, and Health Care." *Journal of Health Politics, Policy and Law* 26 (5): 1145–1163.

Pierson, Paul. 1993. "When Effect Becomes Cause: Policy Feedback and Political Change." *World Politics* 45: 595–628.

———. 2000. "Increasing Returns, Path Dependence, and the Study of Politics." *American Political Science Review* 94 (2) (June): 251–267.

———. 2000. "Post Industrial Pressures on Mature Welfare States." In *The New Politics of the Welfare State.* New York: Oxford University Press.

Piketty, Thomas. 2014. *Capital in the Twenty-First Century.* Boston: Harvard University Press.

Pillay, Yogan. 2001. "The Impact of South Africa's New Constitution on the Organization of Health Services in the Post-Apartheid Era." *Journal of Health Politics, Policy and Law* 26 (4) (August): 747–766.

Pollitz, Karen. 2009. "State High-Risk Health Insurance Pools." *Expert Voices*, NIHCM Foundation (April). www.nihcm.org.

Putnam, Robert D. 2015. *Our Kids: The American Dream in Crisis.* New York: Simon and Schuster.

Quadagno, Jill. 2005. *One Nation Uninsured: Why the U.S. Has No National Health Insurance.* Oxford and New York: Oxford University Press.

Ramjee, Shivani, Tim Vieyra, Matan Abraham, Josh Kaplan, and Richard Taylor. 2014. "National Health Insurance and South Africa's Private Sector." *South African Health Review, 2013/14.* Durban: Health Systems Trust (September) pp. 93–103.

Raylor, Andrew. 2015. "Senate Adopts GOP Budget Targeting 'Obamacare.'" *Washington Post*, May 5.

Reid, T. R. 2010. *The Healing of America: A Global Quest for Better, Cheaper, and Fairer Health Care*. New York: Penguin.

Reinhardt, Uwe E. 2004. "The Swiss Health System: Regulated Competition without Managed Care." *Journal of the American Medical Association* 292 (10) (September 8): 1227–1231.

———. 2011. "The Wyden-Ryan Plan: Déjà vu All Over Again." *New York Times*, December 23.

Rimlinger, Gaston V. 1971. *Welfare Policy and Industrialization in Europe, America, and Russia*. New York: John Wiley and Sons.

Robin Hood tax. www.robinhoodtax.org.uk/.

Romell, Rick. 2006. "Hospital Losses Hit City Heart." *Milwaukee Journal Sentinel*, May 14.

Rotberg, Robert I. 2014. "Overcoming Difficult Challenges: Bolstering Good Governance." *Annals of the American Academy of Political and Social Science* 652 (March): 8–19.

Rothgang, Heinz. 2010. "Conceptual Framework of the Study." In *The State and Healthcare: Comparing OECD Countries*. Heinz Rothgang, Mirella Cacace, Lorraine Frisina, Simone Grimmeisen, Achim Schmid, and Claus Wendt. 10–22. London and New York: Palgrave Macmillan.

———. 2010. "The Converging Role of the State in OECD Healthcare Systems." In *The State and Healthcare: Comparing OECD Countries*. Heinz Rothgang, Mirella Cacace, Lorraine Frisina, Simone Grimmeisen, Achim Schmid, and Claus Wendt. 237–247. London and New York: Palgrave Macmillan.

Rothgang, Heinz, Achim Schmid and Claus Wendt. 2010. "The Self-Regulatory German Healthcare System Between Growing Competition and State Hierarchy." In *The State and Healthcare: Comparing OECD Countries*. Heinz Rothgang, Mirella Cacace, Lorraine Frisina, Simone Grimmeisen, Achim Schmid, and Claus Wendt. 119–179. London and New York: Palgrave Macmillan.

Rothgang, Heinz, Mirella Cacace, Lorraine Frisina, Simone Grimmeisen, Achim Schmid, and Claus Wendt. 2010. *The State and Healthcare: Comparing OECD Countries*. London and New York: Palgrave Macmillan.

Rothstein, Bo. 1998. *Just Institutions Matter: The Moral and Political Logic of the Universal Welfare States*. New York: Cambridge University Press.

Rudowitz, Robin, Samantha Artiga, and MaryBeth Musumeci. 2015. "The ACA and Medicaid Expansion Waivers." Issue Brief. Kaiser Family Foundation (February).

Ryan, Paul. 2008. *A Roadmap for America's Future*.

———. 2010. *A Roadmap for America's Future Version 2.0: A Plan to Solve America's Long-Term Economic and Fiscal Crisis* (January).

———. 2012. "The Future of US Healthcare: Is Rationing Inevitable?" Speech to Milwaukee Press Club. Milwaukee, Wisconsin. March 2.

Ryan, Paul and House Budget Committee. 2011. *The Path to Prosperity: Restoring America's Promise, Fiscal Year 2012 Budget Resolution*. House Committee on the Budget (April 5). budget.GOP.gov.

————. 2012. *The Path to Prosperity: A Blueprint for American Renewal, Fiscal Year 2013 Budget Resolution* (March 20). prosperity.budget.house.gov.

————. 2013. *The Path to Prosperity: A Responsible, Balanced Budget, Fiscal Year 2014 Budget Resolution* (March) budget.house.gov.

Sachs, Jeffrey. 2005. *The End of Poverty: Economic Possibilities for Our Time.* New York, Penguin.

Salganicoff, Alina, Adara Beamesderfer, Nisdha Kurani, and Laurie Sobel, "Coverage for Abortion Services and the ACA." 2014. Kaiser Family Foundation (September).

Sartori, Giovanni. 1976. *Parties and Party* Systems. New York: Cambridge University Press.

Sauerland, Dirk. 2009. "The Legal Framework for Health Care Quality Assurance in Germany." *Health Economics, Policy and Law* 4: 79–98.

Schmid, Achim, Mirella Cacace, Ralf Götze, and Heinz Rothgang. 2010. "Explaining Health Care System Change: Problem Pressure and the Emergence of 'Hybrid' Health Care Systems." *Journal of Health Politics, Policy and Law* 35 (4) (August): 455–486.

Schmid, John. 2015. "Help Wanted: Most U.S. Job Openings Are for Low-skill, Low-pay Workers." *Milwaukee Journal Sentinel*, April 4.

Schmitter, Philippe C. 1979. "Still the Century of Corporatism?" In *Trends toward Corporatist Intermediation*, edited by Philippe C. Schmitter and Gerhard Lehmbruch. Beverly Hills: Sage.

Seedat, Mohaded, Ashley Van Niekerk, Rachel Jewkes, Shahnaaz Fuffla, and Kopano Ratele. 2014. "Violence and Injuries in South Africa: Prioritising an Agenda for Prevention." *Annals of the American Academy of Political and Social Science* 652 (March): 1011–1022.

Sered, Susan Starr and Rushika Fernandopulle. 2007. *Uninsured in America: Life and Death in the Land of Opportunity*, updated edition. Berkeley: University of California Press.

Shisana, O., T. Rehle, LC. Simbaayi, K. Zuma, S. Jooste, N. Zungu, D. Labadarios, D. Onoya, et al. 2014. *South African National HIV Prevalence, Incidence and Behaviour Survey, 2012.* Cape Town: HSRC Press.

Shonkoff, Jack P. and Deborah A. Phillips, eds. 2000. *From Neurons to Neighborhoods.* Washington DC: National Academy Press.

Skocpol, Theda. 1996. *Boomerang: Clinton's Health Security Effort and the Turn against Government in U.S. Politics.* New York and London: W. W. Norton.

Skowronek, Stephen. 1982. *Building a New American State: The Expansion of National Administrative Capacities, 1877–1920.* Cambridge: Cambridge University Press.

South African Medical Association. 2011. *Submission of Comments on National Health Insurance (NHI) Green Paper.* December.

South African Medical Research Council. 2012. *Rapid Mortality Surveillance Report 2012.*

South African Private Practitioner Forum. 2011. *National Health Insurance in South Africa: SAPPF Submission on the Green Paper on National Health Insurance.* December.

Southall, Roger. 2014. "Democracy at Risk? Politics and Governance under the ANC." *Annals of the American Academy of Political and Social Science* 652 (March): 48–69.

Sparks, Allister. 1995. *Tomorrow Is Another Country: The Inside Story of South Africa's Road to Change.* New York: Hill and Wang.

———. 2003. *Beyond the Miracle: Inside the New South Africa.* London: Profile Books.

Specter, Michael. 2007. "The Denialists." *The New Yorker*, March 12, pp. 31–38.

Starr, Paul. 1982. *The Social Transformation of American Medicine.* New York: Basic Books.

———. 2011. *Remedy and Reaction: The Peculiar American Struggle over Health Care Reform.* New Haven and London: Yale University Press.

State Decisions on Health Insurance Marketplaces and the Medicaid Expansion. KFF State Health Facts, updated July 20, 2015. http://kff.org/health-reform/state-indicator/state-decisions-for-creating-health-insurance-exchanges-and-expanding-medicaid.

Statistics South Africa. 2014. *Mortality and Causes of Death in South Africa, 2013: Findings from Death Notifications.* Stat release P0309.3 December 2.

———. 2014. *Poverty Trends in South Africa: An Examination of Absolute Poverty between 2006 and 2011.*

———. 2015. *Quarterly Labour Force Survey, Quarter 4, 2014,* P0211. February 10.

Status of State Action on the Medicaid Expansion Decision. KFF State Health Facts, updated July 20, 2015.http://kff.org/health-reform/state-indicator/state-activity-around-expanding- medicaid-under-the-affordable-care-act/.

Steinmo, Sven and Jon Watts. 1995. "It's the Institutions Stupid! Why Comprehensive National Health Insurance Always Fails in North America." *Journal of Health Politics, Policy and Law* 20:2 (Summer): 329–372.

Stephens, John D. 1979. *The Transition from Capitalism to Socialism.* London: Macmillan.

Stock, Stephanie, Marcus Redaelli, and Karl Wilhelm Lauterbach. 2006. "The Influence of the Labor Market on German Health Care Reforms." *Health Affairs* 25 (4) (July/August): 1143–1152.

Stone, Deborah A.1980. *The Limits of Professional Power: National Health Care in the Federal Republic of Germany.* Chicago: University of Chicago Press.

———. 1993. "The Struggle for the Soul of Health Insurance." *Journal of Health Politics, Policy and Law* (Summer 1993): 286–317.

Streeck, Wolfgang and Philippe C. Schmitter. 1985. "Community, Market, State- and Associations? The Prospective Contribution of Interest Governance to Social Order." *European Sociological Review* 1 (2): 119–38.

Summary of New Health Reform Law. 2011. Kaiser Family Foundation (April 15). www.kff.org.

Summary of Coverage Provisions in the Patient Protection and Affordable Care Act. 2012. Kaiser Family Foundation (July 17). www.kff.org

Survey of Employer-sponsored Health Benefits, 1999–2012. Kaiser Family Foundation and Health Research and Educational Trust. www.kff.org.

Thelen, Kathleen. 2003. "How Institutions Evolve: Insights from Comparative Historical Analysis." In *Comparative Historical Analysis in the Social Sciences*, edited by James Mahoney and Dietrich Rueschemeyer. New York: Cambridge University Press.

Tilton, Tim. 1990. *The Political Theory of Swedish Social Democracy*. Oxford: Clarendon Press.

Timmins, Nicholas. 1995. *The Five Giants: A Biography of the Welfare State* (London: HarperCollins Publishers.

Timse, Tabelo. 2010. "Zuma Reveals His HIV Status." *Mail and Guardian*, April 26.

Tyson, Laura D'Andrea. 2011. "Wyden-Ryan's Unrealistic Assumptions." *New York Times*, December 30.

UNAIDS. 2012. "Regional Fact Sheet 2012."

———. 2015. South Africa. http://aidsinfo.unaids.org.

———. UNAIDS Bulletin.

Unnatural Causes: Is Inequality Making Us Sick? 2008. California Newsreel. www.unnaturalcauses.org.

van den Heever, Alex. 2011. *Evaluation of the Green Paper on National Health Insurance*. Graduate School of Public and Development Management, Johannesburg. December 20.

van Kersbergen, Kees. 1995. *Social Capitalism: A Study of Christian Democracy and the Welfare State*. London and New York: Routledge.

Verba, Sidney and Gary R. Orren. 1989. *Equality in America*. Cambridge: Harvard University Press.

Voce, Anna, Fiorenza Monticelli, Yogan Pillay, Shuaib Kauchali, Rakshika Bhana, Magalagadi Makua, and Gugulethu Ngubane, 2014. "District Clinical Specialist Teams." *South African Health Review, 2013/14*. Durban: Health Systems Trust (September) pp. 45–58.

Vogel, David. 1978. "Why Businessmen Distrust Their State: The Political Consciousness of American Corporate Executives." *British Journal of Political Science* 8 (January): 45–78.

Vogel, Steven. 1996. *Freer Markets, More Rules*. Ithaca and London: Cornell University Press.

Wallerstein, Immanuel. 2004. *World Systems Analysis: An Introduction*. Durham: Duke University Press.

Ward, Andrew. 2015. "NHS to Stop Funding 16 Cancer Treatments." *Financial Times*, January 12.

Webber, Douglas. 1992. "Die Kassenärztlichen Vereinigungen zwischen Mitgliederinteressen und Gemeinwohl." In *Verbände zwischen Mitgliederinteressen und Gemeinwohl*, edited by Renate Mayntz. Gütersloh: Verlag Bertelsmann Stiftung.

Weinbrenner Susanne and Reinhard Busse. 2003. "Proposals for SHI Reform." *Health Policy Monitor* (2) (November) http://www.hpm.org/survey/de/a2/2.

Weisman Jonathan and Ashley Parker. 2013. "Republicans Back Down, Ending Crisis on Shutdown and Debt Limit." *New York Times*, October 16.

——— and Jeremy W. Peters. 2013. "Government Shuts Down in Budget Impasse." *New York Times*, September 30.

Weissert, William G. and Carol S. Weissert. 2012. *Governing Health: The Politics of Health Policy*, 4th ed. Baltimore: Johns Hopkins University Press.

WHO (World Health Organization). 2008. *World Health Report 2008: Primary Health Care (Now More than Ever)* (Geneva).

———. 2010. *Health Systems Financing: The Path to Universal Coverage* (Geneva).

———. 2012. *Achieving Universal Coverage* (Geneva).

———. 2012. *Health Systems Financing: The Path to Universal Health Coverage. Plan of Action* (Geneva).

———. 2014. "The Top 10 Causes of Death." Fact Sheet no. 310, updated May. http://www.who.int/mediacentre/factsheets/fs310/en/;

———. 2015. Countries: South Africa. http://www.who.int/countries/zaf/en.

WHO Commission on the Social Determinants of Health. 2008. *Closing the Gap in a Generation: Health Equity through Action on the Social Determinants of Health. Final Report of the Commission on the Social Determinants of Health.* (Geneva).

Wilkinson, Kate. 2014. "Has Jacob Zuma Hurt the Fight against AIDS More Than Thabo Mbeki?" *Africa Check*, September 23. http://africacheck.org/reports/has-jacob-zuma-hurt-the-fight-against-aids-more-than-mbeki/.

Wolf, Martin. 2012. "Paul Ryan's Plan for America Is Not Credible." *Financial Times,* August 20.

World Bank. 2014. *South Africa Economic Update: Fiscal Policy and Redistribution in an Unequal Society.* 6 (November) no. 92167.

———. 2014. "South Africa Lifts 3.6 Million out of Poverty Thanks to Its Fiscal Policies." 2014. World Bank Press release no. 2015/179/AFR (November 4).

———. 2015. Incidence of Tuberculosis (per 100,000 People).

———. 2015. *World Development Indicators: Health Systems.* http://data.worldbank.org/data-catalog/world-development-indicators.

Wyden, Ron and Paul Ryan. 2011. *Guaranteed Choices to Strengthen Medicare and Health Security for All: Bipartisan Options for the Future.* (December 15). www.budget.house.gov/bipartisanhealthoptions; www.wyden.senate.gov/bipartisonhealthoptions.

Yates, Rob. 2013. "Only Public Funding Can Guarantee Universal Health Coverage." *The Guardian*, October 9.

"Your Friendly Monolith." The Price of Freedom: A Special Report on South Africa. 2010. *The Economist,* June 5, pp. pp. 4–5.

"Your Health Plan Will Now Self-Destruct." 2015. *Businessweek*, November 2–8, 28–29.

Zacher, Mark W. and Tania J. Keefe. 2008. *The Politics of Global Health Governance: United by Contagion.* New York: Palgrave Macmillan.

Zernike, Kate and Megan Thee-Brenan. 2010. "Poll Finds Tea Party Backers Wealthier and More Educated." *New York Times*, April 14.

Zhang, Tie Yuan, Benoit Labonte, Xiang Lan Wen, Gustavo Turecki, and Michael J. Meaney. 2013. "Epigenetic Mechanisms for the Early Environmental Regulation of Hippocampal Glucocortioid Receptor Gene Expression in Rodents and Humans." *Neuropsychopharmacology Reviews* 8: 111–123.

Zimmermann, Melanie. 2006. "Health Financing Reform Idea: Health Fund." *Health Policy Monitor* (7) (June) http://www.hpm.org/survey/de/b7/1.

INDEX

A National Health Plan for South Africa
(1994), 165–6, 168–9
access to health care
defined, 5
and differences by type of insurance,
197
as goal of health care system, 1
accountable care organization (ACO),
65–6, 90–1, 209
Achmat, Zackie, 161
actuarial fairness, 5
Advanced Medical Technology
Association (AMTA), 71–2
adverse selection, 73, 92–3, 118, 196
affordability of health care
defined and measured, 5–7
as goal of health care system, 1
in U.S., 2, 54, 58, 60–4, 80,
90–1
AFL-CIO, 38, 49
African National Congress (ANC)
(South Africa), 143–4, 150
corruption and patronage, 154,
175–6, 179–81, 189
economic strategy (GEAR), 145,
176–9, 205
electoral support and interest group
constituencies, 153–4, 180
health and social policy record,
144–5, 157, 177, 181
HIV/AIDS policies, 152, 157–65,
181

national health insurance proposals,
169–76, 188
Polokwane declaration, 169, 172
Afrikaners, 149, 154
AIDS. *See* HIV/AIDS
all-payer system, 116
Alma Ata Declaration, 31, 178
American Association of Labor
Legislation (AALL), 51
American Association of Retired
Persons (AARP), 19, 49, 57
American Hospital Association (AHA),
37, 49, 71–3, 76
American Medical Association
(AMA), 49
and Health Security, 57
opposition to national health
insurance, 52–3
and PPACA, 71–3, 76
America's Health Insurance Plans
(AHIP), 71–2
antiapartheid movement, 153, 161,
234n1
antiretroviral therapy (ART), 159,
161–5, 181, 188–9, 238n56
apartheid, 149, 188
defined, 143–4
effects on health, 145, 150–1
and HIV/AIDS policy, 158–61
shaping attitudes, 155, 160–1, 188–9
See also "boundary institutions"
Armey, Dick, 75

Association of Social Health Insurance
    Physicians (KV), 104–6, 127, 136,
    138–9
    in physician reimbursement, 115–17,
       133–4, 138

Bill and Melinda Gates Foundation, 33,
    162
biomedical model of health care, 22–3,
    208
Bismarck, Otto von. 96–8, 229n24
block grants (proposed for Medicaid),
    86–7
Blue Cross and Blue Shield, 37–40
Bono, 162
"boundary institutions," 144
    See also apartheid
Brazil and HIV/AIDS policy, 161,
    238–9n59
BRICS (Brazil, Russia, India, China,
    and South Africa), 32, 143
Bundesrat (Federal Council) (Germany),
    107–8, 122, 128, 137
Bundestag (Federal Diet) (Germany),
    107, 137
bundled payments
    See diagnosis related group, payment
    reform
Bush, George W., 74–5, 164

"Cadillac plan" tax, 64
Campaign for Essential Medicines, 33,
    162
Cancer Drugs Fund, 202
capitation, 57–8, 65–6
Catholic social teaching. *See* social
    Catholicism
Center for Medicare and Medicaid
    Innovation, 66
Center Party (Germany), 97–8, 111
challenges in health policy, 2, 20–34
    in Global South, 20, 23–34
    in industrialized democracies,
       20–3
Chamber of Commerce (U.S.), 57

Children's Health Insurance Program
    (CHIP), 42, 59, 86
Christian Democratic parties,
    14–15
Christian Democratic Union (CDU)
    (Germany), 120–2, 128, 139–40,
    233n79
    electoral and interest group
       constituencies, 109–10
    and social market economy,
       111–12
Christian Social Union (CDU)
    (Germany), 109, 139–40
Chrysler, 54, 59
citizens' insurance
    (Bürgerversicherung), 136–9
Citizens United, 48
CLASS Act (Community Living
    Assistance Services and Supports),
    79
clinical guidelines, 57–8, 68, 118, 120,
    123–6, 201–3
    See also comparative effectiveness
       research, Federal Joint Committee,
       National Institute of Health and
       Care Excellence, Patient Centered
       Outcomes Research Institute
Clinton, Bill, 54–6, 70, 163
Clinton Plan. *See* Health Security
commercial insurance. *See* for-profit
    insurers
Commission for Financial Sustainability
    of Social Security Systems
    (Germany). *See* Rürup Commission
community health centers, 66
community health workers, 167, 170,
    174, 203, 209
community rated premiums, 55, 93
    defined, 37
    in Germany, 140
    history of in U.S., 37–40
    modified community rating in
       PPACA, 61–2, 73, 93
    in Patient CARE Act, 86–8
    in Ryan Medicare plan, 83

comparative effectiveness research, 199–203
in Germany, 123–4
in U.S., 66–8
See also clinical guidelines, Federal Joint Committee, National Institute of Health and Care Excellence, Patient Centered Outcomes Research Institute
compulsory licensing, 162–4
Concerted Action in Health Care, 116, 233n76
Congress (U.S.), 12, 164
blocking national health insurance, 52, 56
and IPAB, 67, 81, 86
powers of, 47
Congress of South African Trade Unions (COSATU), 153
Congressional Budget Office (CBO) (U.S.), 65, 86
cooperative, health insurance, 70
coordinated care
See accountable care organization, disease management program, gatekeeper model, integrated care contract, integrated delivery system, patient centered medical home
copayment. See cost sharing in health care
corporatism, 16–17, 229n25
in German health care system, 103–6, 141, 186–7, 203
and Health Care Restructuring Act, 120
and Health Insurance Modernization Act, 123–5
problems with, 115–19
cost sharing in health insurance
in Germany, 121, 127–8
in U.S., 41, 58, 60–1, 84, 88, 91
cream skimming (risk selection)
in Germany, 131
in U.S., 39–40, 62

DALE (disability adjusted life expectancy), 8
DATA (Debt, AIDS, Trade, Africa), 33, 162
deindustrialization, effects on health insurance
in Germany, 114–15
in U.S., 43
Democratic Alliance (South Africa), 154
Democratic Party (U.S.)
and Health Security, 54–6
and national health insurance, 52–6
and PPACA, 68–70, 72–4, 76–8, 91, 92–4, 185
Department of Health (South Africa), 147, 166, 172, 174
Department of Health and Human Services (U.S.), 77
diagnosis related group (DRG), 45, 102–3, 120, 171
Discovery Health, 173–4
disease
burden in South Africa, 144–5, 150–2, 157–8, 187–8, 211n4
communicable (infectious) vs. chronic noncommunicable, 21, 24, 27, 144–5, 157–8
disease management program (DMP), 126, 209
district clinical specialist support team, 170, 174, 203, 209
Doctors Without Borders, 33
Doha Declaration on TRIPS and Public Health, 163
See also World Trade Organization
DOTS (directly observed treatment, short course). See tuberculosis
DRG. See diagnosis related group
Drugs for Neglected Diseases, 33
dual health care system in South Africa, 145–6, 187–8, 197–8, 203–5
origins of, 149–50
See also for-profit health sector in South Africa, public health sector in South Africa
Duesberg, Peter, 159–60

Economic Freedom Fighters (South
  Africa), 179
electoral system
  proportional representation, 13–14,
    107, 152, 230n32
  single member district simple
    plurality, 13–14, 75, 230n32
electronic medical records, 66, 174, 200,
  202–3
employer mandate
  in Germany, 99, 196
  small business exclusion under
    PPACA, 63
  in U.S., 54, 63–4, 78, 196
employers (Germany)
  concerns over contribution rates, 114,
    128, 129–30, 138, 233n76
  in financing SHI, 99, 129, 131–2, 140,
    196
employers (South Africa)
  in health care reform debates, 153
  offering health insurance, 149
employers (U.S.)
  concern over rising health insurance
    costs, 54
  and Health Security, 56–7
  and managed care, 57–8
  opposition to national health
    insurance, 52–3, 57
  and PPACA, 72–4
employment-based insurance in U.S.
  erosion of, 43, 54
  origins and development, 37–40
  problems for small business, 39–40,
    43
Enthoven, Alain, 55
epigenetics, 207
equity in health care
  different definitions of, 5
evidence based medicine. *See*
    clinical guidelines, comparative
    effectiveness research, Federal Joint
    Committee, National Institute
    of Health and Care Excellence,

Patient Centered Outcomes
  Research Institute
exchanges, health insurance
  and PPACA, 60–3, 77–8
  in Ryan's Medicare reform proposal,
    83
experience rated premiums
  defined, 5, 39
  in Germany, 101
  in Health Security, 55
  history of in U.S. 37–40
  in PPACA, 61–2, 73
  in Republican reform proposals, 87–8

family doctor model (Germany). *See*
  gatekeeper model
Farmer, Paul, 27, 207
Federal Association of Social Health
  Insurance Funds (GKV-SV),
  104–6, 136, 187
Federal Association of Social Health
  Insurance Physicians (KBV),
  104–6, 136
Federal Constitutional Court
  (Germany), 108, 138
Federal Joint Committee (FJC), 103–6,
  123–5, 136, 138, 186, 191, 203
Federal Ministry of Health (BMG)
  (Germany), 109
  in Health Fund, 131–3, 141, 187
  role in corporatism, 103–6, 125
  in setting budgets, 120
  in setting uniform contribution rate,
    131–3, 187
federalism, 12
  in Germany, 102, 107–8, 122, 128,
    137
  in South Africa, 147, 152–3
  in U.S., 46, 55, 60, 79–82, 86, 92–3
  See also Bundesrat
fee-for-service, 45, 57, 102, 116, 134
filibuster, 47, 70, 93
financial transaction tax, 204, 205
  See also Robin Hood tax

flat-rate premium (Gesundheitsprämie), 137

for profit health sector, South Africa. *See* dual health care system in South Africa, private health sector, South Africa

for profit insurers (Germany), 100–1, 129–30, 135, 139, 197

for profit insurers (U.S.)
  and opposition to national health insurance in the U.S., 37–40
  and opposition to public option, 73–4
  and PPACA, 61–2

for-profit insurers, 5

Free Democratic Party (Germany), 120–2, 128, 139
  electoral and interest group constituencies, 109–10

FreedomWorks, 75

gatekeeper model, 125–6, 203, 209

Gates Foundation. *See* Bill and Melinda Gates Foundation

GEAR. *See* Growth, Employment and Redistribution

General Motors, 59

German Democratic Republic (GDR) (East Germany), 102, 107, 228n10

German Hospital Federation (DKG), 103–5

German unification
  effect on contribution rates, 114
  and polyclinics, 102, 127

Global AIDS Alliance, 162

Global Fund to Fight AIDS, Tuberculosis, and Malaria, 164

globalization, economic, 21–2

goals of health care system, 1, 5–10, 184

Great Recession, 58–60, 75, 204, 177

Green Party (Germany), 114, 123, 128, 233n78

Growth, Employment, and Redistribution (GEAR), 145, 176–9, 205

HAART (highly active antiretroviral therapy), 161, 165, 238n56
  See also antiretroviral therapy

Hartz reforms, 114, 122

HCAN (Health Care for America Now), 74

Health Care Cost Containment Act of 1977 (Germany), 116–18

Health Care Restructuring Act of 1993 (Germany), 120–3

health care system goals. *See* goals of health care system

Health Fund (Germany), 131–3, 187, 190

health insurance marketplaces. *See* exchanges

Health Insurance Modernization Act of 2004 (Germany), 123–8

health policy challenges. *See* challenges in health policy

health savings account (HSA), 87, 91

Health Security, 54–7, 63

Health System Financing: The Path to Universal Health Coverage, 31

Helen Suzman Foundation, 172–3

Heritage Foundation, 84

Heywood, Marky, 161

high-risk pools in insurance, 88, 91, 196–7

Hill-Burton Act of 1946, 44

HIV/AIDS (Human immunodeficiency virus/acquired immunodeficiency syndrome), 24, 27–8, 31, 168, 178–9
  ANC policies toward, 145, 157–65
  Brazil's policy, 161, 238n56
  prevalence and mortality rates in South Africa, 2–4, 144, 150–2, 157–8, 164–5, 211n4
  and South Africa's health care system, 148, 165, 167, 188

Iacocca, Lee, 54

ideology, shaping health policy, 17–18
  See also liberalism, national liberation movement, social market economy ideology

imperialism, 25–8
Independent Patient Advisory Board
    (IPAB), 67–8, 83–5
individual insurance, proposals for, 64,
    137
individual mandate
    in Germany, 99, 135, 191, 196
    in U.S., 63–4, 79, 185–6, 191, 196
inequality
    effects on health, 207, 210
    in South Africa, 177–8
    in U.S., 210
    See also poverty, social determinants
        of health
infectious disease. *See* disease,
    communicable
informal sector, 174, 178, 198
Institute for Quality and Efficiency in
    Health Care (IQWiG) (Germany),
    123–4
institutions, political, 10–13
insurance reforms in PPACA, 61–2,
    73
integrated care contract (ICC), 125–6,
    135, 209
integrated delivery system (IDS), 45,
    202–3
interest groups, 16–17
Internal Revenue Service (IRS), 38,
    92
International Monetary Fund (IMF),
    29, 32–3
international organizations, 28–33

Johnson, Lyndon B., 53, 56

KBV. *See* Federal Association of Social
    Health Insurance Physicians
Kennedy, Edward (Ted), 71
Kennedy, John F., 53
King v Burwell, 92–3
Koch brothers, 75
Kohl, Helmut, 116, 120
KV. *See* Association of Social Health
    Insurance Physician

labor unions, 16
    in Germany, 97–100, 109–10, 128,
        136, 138, 233n78
    in South Africa, 153, 172, 179
    in U.S., 51–2, 57, 64, 71–2, 74
    See also AFL-CIO, African National
        Congress, American Association
        for Labor Legislation, Congress
        of South African Trade Unions,
        Democratic Party, Social
        Democratic Party
Lauterbach, Karl, 136
liberalism, ideology of (United States)
    in health care reform debates, 52–3,
        57, 68–9, 74–5, 78, 81
    origins and components of, 49–51

Malema, Julius, 179, 237n39
managed care, 57–8, 201–2
managed competition
    in Germany, 120–2, 129–33, 141,
        186, 198–9
    theory of, 55
    in U.S., 60–3, 198–9
Mandela, Nelson, 147, 155, 159, 237n37
Massachusetts Health Plan, 63
Mbeki, Thabo, 159
    and HIV/AIDS policy, 154, 156,
        159–62, 164
McCain, John, 59, 64
Medicaid, 9, 53, 197
    expansion under PPACA, 60–1,
        79–81, 89–90, 185, 192
    and Patient CARE Act, 86, 91
    and Paul Ryan's reform proposal,
        86–7
    program description, 40, 42–3
    and Republican Party reform
        proposals, 86–7, 91
Medicaid expansion. *See* Medicaid
medical home. *See* patient centered
    medical home
Medicare, 49, 76, 90, 203
    description of, 40–2
    diagnosis related groups (DRGs), 45

doughnut hole in Part D drug
program, 41–2, 72
and PPACA, 61, 64, 86, 90, 203
and Ryan's reform plan, 82–5, 91
Medicare Advantage plans, 42, 64
Medicare Modernization Act of 2003,
41
Medicines and Related Substances
Amendment Act of 1997, 162–3
Merkel, Angela, 129, 137
Millennium Development Goals
(MDGs), 31, 33
Moveon.org, 74
multinational corporation (MNC),
21–2, 32, 153–4, 189

National Federation of Independent
Business (NFIB), 57, 74
National Health Act of 2004 (South
Africa), 166
national health insurance (NHI),
95, 97
proposals for in South Africa, 168–76,
193–4
National Health Insurance Fund (South
Africa), 171
National Health Insurance in South Africa
(2011), 188
content of, 169–72
critiques of, 172–6
fate of private sector health care,
173–5
financing issues, 174–6, 205–6
National Health Planning and Resource
Development Act of 1974, 45
National Health Service (NHS), 15,
199, 201, 243–4n18
in South Africa, 97, 147, 150, 165–6
National Health Service Commission
(Gluckman Commission), South
Africa, 168–9
National Institute for Health and Care
Excellence (NICE), 201
National Labor Relations Board
(NLRB), 38

national liberation movement (NLM)
ideology within the ANC, 154–6,
180
National Party (South Africa), 143, 149,
154, 158–9, 169
Nazi regime, 98, 107–8, 111
NFIB v Sibelius, 79–81
NGO (nongovernmental organization)
defined, 33
in health care provision, 167
in health policy, 28–9, 33–4, 153–4,
161–4

Obama, Barack, 65, 185
and Congress, 69, 185
and health care interest groups, 70–4,
185
and individual mandate, 64
and public option, 69–70, 73
OFA (Organizing for America), 74
Office of Health Standards Compliance,
171, 173
ONE Campaign, 33

parallel importation, 162–3
parliamentary system, 11
in Germany, 107–8
in South Africa, 152
path dependence, 19
The Path to Prosperity, 224n79
The Path to Universal Coverage (2010), 194
Patient CARE (Choice, Affordability,
Responsibility, and Efficiency) Act,
86–8, 91, 93–4
patient centered medical home, 65, 90,
203, 209
Patient Centered Outcomes Research
Institute (PCORI), 67–8, 201, 203
Patient Protection and Affordable Care
Act (PPACA), 2010 (U.S.), 35–6,
169, 185–6
assessment of, 90–1, 191–2, 201, 198
background to, 59–60
and comparative effectiveness
research, 66–8, 203

Patient Protection and Affordable Care
    Act (PPACA)—*Continued*
    compared to Republicans alternatives,
        89–92
    content of, 60–8, 191–2
    implementation of, 77–81
    and public opinion, 196
    reform politics, 68–77
payment reform, 65–6, 90–1
    lump-sum payments, Germany, 134,
        102
    See also diagnosis related group
peer review. *See* physician practice
        reviews
PEPFAR (President's Emergency Plan
        for AIDS Relief), 164
pharmaceutical companies
    and HIV/AIDS, 160–3, 189
    in U.S., 49, 71–2
PhRMA (Pharmaceutical Research and
        Manufacturers of America), 49,
        71–2
physician practice reviews, 57–8,
        117–18, 120, 123–5, 126, 201–3
play or pay. *See* employer mandate
pluralism
    in interest group systems, 16
    in U.S., 47–9
policy change
    in health care reform, 189–94
    types of, 18–20
policy feedback, 18
policy legacies, 18–20, 51
political action committee (PAC), 48
political parties, 13–15
Polokwane declaration. *See* African
        National Congress
polyclinic, 102, 126–7, 138, 202
poverty
    different levels defined, 23
    effects on health status, 22–3, 27,
        150–2, 210
    in South Africa, 177–8
    See also inequality, social determinants
        of health

preexisting medical condition, 39, 61–2
premium subsidies in PPACA, 63–4,
        92–3, 135, 195–6
premium support. *See* voucher
presidential system. *See* separation of
        powers
Primary Health Care (Now More than Ever)
        (2008), 194
private health sector (South Africa), 145
    as compared to public sector health
        care system, 146–8
    problems with, 148, 204
private insurance. *See* for-profit insurers,
        private health sector (South Africa)
proportional representation. *See*
        electoral system
provider reimbursement reform. *See*
        payment reform
public opinion
    and health care reform in U.S., 55, 196
public option, 69–70, 73, 76–7, 186, 196
public sector health care in South Africa
    organization of, 146–7, 149–50
    in relation to private sector, 145–9
    structural problems with, 166–8
    See also dual health care system in
        South Africa

QALY (quality adjusted life year), 8,
        200–1
quality of health care
    defined and measured, 8–9
    as goal of health care system, 1
    in U.S., 65–8, 90

rationing, 201–2
Reagan, Ronald, 45, 51
reconciliation, 93
Republican Party (U.S.)
    and Health Security, 56–7
    and individual mandate, 63–4
    and national health insurance, 52–3,
        56–7
    and political strategy after PPACA,
        92–4

and PPACA, 69–70, 74–5, 80–1, 185
  reform proposals, 81–91, 196
  and Tea Party, 74–5, 81
responsiveness of health care system, 9
  in choice of insurer in Germany,
    118–19, 199
risk adjustment
  in German health insurance, 121,
    131–3, 135, 185, 196–7
  in U.S. 55, 62, 73, 195–8
risk equalization. *See* risk adjustment
risk pooling in insurance
  under Blue Cross and Blue Shield,
    37–40
  defined, 37
  insurance industry position (U.S.), 73–4
  under PPACA, 62–4, 93
  as requirement for equitable access to
    insurance, 5, 195–8
risk selection. *See* cream skimming
Rivera, Dennis, 72
A Roadmap for America's Future, 224n79
Robin Hood tax. *See* financial
  transaction tax
Romney, Mitt, 63
Roosevelt, Franklin, 52
Rürup, Bert, 136–7
Rürup Commission (Germany), 136,
  233n79
Ryan, Paul
  criticism of IPAB, 83–4
  health care reform proposals, 82–6
  Medicaid reform proposal, 86
  and Patient CARE Act, 86
  premium support (voucher) for
    Medicare, 83–4
  trajectory of political career, 92
  See also *Path to Prosperity, Roadmap for
    America's Future*

Schmidt, Ulla, 125, 136
Schröder, Gerhard, 123
Seehofer, Horst, 122
SEIU (Service Employees' International
  Union), 71–2

selective contracting between insurers
  and providers, 138–9
Self-Governance Act of 1951
  (Germany), 98–9
separation of powers, 11, 82
  in blocking national health insurance,
    52, 56
  and Medicaid expansion, 81
  in U.S. political system, 46–7
  See also Congress, Supreme Court
sickness funds. *See* social health
  insurance funds
single member district simple plurality.
  See electoral system
single-payer national health insurance.
  See national health insurance
social assistance vs. social insurance,
  42–3
social Catholicism, 14, 97, 111
Social Democratic Party (SPD)
  (Germany), 114, 122–3, 128,
  136–8, 140, 233n78
  electoral and interest group
    constituencies, 109–10
  and social market economy, 111–12
social determinants of health, 22–3, 27,
  206–10
  in South Africa, 150–2, 167–8
social health insurance (SHI)
  (Germany), 15
  contribution rates, 100, 114, 128, 129,
    131–2, 138, 139–40
  expanding base of financing, 129,
    204–5
  financing debate, 113–15, 129, 136–9,
    141
  lack of choice of insurer, 118–19
  organization and financing, 99–103,
    186
  origins, 95–9
Social Health Insurance Competition
  Strengthening Act of 2007
  (Germany)
  content, 129–36
  reform politics, 136–9

social health insurance funds (Germany)
in corporatism, 104–6, 115–18, 120
and managed competition, 118–19,
121, 130–3
types of, 99–100
social market economy (SME), ideology
(Germany), 110–12, 187
solidarity principle in health care
financing, 5, 141
South African Communist Party, 154
South African Medical Association, 173
South African Private Practitioner
Forum, 173
Stern, Andy, 72
structural adjustment, 29–30, 177–8,
189
"structural violence," 27
subsidiarity in German health care and
welfare state, 111–12, 186–7
Supreme Court (U.S.), 48, 79–81, 92–3,
185

Tea Party (U.S.), 74–5, 81
toxic stress, 207, 212n11, 245–6n31
See also social determinants of health
Treatment Action Campaign (TAC),
153, 161–3, 172
TRIPS (Trade Related Aspects of
Intellectual Property Rights),
162–4
Truman, Harry, 52
Truth and Reconciliation Commission,
237n37
Tshabalala, Msimang, 159, 161
tuberculosis (TB)

in Global South, 24, 27, 30
in South Africa, 4, 144, 147, 157–9,
164–5, 178–9, 211n4
treatment of, 30, 159, 237–8n49
Tutu, Desmond, 237n37

UNAIDS, 30, 164
UNICEF, 30, 153
uninsured
in Germany, 114–15
in U.S., 2, 52, 54, 58–60, 80–1,
89–90
unitary government, 11–12

van den Heever, Alex, 173
Veterans Administration, 43
Vilakazi, Herbert, 160
voucher
in Medicare, 83–4

World Bank (WB), 29
World Health Organization (WHO)
on HIVAIDS and TB, 159, 164,
237–8n49
and primary care, 31, 178, 194
role in global health, 30–1, 153, 174,
194
and social determinants of health,
209
and universal coverage, 194–5,
204–5
World Trade Organization (WTO), 29,
162–4, 166

Zuma, Jacob, 164, 177, 180, 237n39

Printed in the United States
By Bookmasters